ANTHROPOLOGY AND INTERNATIONAL HEALTH

CULTURE, ILLNESS, AND HEALING

MARK NICHTER

*Department of Anthropology, The University of Arizona,
Tucson, Arizona, U.S.A.*

ANTHROPOLOGY AND INTERNATIONAL HEALTH

South Asian Case Studies

KLUWER ACADEMIC PUBLISHERS

DORDRECHT / BOSTON / LONDON

Library of Congress Cataloging-in-Publication Data

```
Nichter, Mark.
    Anthropology and international health : south Asian case studies /
Mark Nichter.
      p.   cm. -- (Culture, illness, and healing ; 15)
    Bibliography: p.
    ISBN 0-7923-0005-X
    1. Medical anthropology--India, South.  2. Medical anthropology-
 -Sri Lanka.  3. Health behavior--India, South.  4. Health behavior-
 -Sri Lanka.  5. Health education--India, South.  6. Health
 education--Sri Lanka.   I. Title.  II. Series.
 RA418.3.I4N53  1989
 610'.954--dc19                                        88-8448
```

ISBN hardback: 0-7923-0005-X
ISBN paperback: 0-7923-0158-7 (U.S. paperback only)

Published by Kluwer Academic Publishers,
P.O. Box 17, 3300 AA Dordrecht, The Netherlands.

Kluwer Academic Publishers incorporates
the publishing programmes of
D. Reidel, Martinus Nijhoff, Dr W. Junk and MTP Press.

Sold and distributed in the U.S.A. and Canada
by Kluwer Academic Publishers,
101 Philip Drive, Norwell, MA 02061, U.S.A.

In all other countries, sold and distributed
by Kluwer Academic Publishers Group,
P.O. Box 322, 3300 AH Dordrecht, The Netherlands.

Printed on acid-free paper

All photographs made by Mimi Nichter

TABLE OF CONTENTS

v

ACKNOWLEDGEMENTS

I would like to acknowledge the support and research assistance of several individuals. Mimi Nichter worked with me as a co-researcher in both India and Sri Lanka. In addition to co-authoring four essays in the volume and contributing photographs, she offered me constructive criticism on numerous drafts of each of the other chapters. In India, Srinivas Devadiga worked close with me as a research assistant. I owe many of my insights on popular health culture and communication dynamics to him. His mother (deceased) was one of my best informants on subjects related to maternal and child health. K. H. Bhat assisted me in the collection of survey data introduced in chapters two and five. Amrith Someshvar served as my resident expert on Tuluva folk culture. Poet, folklorist, and participant in South Kanara's rich cultural life, Amrith shared his knowledge with me, never tired of my questions and always encouraged me in my studies. Vaidya P. S. Ishvara Bhat (decreased) served as my local expert on ayurvedic theory and Vaidya P. S. Ganapathy Bhat (deceased) and Kangila Krishna Bhat served as my advisors on practitioner-patient communication and medicinal herbs.

The Poogavana household of Vitla, the Daithota and Kalpana households of Panaje, and the G. N. Bhide household of Mundaje literally adopted my family and allowed Mimi and I to carefully observe village life from their porches and family life from their kitchens. My gratitude to these households and especially Venkatramana and Jaya, Shampa, Shankar Bhat, Sumathi and Amma is beyond words.

I owe much thanks to the people of Vittal, Puttur, Panaje, Bettampady (South Kanara) and Belse (North Kanara) for sharing with us their lives and interpretations of reality. I would also like to acknowledge the primary health center staff, the medical practitioners and chemist shop owners who afforded me the opportunity to observe and interview them on the job. Confidentiality prohibits my mentioning these people by name.

In Sri Lanka, I would like to acknowledge the assistance of Shantha Veragowda who periodically served as my research assistant and the eleven health education masters degree candidates with whom I lived and worked. Virtually all of my research findings were discussed with this group of seasoned field staff assigned to the Health Education Bureau. They broadened my understanding of Sinhalese health culture and assisted me in conducting research on many of the issues discussed in Chapters one, three, six and eleven. I would especially like to thank B. A. Ranaveera.

Research in India was supported by a Radcliffe Brown award (UK) in 1974—1976 and an Indo-US Subcommission on Education and Culture

Award in 1979—80. During this time I was sponsored by the National Institute of Mental Health and Neurosciences, Bangalore. A Fulbright Fellowship supported research in Sri Lanka in 1984 and a WHO assignment facilitated research conducted in 1985. I was affiliated with the Postgraduate Institute of Medicine, University of Colombo and the Bureau of Health Education. Subsequent short field trips to South Asia have been indirectly funded by consultant activities.

Finally, I would like to thank Charles Leslie for his continued support and encouragement over the years.

SOURCE REFERENCES

Chapter 1:   Published in *Human Organization 46*: 1, pp. 18—28, 1987.
Chapter 2:   Published in *Human Organization 42*: 3, pp. 235—246, 1987.
Chapter 3:   New.
Chapter 4:   New. Includes material published in 'The Language of Illness', *Anthropos 74*: 181—201, 1979.
Chapter 5:   Expanded and edited version of paper published in *Medical Anthropology 5*: 25—48, 1984.
Chapter 6:   Published in *Social Science and Medicine*, as 'From Aralu to ORS: Sinhalese Perceptions of Digestion, Diarrhea and Dehydration.' 27: 1, 39—52, 1988.
Chapter 7:   Expanded and edited version of paper 'The Layperson's Perception of Medicine as Perspective into the Utilization of Multiple Therapy Systems in the Indian Context' *Social Science and Medicine 14b*: 225—233, 1980.
Chapter 8:   Revised version of paper 'Paying for What Ails You: Sociocultural Issues Influencing the Ways and Means of Therapy Payment in South India', *Social Science and Medicine 17*: 14, 957—965, 1983.
Chapter 9:   New.
Chapter 10: Published in *Social Science and Medicine 21*: 6, 667—69, 1985.
Chapter 11: New. Contains material from an article entitled 'Health Education by Appropriate Analogy: Using the Familiar to Explain the New' published in *Convergence, Journal of Adult Education*, Vol. XIX, No. 1, 1986 and *An Anthropological Approach to Nutrition Education*. International Nutrition Communication Service, Education Development Center, Newton, Ma. 1981.

INTRODUCTION

In this book I present a series of eleven essays written between 1978 and 1987 on subjects relevant to the anthropology of health and international health. The issues addressed in these essays were investigated during 38 months of fieldwork in rural southwest peninsular India (1974—86) and 15 months of fieldwork in southwest Sri Lanka (1983—84). During various periods of this time I conducted ethnographic fieldwork, explored the feasibility of participatory community research, facilitated the development of a postgraduate health education training program, and served as a consultant to various international health organizations. The essays document my ongoing attempts to integrate academic interests in the anthropology of health with applications of anthropology for international health and development.

The volume is divided into four sections structured around the themes of: ethnophysiology, illness ethnography, pharmaceutical related behavior, and health communication. Included are studies of fertility and pregnancy (Chapters 1 and 2), states of malnutrition and approaches to nutrition education (Chapters 5 and 11), diarrheal disease and water boiling behavior (Chapters 6 and 10), and lay perceptions of fertility control methods and medicines (Chapters 3 and 7). Emerging from these studies is a recognition that perceptions of ethnophysiology and contingent health concerns significantly influence health behavior and the use as well as demand for traditional and modern health resources.

In several of the essays, I explore health as it is culturally constituted and risk to illness as it is culturally interpreted (Chapters 2, 3, 5 and 7). The 'at risk' concept is central to international health. A cultural understanding of how vulnerability to illness is interpreted in general, and what constitutes a state of risk to particular types of illness is essential for an understanding of household health behavior. It is vital to the success of primary health care programs which endeavor to engage the community in preventive health activities as well as efforts to adapt biotechnology to culture.

Also considered in the volume are notions of illness causality, the dynamics of illness classification, and symptom reporting to practitioners (Chapter 4). Emphasized is the fluidity of the doctrine of multiple causality, specificity and ambiguity as features of folk classification, and the social relations of describing illness. Attention is directed toward perceived dietary and medicine needs in relation to native illness categories (Chapters 5, 6 and 7). A study of the manner in which the qualities of medicines are assessed (Chapter 7) is complemented by a study of the ways in which practitioners in a competitive marketplace meet client demands and collect fees for services (Chapter 8).

Highlighted in the essays are both patterns of normative health behavior and diversity in health practice. I point out that popular health culture contains elements of both folk and pluralistic medical traditions (Chapters 4 and 5). Many health ethnographies which describe cultural health beliefs and practices convey a sense of consensus. I draw attention to the range and variation of interpretations afforded by generative conceptual schema. In ethnographic studies of fertility and pregnancy (Chapters 1 and 2), I illustrate intraregional differences in dietary and fertility related practice which impact on health status. Ideas about health and illness are not static. In a discussion of the introduction of biotechnical fixes (Chapters 3, 7, and 9), I argue that new ideas and health products are interpreted in relation to familiar frames of reference. Traditional knowledge is at once reproduced as well as modified by new experiences.

In several esays I identify issues to be addressed by health educators and suggest courses of action to be explored by health planners. These suggestions emerge from my practical involvement in primary health care. They should not be taken to mean that I view education or the provision of better health services to be a panacea for good health. I take it as a given that household and community health requires that basic human needs be met, issues of equity be addressed and decentralized problem solving be engendered. Moreover, a population-based approach to the practice of medicine needs to be fostered and made responsive to the community. I am critical of conventional health education based on didactic teaching and place emphasis on the negotiation of meaning and empowerment through knowledge. The approach to health education which I advocate entails an analysis of community health behavior and communication patterns, an assessment of practitioner treatment patterns, the promotion of participatory research experiences, and consumer education.

At a time when the social marketing of health products has become popular and the media has reached all but the most remote regions of the world, I argue that underdevelopment in health communication persists (Chapters 3, 5, 6 and 11). Without enhancing popular understanding of such basic health concepts as the fertility cycle and dehydration (Chapters 1 and 6), the role of health education is limited to fostering community compliance and participation in a market economy where public health fixes are available at a subsidized price. In an essay examining the ramifications of the rising trend toward health commodification (Chapter 9), I argue that those in international health must look beyond the effect of medical fixes to the ideology and approach to health embodied by the consumption of medicines. Emphasis is placed on the social relations of health care inclusive of a sense of responsibility for community and environmental well being.

Many of the essays in this volume focus attention on cultural perceptions of health and illness as predisposing factors which influence health care practice. Absent is a presentation of survey and ethnographic research which I have conducted on enabling and service related factors effecting patterns of practitioner utilization and household expense accounted for by health care seeking. While occasionally referred to in the present set of essays, these subjects lie outside the scope of this volume. The ethnographic accounts presented here largely constitute what I would describe as stage one micro level research in an anthropology of international health. I may briefly describe how this research fits into a broader research framework which I divide into a series of stages.

Stage one health ethnography is represented in this volume by studies of fertility, childrens' malnutrition and diarrhea. These exploratory studies identify pertinent questions and topics for stage two population-based research such as the study of pregnancy related dietary behavior found in Chapter 2. Stage two studies consider the distribution of health beliefs and behaviors in populations defined by specific social factors (e.g. caste, class, household dynamics, educational status). Complemented by epidemiological research, stage two anthropological research identifies groups at special risk by measuring the impact of sets of behaviors on the health status of individuals, households or larger social networks.

Stage one research also generates proposals for "action research" which tests the viability of alternative health care approaches through active experimentation. This is exemplified by the education by analogy approach to nutrition education described in Chapter 11. Stage one research also provides baseline data against which community response to existing health interventions and programs may be assessed. Examples are provided by the study of ORS (Chapter 6) and fertility control methods (Chapter 3), as well as studies of vaccination programs (Nichter 1989) and villagers' perceptions of the work of primary health care workers (Nichter 1984).

Stage three research is prospective and considers the broad ramifications of health interventions overtime through both household and community based studies. This is illustrated by the study of health commodification found in Chapter 9 which explores the changing use of commercial pharma-ceutical products in home care. It is complemented by research on the delivery of health care by practitioners (Chapter 8) and a social systems analysis of the health delivery system (Nichter 1986). While the former explores the practice of medicine as it is influenced by social and economic factors, the latter considers the political and bureaucratic aspects of health care delivery programs at the local level. These micro level studies are interlinked to macro level studies of health and development bureaucracies (e.g. Foster 1987, Justice 1987). Macro level studies of structural, processual, and political-economic aspects of health programs inform and are informed by micro level studies.

The research agenda of medical anthropologists, as I illustrate in this volume, is at once responsive to international health objectives yet critical of conventional approaches to health provision and promotion. Research topics are emergent and based as much on observations of social life and cultural interpretations of meaning as on patterns of sickness. This is clearly evident in the studies of biotechnological fixes presented. Fixes, be they medications, contraceptives, vaccines, or ORS, are resources, not answers, to international health problems. The acceptance and manner of use of such resources in large measure depends on social and cultural contingencies, issues of cost which extend beyond direct cash expenditure, and notions of risk dictated by cultural common sense.

REFERENCES

Foster, G.
  1987 Bureaucratic aspects of international health agencies. *Social Science and Medicine* *25*: 9, 1039—1048.
Justice, J.
  1987 The bureaucratic context of international health: A social scientist's view. *Social Science and Medicine 25*: 12, 1301—1306.
Nichter, M.
  1984 Project Community Diagnosis: Participatory research as a first step toward community involvement in primary health care. *Social Science and Medicine 19*: 3, 237—252.
  1986 The Primary Health Center as a social system: PHC, social status and the issue of teamwork in South Asia. *Social Science and Medicine 23*: 4, 347—355.
  1989 Vaccinations in South Asia: False expectations and commanding metaphors. *In* J. Coreil and D. Mull (eds.) *Anthropology and Primary Health Care*. The Netherlands: Kluwer Academic Publishers.

SECTION ONE

ETHNOPHYSIOLOGY

INTRODUCTION

Highlighted in this section which is coauthored by Mimi Nichter, are lay perceptions of physiology. Documented are perceptions of bodily processes which influence women's health practices during pregnancy, fertility related behavior during the month, and the demand for fertility control methods. The importance of ethnophysiology is noted in several other essays in this volume where medicine taking behavior and folk dietetics are examined. Much popular knowledge of how the body functions is tacit. It is embodied, known through health practice and habit as distinct from being objectified and abstract. Notions of ethnophysiology and contingent health concerns index key cultural values as well as images inspired by analogical reasoning. We demonstrate that health practices associated with metaphorical models of ethnophysiology have profound public health ramifications.

5

1. CULTURAL NOTIONS OF FERTILITY IN SOUTH ASIA AND THEIR IMPACT ON SRI LANKAN FAMILY PLANNING PRACTICES

In this paper we address a topic crucial to the field of family planning, yet rarely identified as a subject for research: cultural perceptions of fertility. Data from two ethnographic contexts will be presented: South Kanara District, Karnataka State, India and Low Country, Southwest Sri Lanka. A case study which sparked our curiosity in the cultural perception of fertility will initially be introduced, followed by a general discussion of the anthropological literature on fertility and conception in India. In most of this literature, conception is discussed in relation to systems of descent. Moving beyond textual sources, we will present field data on folk notions of fertility collected in both South India and Sri Lanka during the course of medical anthropological research. In the Sri Lankan context, attention will additionally be paid to how health ideology affects family planning behavior; more specifically, for whom a "safe period" constitutes a popular traditional mode of fertility control.[2] Turning to family planning programs in Sri Lanka, we will suggest that the provision of fertility cycle education for the 25-35 year old age cohort could result in a more effective usage of safe period with condoms as a popular means of birth control. While most members of this group have expressed a marked desire for birth postponement and spacing, they presently underutilize modern family planning methods (Contraceptive Prevalence Survey 1983).

THE INDIAN STUDY

In 1974 while conducting ethnographic research on health culture in South Kanara, we became intrigued by the numerous references in local folklore to a woman's heightened fertility after her purification bath taken on the fourth day of menses. Some of these references described a woman as being so fertile at this time, that the mere sight of a man was enough to influence the features of a child conceived during that month. Inasmuch as the region was predominantly matrilineal, we initially interpreted such references within the context of matrilineal kinship and descent. Later, however, while studying laypersons' notions of physiology, we found members of both matrilineal and patrilineal castes who considered the first week following menstruation to be particularly fertile. Moreover, similar references to times of peak fertility were noted in the folklore of patrilineal caste groups inhabiting the nearby Deccan Plains.

7

A case which highlighted the importance of cultural notions of fertility to us involved a middle-aged Brahman couple who frequented a traditional ayurvedic practitioner for fertility medicines. The husband and wife both had college educations and resided in a rural village. They had been married for seven years and family members described their marital relationship as close. Not having conceived a child in the first three years of marriage, they had initially consulted a relative who was a qualified doctor. They were both tested thoroughly and found biologically capable of having children. The doctor did not, however, discuss with the couple their sexual behavior. After consultations with three other doctors, the couple visited numerous temples where vows were made. Additionally, the woman underwent two dilatation and curettage procedures. She had these procedures performed because she felt that perhaps her womb was "unclean or blocked." Dilatation and curettage procedures are popular among the middle class in India as a perceived means of increasing fertility (Nichter 1981a). Finally, the couple sought the advice of a renowned ayurvedic practitioner who prescribed special dietary practices and herbal preparations. In addition to the balancing of body humors, these regiments were taken to increase, strengthen and thicken the husband's *dhatu* (the vital part of semen and to cool the wife's overly hot body, purify her blood, and stop *dhatu* loss manifest as leucorrhea (Nichter 1981b). Despite these efforts, the woman had not conceived.

We came to know this couple quite well and on one occasion we questioned them individually about their sexual behavior — a matter of utmost intimacy. To our astonishment, we found that for seven years the couple had been engaging in coitus only for the first three days following the menstruation purification bath. Having a child was of such importance to this couple that they had abstained from sexual activity during most of the month in an effort to save enough *dhatu* to afford them "the best chance of having a strong child at the easiest time for conception." When we discussed this case with three middle-aged local ayurvedic practitioners, we found that two out of the three considered this time period to be particularly fertile. Two of the practitioners noted additionally that they had learned from books that mid cycle was "also" a fertile time. Traditional and modern knowledge had been incorporated into an eclectic knowledge base.

Returning to the region's oral tradition, we found references associating the fourth day after menstruation with both purity and fertility.[3] We questioned whether it was just purity in itself which was associated with the power of fertility or perhaps some set of contingent factors. With respect to contingent factors influencing states of fertility, we noted that menstrual blood is not only deemed impure, but also heating. During interviews, informants placed emphasis on the heating nature of menstrual blood, not its impurity, when discussing menstruation as a state of non-fertility. An image commonly offered was that contact with menstrual blood was so "heating" as to dry a man's semen, just as the touch of a menstruating woman was heating enough to "cause a vine of cooling betel leaves to wilt."

Following up on the latter idea, we questioned a local ayurvedic scholar (pandit) about conception among animals who are fertile ("in heat") during menstruation. Conception among humans and animals was contrasted by the pandit. He described animals, creatures of the wild, as conceived from a state of heat. Heat constituted a state of uncontrol, "unbound desire ruled by hunger." Humans as higher, more controlled, "purer" beings were conceived through the containment of heat during coitus.[4] This image was elaborated upon in relation to metamedical dimensions of Brahmanic Hinduism, an analysis of which lies outside the scope of this paper.[5]

Closer to popular Brahmanic Hindu thought were analogical descriptions of conception made by the pandit which employed agriculture as a referential framework. Agricultural analogies for conception are widely reported throughout India (Das 1976; Dube 1978; Fruzzetti and Ostor 1976; Inden and Nicholas 1977; Mayer 1960).[6] They are found in the Ramayana and Dharmasastra (Trautmann 1981), as well as in such Ayurvedic texts as the Charaka Samhita (Inden and Nicholas 1977). Moreover, they play an important part in the marriage rituals of several patrilineal castes (Dube 1978). The most prevalent analogy describes conception in terms of the "male seed" and "female field." Reference to this image of conception has most often been cited by social scientists in the course of examining patrilineal descent. The following quote is illustrative:

The quality of the field can affect the quality of the grain, but it cannot determine the kind. . . . The seed determines the kind. The offspring belongs to one to whom the seed belongs. In fact he also owns the field. . . . By equating the woman's body with the field or earth, and the semen with seed, the process of reproduction is equated with the process of production and rights over the children with the rights over the crop. . . . The language of the seed and the field is used for stressing the woman's lack of rights over her children in the event of separation or divorce (Dube 1978: 8—9).

The importance of the seed-field analogy extends beyond its use as a charter for partilineal descent in particular caste cultures. Data from South Kanara District are illustrative. A common way to note that a woman is pregnant in the Tuḷu language is to say *alena bangida onji bittu koddyondundu*, literally, in her stomach a seed sprouts. While this expression could lead one to ponder whether the agricultural analogy noted above is a pervasive feature of popular thought about conception in South Kanara, such is not the case. Indeed, an analogical model linking descent to notions of conception is notably absent in this region's rich oral tradition. This is not to say, however, that agricultural imagery is absent from, or is not being incorporated within, popular thought about conception.

Living in a region of intensive rice cultivation, people have found agricultural imagery appealing when employed as a referential framework by ayurvedic practitioners. Practitioners use such imagery in their efforts to explain to clients health issues including those related to fertility and infertility. Agricultural imagery once introduced is often generalized, extended, and incorporated within the region's popular health culture. For example, we documented one instance wherein a villager extended an analogy about conception in a way not envisioned by the ayurvedic practitioner he had consulted. The practitioner had in passing compared the informant's wife to a dry rice bed when explaining the action of a fertility medicine prescribed for the woman during the first 16 days of her cycle. When we later asked the informant about times of fertility during a woman's monthly cycle, the informant noted that after a rice field is plowed and manured, it is left standing for three days before seed is sown. On the third day "the soil is soft, moist and easily able to sprout fertile seed. Then, day by day, the soil becomes more and more difficult to penetrate." The informant stated that this was also the case with women who "after three days of menstruation are wet, soft and most capable of conceiving." According to the informant, a woman's condition was less and less favorable for conception as her cycle progressed. After 15 or 16 days (from the onset of menstruation) conception became unlikely as the woman, like the field, became dry. The informant was quick to note, however, that when reckoning the likelihood of conception one also had to consider the strength of the man's seed to "take root." A strong seed might root even under less opportune conditions. This idea was echoed by the advice offered to couples desiring progeny by a local ayurvedic practitioner. The practitioner's notion was that stronger, healthier seed would sprout seven to twelve days after the onset of menstruation, whereas any seed might sprout four to six days after onset. The practitioner therefore advised couples to engage in sex for strong progeny only during the latter fertile days of a woman's cycle.

An analysis of the practitioner's patterns of treatment revealed an implicit assumption about a woman's cycle being divided into two 15-day sectors. For women who wanted to conceive he prescribed two kinds of herbal decoctions, *kashaya*, the first to be taken the day after the onset of menses to day 15, and the second from day 16 to menses onset. The first of these "family" medicines functioned to prepare the womb, *garbha kosha*, to accept seed and reduce the possibility of *sutaka vayu* (literally pollution wind, an ailment linked to seed rejection). The second medicine was taken to make the womb strong enough to hold the seed. A local proprietor of a commercial ayurvedic medicine shop with whom we discussed this idea noted that it was reflected in a popular prescription pattern by practitioners using commercial ayurvedic products. The medicine *Ayapan* would be prescribed during the first 15 days of a woman's cycle, followed by "Loes Compound" during the next 15 days.

While analogical thinking linking conception to agriculture was revealed during our interviews, it would be misrepresentative to describe the seed-field analogy as a pervasive cultural model for conception in South Kanara. Conception is not a widely thought about or elaborately worked out cultural concept among the non-Brahman, largely matrilineal castes of South Kanara. The most common idea expressed was that in order for conception to occur the mingling of both male and female semen, *dhatu*, was required at the proper time of the month. More emphasis was placed on the time of the month when a woman is fertile than details about why this time is physiologically fertile. A notion of the mixing of *dhatu* would seemingly endorse a more cognatic theory of descent. We found, however, that an ecletic body of ideas linked blood as life force to descent. Some informants spoke of all children conceived by a couple as sharing a mixture of both parents' blood. Others spoke of girls sharing their mother's blood and boys their father's blood. Many informants found the subject of conception troublesome to think about abstractly. They shifted between references to blood which incorporated ideas about descent, ideas about health and illness. Ideas were diffuse and not well integrated. It might be argued that such an eclectic body of ideas about conception better serves the prevailing pattern of discerning descent. The latter is more determined by pedigree (family fame, property, etc.) than strict interpretations of descent by blood line.

LAY NOTIONS OF FERTILITY: CROSS-CULTURAL REFERENCES

On returning to the West we conducted a literature search on cultural ideas pertaining to fertility. Despite the existence of a voluminous literature on cultural aspects of family planning attitudes and practices, very little data were available on the subject of cultural notions of fertility.[7] In India, Nag (1968:83) reported that some West Bengali women consider the 4th to 12th days following the onset of menstruation to be favorable for conception. A reference to lay perceptions of "safe period" was found in Mandelbaum's (1970) book on social and cultural dimensions of human fertility in India. Mandelbaum devoted one paragraph to this subject while making note of the implications of post menstruation taboos:

There is one kind of abstinence that paradoxically may result in higher rather than lower fertility. It is popularly believed that a woman's most fertile period comes in the days immediately following the cessation of menstruation and that the rest of the menstrual cycle is "safer." Sexual relations are forbidden during menstruation and almost all couples rigorously observe this taboo. But in a number of groups a postmenstrual taboo period is also favored. In a sample of women from a Mysore village, 66% reported abstinence for at least 8 days after onset, as did 40% of the women in a sample from a middle-class part of Delhi. Some women reported up to 15 days of abstinence after onset. As C. Chandrasekaran points out, with such abstinence periods, "the timing of coitus appears to coincide with the days of the woman's ovulation" (Mandelbaum 1970:64).

No indication is given by either Nag or Mandelbaum as to why the time period immediately following menstruation should be considered fertile, or what ramifications such a conceptualization might have on family planning practices. Indeed, it is not clear from the data presented by Mandelbaum as to why a formal prohibition on coitus exists during the most fertile time of the month. Is it related to ritual impurity health concerns (for the woman or man), or perhaps to a deliberate, but unstated, practice of birth control?

Gould (1969) goes a step further in speculating on the ramifications of existing ideas about fertility and suggests that fertility education might have a positive impact on the practice of family planning.

Villagers are interested in and do practice a folk based rhythm method. The problem is that their conception of the fertility cycle is inaccurate. They believe that the safe period embraces the middle fifteen days of the menstrual cycle. Rhythm practiced in accordance with this idea must increase rather than decrease fertility. But if family planning workers concentrated on teaching the villagers the correct safe period, plus coitus interruptus, I feel these methods would prove to be more acceptable at this stage than more sophisticated approaches. In the West, after all, the birth rate began to drop through the adoption of methods like this (Gould 1969:549).

Our literature search revealed that the Indian subcontinent is not the only ethnographic region where the period of time immediately following menstruation is thought to be particularly fertile. Historically, references to this perception of fertility are abundantly found in the writings of classical Greek physicians (Finch and Green 1963), as well as English physicians during the 19th century (McLaren 1984).[8] Rubel et al. (1975) note that in Cebu, Philippines, it is believed that conception is facilitated if coitus takes place on the fourth day after the onset of the menstrual cycle. In Afghanistan, Hunte (1985) has noted that the practice of a folk rhythm method involves abstinence from intercourse directly before and after the menstrual period. These are times in a woman's cycle that are perceived as fertile. Likewise, Hansen (1975), in his book on the Polynesian island of Rapa, notes:

Most Rapans would like to limit their families to two or three children. To this end, they practice a rhythm method of birth control, but they find it most ineffective. "I don't understand it," remarked one woman, then expecting her eighth child. "We abstain from intercourse for three or four days right after my period every month, but I keep getting pregnant. . . .". Further checking revealed it to be the general opinion on Rapa that conception occurs during the few days immediately following menstruation (Hansen 1975: 52).

Hansen is the only scholar whom we identified as having investigated why an indigenous population perceived the time period following menstruation to be fertile.[9] His research led him to consider the "mechanics of the uterus," what we prefer to call the "ethnophysiology of fertility".

The uterus is conceived to be a mechanical organ which opens and closes. Remaining tightly closed most of the time, it opens for several days each month to allow the stale blood to run out. Rapans support their concept of a mechanical uterus with their belief that blood is harbored in the uterus in liquid form, like water in a bottle. If the uterus did not open and close but remained perenially open, they argue, then instead of regular menstrual periods there would be a constant seepage of blood. Just as blood cannot escape a closed uterus semen cannot enter it, so there is no possibility of conception during the greater part of the cycle. [Hence one can understand their incredulity at our assertion that conception is most likely to occur about midway between menses.] Conception could occur during menstruation but ideas that menstrual flow is contaminating led them to avoid intercourse at this time. However, the uterus remains open for a few days after menstruation, and this is the time when, in Rapan eyes, conception occurs (Hansen 1975: 53).

We will see shortly that Rapan ideas about conception are not far removed from lay ideas expressed by some Sri Lankans. Before turning to the Sri Lankan context, however, it is insightful to briefly present some data collected by Johnson et al. (1978) about knowledge of reproduction in a central Michigan prenatal clinic for multi-ethnic, low income clientele in the United States. This data may serve to illustrate that lay knowledge of fertility is an issue in need of study in developed as well as developing countries.

The majority of women interviewed in the prenatal clinic did not understand reproductive physiology. Sixty-one percent could not correctly answer questions as to why their menstrual periods occurred, the source of menstrual blood, or why the menstrual flow stopped. . . . One of the most prominent misconceptions about menstruation involved uterine anatomy. Many of the women seemed to perceive it as an organ which was closed between menstrual periods and which had to open up to allow the blood to get out. They were greatly concerned that nothing impede this process. . . . Sixteen percent believed that pregnancy was most likely to occur during menses because the uterus was open, allowing the sperm to enter. Conversely, it is logically closed at mid-cycle and therefore thought safe for intercourse without risk of pregnancy (Johnson et al. 1978: 860-861).

In a follow-up study of 200 undereducated Black inner-city women, Johnson and Snow (1982) found that 64% of their informants were unable to answer when in their cycle they could become pregnant, 79% did not know of a safe period for intercourse, and 60% did not know they could become pregnant while breastfeeding infants.

THE SRI LANKAN STUDY

What difference, if any, do ethnophysiological notions of fertility have on the layperson's family planning related behavior? We had the opportunity to look into this issue in 1984 while conducting anthropological fieldwork in southwest Sri Lanka. With respect to existing data on lay notions of fertility in Sri Lanka, Nag (1968: 43) has summarized the observations made by Ryan in the early 1950s in a low country Sinhalese village. "According to folk physiology, conception is not likely to occur during the period of 14 days preceding menstruation. People, however, have little faith nowadays in this theory, probably because they have noticed many exceptions." The implication of this statement is that folk ideas about fertility have little impact on family planning related behavior. McGilvray (1982: 52), in a more recent study, notes that among Tamils in the Batticaloa region of eastern Sri Lanka the 12—14 day post-menstruation fertility idea continues to be prevalent. McGilvray did not comment on Ryan's statements regarding the degree of faith the lay population places in traditional ideas of fertility, nor how their ideas about fertility influence their family planning behavior. His more general impressions of folk health behavior are, however, suggestive of possible family planning related behavior:

There is quite a bit of skepticism about many aspects of traditional ethnomedical doctrine, just as there is skepticism about the gods and penicillin. You can be skeptical but still want to cover your bets. The entire pluralistic domain of healing strategies reflects this sort of pragmatism and lack of concern with adherence to one specific doctrine (McGilvray, personal communication).

Among the rural low country Buddhist population we interviewed, there co-existed numerous ideas about when a woman is fertile during her monthly cycle. These ranged from a few days prior to menstruation to the first 15 days of the cycle calculated either from the day menstruation started or the day a woman took her fourth day purification bath. Figure 1 summarizes the ideas of 100 literate, rural Sinhalese women under the age of 45.[10] Data are presented by way of two to three day time frames which enable the presentation of responses which denote the informant's own time divisions. The first time frame depicted is a two day frame prior to menstruation. The next time frame consitutes the three day period a woman is culturally perceived to be menstruating. It is important to note that the following two time frames were cited by over 80% of the sample:

1. From the fourth day following the menstruation purification bath until the 11—12th day of a woman's cycle.

2. From the fourth day following the menstruation purification bath until the 14—15th day of a woman's cycle.

Evoking responses to the question of when one is most/least fertile required tact and innovative interviewing techniques. In Sri Lanka, fertility is not a subject easily spoken about through direct questioning. When we talked with interviewers who had worked on the World Fertility Survey (1978) and the Contraceptive Prevalence Survey (1983), we asked how survey respondents had discussed "safe period" as a method. Interviewers remarked that when probed about traditional methods, women respondents spoke of "being

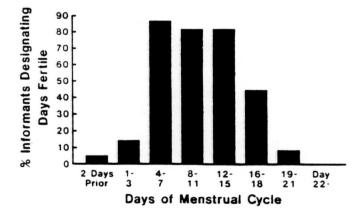

Figure 1. Days Perceived as Fertile (N = 100)

careful", *api paressam venava*. This was ticked on the survey form as indicative of "safe period."

In our own interviews we spent considerable time engaging in cultural free association with informants about a wide range of subjects spanning the dynamics of how they met their partners to issues involving health and the economics of family life. When introducing the topic of fertility we did not present ourselves to informants as authorities on the subject, but rather as people trying to learn from folk wisdom and their individual experiences. Moreover, we worked with Sri Lankan co-interviewers to develop a metaphorical interview style to be used with informants who responded poorly to direct questioning. Although the metaphorical interview was used with approximately one quarter of our informants, this interview method generated some of the most insightful data pertaining to why specific time periods were considered particularly fertile.

To engage in metaphorical interviewing, the interviewer needs to identify a familiar referential framework within which a sensitive topic can be addressed while maintaining an acceptable degree of social distance. Interviews within the metaphor, a convergence communication technique (Mimi Nichter 1982; Buck et al. 1983) move back and forth from analogy to specificity in an accordian-like fashion. An example of a metaphor developed for interviews on fertility is cited below and leads into a discussion of lay ideas underscoring the notions of fertility noted above.

When we first began our interviews about fertility, we found that most informants had a far more difficult time initially replying to a direct question about "safe period" as a family planning practice, than to the question "when in the month is it easiest to become pregnant?" Direct questions focusing on fertility evoked the responses noted earlier, with little idea gained as to why these times of the month were considered fertile. Informants commonly stated that this was what others had told them or what they had heard. At this point, we engaged a select group of key informants in metaphorical interviews.

One of the most effective referential frameworks that was utilized evoked the image of the womb as like a flower. This image was suggested by our senior co-interviewer, a retired rural development research officer who was also a popular local poet. Poetic expression is commonplace in Sinhala culture and the image of a flower is pervasive in Sinhala poetry as a symbol of fertility, a symbol utilized in the ritual marking of a girl's first menstruation.[11] After the image of the flower was introduced, informants were given a chance to free associate, eventually being asked a question such as "When in the month is the bud most ready for the bloom of conception?"

One image which emerged from this question frame was quite similar to the ideas expressed by the Rapan islanders. The flower was most "open" to conception during and following menstruation. Ideas varied as to how long the flower stayed open following menstruation, indicative of the variety of ideas reported about fertility duration. Ideas also varied as to whether one could become pregnant during menstruation. While no Sri Lankan informant spoke of a woman being too hot to conceive during menstruation, as informants had noted in South India, most informants pointed out that the flow of blood outwards would prevent conception.[12] Reference would inevitably be made to a woman being impure, *killi*, at this time, but the latter was not explicitly linked to infertility. Fifteen of our 100 informants noted that having intercourse during menstruation could lead to conception, and two informants specifically mentioned that newlyweds anxious for a child engage in intercourse during menstruation as the chances of conceiving at that time were high. Six informants believed that the uterus opened a few days prior to menstruation and that conception was possible at this time.

Two other ideas associated with fertility behavior emerged from cultural free association about the image of a uterus opening and closing. The first was that following delivery a woman is at high risk of becoming pregnant while she is still bleeding—a period of time ranging from two weeks to three months. During this time her womb is spoken of as an "open" healing wound. The first 14 days following delivery are considered to be high risk days when a woman is 'open' to become pregnant. Many women expressed the idea that abstention from intercourse was necessary until a woman's periods became regular for reasons relating to both general health and the prevention of pregnancy.[13] Other women viewed amenorrhea after the third month follow-ing delivery as a "safe period" if a woman was breastfeeding. Although not expressed directly, the underlying idea here may well be that the uterus remains closed "after the wound healed" and until menstruation reoccurred. Ideas directly expressed by women subscribing to the latter notion took the form of a chain complex: strings of events considered contiguous. It was noted that menstrual blood is utilized in the formation of breastmilk and that indulgence in sex results in both a reduction of breastmilk and a resumption of menstruation. Some Sinhala informants perceived the birth rate of Muslims to be higher because "coitus was resumed early after delivery, babies were weaned-bottlefed early and therefore menstruation returned early."[14] Underscoring such a chain complex could well be ethnophysio-logical notions incorporated from ayurvedic humoral ideology. According to the latter, food is progressively transformed into a series of body substances from blood, flesh and bone to breastmilk and semen, *dhatu*. According to lay interpretation, as *dhatu* reserves in the form of semen become depleted through sexual activity, the body attempts to replenish these reserves. This leads to a reduction of the amount of *dhatu* available for breastmilk production.

Government midwives noted that there was widespread belief that a woman could not become pregnant after delivery before the resumption of menstruation if she was breastfeeding.[15] This belief, compounded by a fear of reduced breastmilk if one used "heaty" birth control pills, resulted in a pronounced decrease in the use of family planning methods during post-partum amenorrhea even when menstruation was delayed as long as one year. All women interviewed noted that if a woman became pregnant while breastfeeding she must stop breastfeeding for both the health of her fetus and her breastfed child. *Mandama dosa*, a folk illness often manifest as acute protein calorie malnutrition, was derectly linked to breastfeeding while pregnant. Inasmuch as most mothers considered one-and-a-half years as an optimum amount of time to breastfeed children, there was considerable concern about not becoming pregnant before this time had passed. For cultural reasons associated with notions of ethnophysiology, this concern was chiefly expressed during the first three months following delivery.

Analogical associations comparing a woman to an agricultural field were less prominent in Sri Lanka than in India. Two agricultural analogies evoked during interviews were, however, noteworthy. The first was elicited while interviewing women about how modern family planning methods were perceived to work. Birth control pills are considered by Sri Lankan women to have heating and drying properties. These properties are not perceived as "side effects" of the pill, but rather the very properties which constitute the means by which the pill effectively prevents fertility. In the context of articulating this, one female informant noted that the uterus is dried by the heating effect of the pill so the seed cannot take root. She went on to note that a woman taking the pill was as dry as she would be in the later days of her cycle before menstruation. She then warned that being in this hot, dry state for a long period of time led to the uterus "crumbling" like a piece of wood disintegrating when left out in the sun. This rendered a woman incapable of conception. The latter image reemerged in subsequent inter-views about the properties and dangers of using birth control pills. These interviews led us to question whether a wetness-dryness folk model of conception might not be more prevalent than our interviews had revealed. What needs to be researched is whether this model is context specific to thinking about the pill, or constitute a more general model. A more sensitive set of research questions need be developed.

Cultural free association led to a second analogy being made between the fertility of women and the land. During a conversation with a male agricul-turist, a woman's menstrual cycle was offhandedly compared to that of the moon cycle. Follow-up research on qualitative aspects of moon phases led to a string of references being made about such subjects as crop sowing, hair cutting and signs of a good and bad death. A brief consideration of this data is insightful. In Sri Lanka, all crops with the exception of tubers are sown prior to the full moon. Plants are sown as the moon is waxing, a time known in Sinhala as *puru paksha*, and in Tamil as *valar pirai*.[16] Concordantly, during this time of development, weddings are planned as are house warming ceremonies and the laying of foundations. Hair is cut during this time in the belief that a longer healthier quantity will grow back. Birth and death during this time are deemed auspicious. To the contrary, occurrence of death during the waning of the moon is deemed inauspicious. Only yams are planted while the moon is waning, inasmuch as tubers grow downward.

Accordingly, the informant associated the waxing of the moon with the first 16 days of a woman's cycle, a time of fertility and growth. The waning of the moon was associated with the latter half of a woman's cycle, a time of decreasing fertility. This conceptualization evoked through a set of images during cultural free association may well constitute a meta dimension to lay ideas about the first 15—16 days of a woman's cycle being her fertile period. It is also feasible that the second most common fertility duration range cited by informants, 14—15 days from the menstruation purification bath, constitutes a variation on this theme. There was considerable confusion among many informants as to whether one calculated fertile days from the first day of the cycle or the day of the menstruation purification bath.

IMPLICATIONS FOR FAMILY PLANNING

Two broad family planning related issues arise in light of the data presented from Sri Lanka. The first involves research on the prevalence and effectiveness of traditional fertility regulation practices in Sri Lanka, while the second involves family planning education. Sri Lanka is a rapidly developing country which boasts a high literacy rate for both men (90%) and women (82%); a low infant mortality rate (37/1,000); good access to medical services; and an island-wide transportation and mass media network (Pollack 1983). With respect to family planning, data from both the World Fertility Survey (1978) and the Contraceptive Prevalence Survey (1983) reveal that a large number of Sri Lankans are in favor of population control. Indeed, almost all our informants were interested in limiting their family size in response to economic pressures and changes of "wealth flow" within the family (Caldwell 1980). Despite family planning as a documented felt need, the Contraceptive Prevalence Survey (CPS) showed that only 23% of women who did not want more children were using a modern method, 40% were using a traditional practice and 36% were using no method at all.[17] According to the results of the World Fertility Survey (WFS) and CPS surveys, low utilization of modern methods could not be attributed to lack of familiarity with these methods. Knowledge, or what may more accurately be termed familiarity with methods, was noted in 91% of the WFS and 99% of the CPS survey populations. Quantitative data collected on the practice of safe period (when people are "careful") may, at best, be considered impressionistic because surveys to date have neglected to follow up on "when people are careful and how."[18] This limitation aside, it is evident that in Sri Lanka traditional practices are clearly popular and that barriers to the adoption of modern methods exist for reasons which go beyond literacy and familiarity with modern methods.

It is beyond the scope of this paper to consider why modern methods are not more popular. This is addressed in detail in Chapter three. Highlighted will be both lay perceptions of how modern family planning methods work and ideas about side effects in the context of popular health culture. What may be noted at present is that ideas about how modern methods work impact on when couples adopt methods and what couples choose to use as birth control. Let us consider this point in relation to CPS data. According to CPS data (1983: 67—71), the rhythm method (more appropriately labeled safe period) is clearly the *temporary* fertility control practice of choice for women aged 15—49. In respect to *all forms of* birth control, rhythm is the most popular mode until age 24. In the 25—34 year old age groups, sterilization takes a slight lead in popularity, with this lead becoming prominent after age 35.[19] These data suggest that women who want to space their children or postpone childbirth prefer traditional practices of fertility control to modern methods, while those women who no longer desire conception opt for sterilization.

How common is the use of traditional practices of birth control? According to the CPS (1983: 67) of ever-married women aged 30—34 who had ever used contraception, 47% had used traditional methods (safe period and withdrawal). This is significantly higher than the findings of the WFS which estimated that 21% of this cohort had at some time used traditional practices. Our impression is that the practices of "safe period" and withdrawal are far more pervasive than indicated by either of these two surveys. In defense of this impression let us cite data from both our own research and that of a health educator graduate student (Chullawathi 1985) who conducted a village study in an effort to validate and expand upon our findings. During our ten months of research, we felt close enough to 35 of our married female informants aged 25—35 to interview them about their traditional birth control practices. Each of these women was literate, had one to two children and was considering the possibility of having another child. Of this group, two-thirds were using or had used in the past two years, safe period and/or withdrawal as a birth control method. Only five of these women had tried the pill and two had tried the loop. Six reported that their husbands sometimes used condoms in conjunction with their ideas of the unsafe period. Two took birth control pills "only" during the perceived unsafe period.

Chullawathi followed up on the impressions cast by these interviews with women from three different districts in low country Sri Lanka. She conducted a more rigorous cluster survey in three villages of Galle District. With the assistance of two local field assistants she interviewed all mothers under 35 years of age. Of the 95 women interviewed, 97% were literate and 52% were educated to the 10th standard. Among these women she found that 65% had used safe period as a primary means of birth control, with 44% of the women using this practice currently. Fifty-six percent of her sample reported that they had experienced an unexpected pregnancy. Of those in her sample who had specifically used safe period, 31% reported conceiving while using this practice. Of the 42 women currently using safe period, only 7 stated that their husbands used this practice in conjunction with condoms. Chullawathi further noted that 87% of her informants noted that they had a regular menstrual cycle. With respect to the probable effectiveness of their practice, 13% of her sample engaged in coitus only between the 20—28th days of the cycle yielding a high probable efficacy. Another 18% engaged in coitus after the 15th day of the cycle. The remaining women reported a wide range of ideas about safe period which indicated that the 14—18th day of the cycle was considered safe.

The question may be asked how is it that the lay population has not caught on that their ideas about fertility do not accord with their experience of conception? In the first instance, folk ideas of fertility do in some case cover peak fertility periods.[20] Further, it must be recognized that interpretation is a hermeneutic process and common sense has a cultural dimension. Three points may be made in this regard. First, communication between husband and wife about perceived fertility is often minimal inasmuch as it entails discussion of a personal practice as opposed to a publicly sanctioned method.[21] Moreover, many women feel that they must succumb to their husband's sexual demands if not wishes. This is not to say, however, that women do not have available to them means by which to distance themselves from sexuality, for cultural institutions such as religion provide such means. What we would emphasize is that there are slips in the practice of safe period regardless of the scientific validity of this practice. Humans are as much rule breakers as rule makers and obeyers. Pregnancy attribution is often interpreted in relation to slip-ups during the first 16 days of a woman's cycle when she is culturally perceived to be fertile.

A second point involves menstrual irregularity and the range of factors from diet to physical activity and stress which impact on the frequency and duration of a woman's cycle (Harrel 1981). Menstrual irregularity, particularly amenorrhea, contributes to confusion about a woman's fertility and raises doubts as to whether a woman is pregnant or not. The latter point has important ramifications. Periodic amenorrhea is not uncommonly suspected to be pregnancy in both rural southwest India and Sri Lanka. Many women, experiencing amenorrhea, engage in activities to "bring back menstruation" as soon as they feel that their cycle is past due and that they might be "becoming pregnant." Their use of dietary manipulation, herbal decoctions, and hard work to bring back their menses is not viewed as causing an abortion. It is rather a form of menstrual regulation.[22] Menstrual regulation is particularly common among lactating women wishing to continue breastfeeding, but who think they may be "becoming" pregnant. As previously noted, there are cultural sanctions against breastfeeding a baby while a woman is pregnant.

Lay interpretation of a delayed menstrual cycle followed by its return after dietary manipulation and the like leads some women to interpret that they were indeed in the process of becoming pregnant. Retrospective thinking is often more influenced by ideas about fertility than safe period. While many women entertain some measure of doubt as to the validity of their ideas about a non-fertile period, they still maintain traditional ideas about when they are most fertile. These women tend to associate their perceived state of pregnancy, prior to bringing back their menses, with an act of coitus during the first 16 days of their cycle. For others who have not experienced coitus within this time frame, or for whom pregnancy continues despite alterations of diet and the taking of herbal decoctions, there is always a fatalistic theme to fall back on. Among Sinhalese Buddhists, a common expression noted at this time is "the child that is meant to be born will be born."

EDUCATION ABOUT FERTILITY

In the Yucatan, as in many parts of the world, women believe that the most fertile time is immediately before and after menstruation, because at that time "the uterus is open." Women who want to avoid pregnancy will have intercourse in mid cycle when they believe the uterus to be closed — exactly at the most fertile time. The medical staff, however, were not aware of this belief. So the family planning course failed to impart the single piece of information which could be expected to have a real impact on contraceptive behavior.

(Jordan 1987: 6)

Fertility is not a subject discussed with lay people by family health workers, public health midwives or hospital staff. Reasons why this subject is not introduced involve both the sensitivity of the topic and the attitude that "to talk to lay people about such things will only reduce their interest in accepting scientific family planning methods." The latter argument was commonplace in our discussions with health staff. The argument complements the strong position which Sri Lankan politicians take against sex education which they feel will lead to premarital sex among youth. Proponents of both arguments underestimate the potential for miseducation when appropriate education is not provided. They fail to appreciate existing fertility regulation and sexual behavior. In regard to family planning knowledge and behavior, the following points may be emphasized:

1. The belief of health planners that literacy in itself will "correct false and superstitious beliefs about the body" is naive. Most of our literate informants continued to entertain traditional ideas about fertility at times incorporating these with modern ideas. Less than 15% of our 100 literate informants had a correct, scientific idea of safe period.

2. Literacy in itself provides one with an equal opportunity to both education and miseducation, in accord with the range of information available to read. In the Sri Lankan context, more information of dubious scientific merit is available on sexuality than information on fertility which addresses lay concerns in a manner which is culturally responsive and understandable. According to one Sri Lankan sociologist, some 153 sex

magazines are available in the streets of Sri Lanka spreading spurious information about human sexuality.[23]

3. By not addressing lay ideas about the ethnophysiology of fertility,
current family planning education is less effective than it could be. This is
illustrated by women failing to heed government midwives' advice about
adopting family plannning methods after delivery before menstruation re-
sumes. As noted, many women feel it is unnecessary to adopt contraceptive
behavior until 12—18 months after delivery.

4. There is a marked reluctance to adopt temporary modern family
planning methods among many recently married couples having no or only
one child. This reluctance is related to an expressed concern that the use of
modern methods may interfere with their ability to have healthy children in
the future. Based on our interviews, we suspect that many such couples
practice a combination of safe period and withdrawal, or safe period and
condom use. Indigenous and eclectic notions of fertility affect practice as well
as efficacy of practice.

The latter point needs to be considered in light of present international
interest in identifying potential user groups for natural family planning
methods and a combination of natural and modern methods.[24] From the
interview data gathered it would appear that literate, young Sri Lankan
couples having no or only one child, wishing to postpone or space childbirth,
would consitute ideal candidates for such programs. Many of these couples
are not current users of modern methods and many of those who use
condoms do so in combination with an idea of fertility which is unscientific.
A culturally sensitive program which educates about fertility, both in respect
to the planning and prevention of conception, would constitute a visible
example of family planning, not just a program to lower population growth.
In order for such a program to be successful it will be necessary to generalize
the recommendations made by Johnson et al. (1978) on the basis of research
in the U.S. clinical context:

Most educational schemes in clinical settings are based on the premise that the presentation of
proper information is what is required to improve patient knowledge and behavior. This is the
case only where patients lack information. A very different sort of problem is the replacement
of incorrect information. A patient who is presented with a fact which conflicts with what she
believes to be true culturally is not necessarily going to reject the old and take on the new
because the correctness of the new is scientific fact. To deal with this problem, health care
personnel must learn to ask other sorts of questions, to elicit information which may seem to
them ridiculous and to do so in a nonjudgemental and noncondescending manner. They will
then have to develop educational programs in an individualized manner to allow for the
variety of beliefs among their patients (Johnson et al. 1978: 853).

Broadening these recommendations in the development context will entail
the coordination of interpersonal and mass media health communication
approaches responsive to ongoing ethnographic research incorporated within
the health education process.[25]

NOTES

1. The population studied in South Kanara was a multi-case mix of Tuḷu and Kannaḍa speakers residing in Bantval, Puttur, and Beltangadi Taluks. In Sri Lanka the population studied consisted of multi-caste Sinhalese Buddhists. Fieldwork was conducted in Ratnapura, Horana, Galle, and Matara Districts.

2. "Safe period" is a term designating a time during a woman's monthly cycle which she perceives as a time of low fertility. By the "practice of safe period" we mean either that a woman engages in sexual activity only during the time associated with low fertility, *or* that she avoids times she associates with high fertility.

3. The fourth day following the onset of menstruation is marked by a bath which denotes that a woman is ritually pure whether or not she is still bleeding. In keeping with anthropological theory involving purity and danger (Douglas 1966), it could be argued that a woman is open to forces of transformation at a transitional time of *rite de passage*. This might explain legends linking the time of the fourth day bath to immaculate conception from the gods (children being "born in truth") and children taking on the characteristics of those whom a woman's eyes first befall. What it does not explain is why the first half of a woman's cycle (following menses) is deemed more fertile than the second half of her cycle.

4. The ayurvedic concept that heat is contained during coitus leading to conception is underscored by an epistemology regarding the creation of the universe. With regard to human conception, the idea is that "*dhatu ojus*," the potent factor within semen, is a "cooling-light substance" capable of containing heat. Contained heat is a creative force, while uncontained heat is a power of the "wild." (Personal communication from Vaidya P. S. Ishvara Bhat, Vittal, South Kanara District, Karnataka, India.) According to ayurvedic texts, a women's fertility extends to the 16th night of her cycle, or the 12th night after cessation of her menstrual flow (Dash 1975: 11). Coitus during menstruation can lead to conception but results in fetus malformation. The idea that copulation during menstruation can lead to conception but results in ill health is not limited to the Indian subcontinent. According to Talmudic Judaism, a sexual taboo at menstruation is due to a belief that children conceived at this time would be lepers (Spivak 1891, noted in Snowden and Christian 1983: 233).

5. For example, the informant described the Havik Brahman ritual of *oupasana* as symbolizing the union of man and woman through the bonding of heat, a metaphor for conception and creativity. During Havika and other Brahman caste marriage rituals, the couple attends to a ritual fire. Following this act the couple is given a bamboo tube. Placed in this tube by the priest with his left hand are 68 pieces of *durbe* grass, *Cynodon dactylon*. This grass is a symbol of purity which is used as a sacred perimeter to contain the ritual fire. With the right hand the priest places into the tube a branch of *ati, Ficus glomerata*, a symbol of fire, wrapped in sacred thread symbolizing a twice born Brahman male. At the death of either partner the *oupasana* tube must be burned in the funeral pyre signifying the non-bound nature of heat on the part of the remaining partner. If the remaining partner is a male under the age of 50, he is immediately advised to become remarried "for the sake of controlling his heat." If female, the partner is subject to a series of biosocial restrictions to control her state of heat manifest as sexuality.

6. The field-seed image of conception is noted elsewhere in South Asia. For example, Maloney et al. (1981: 119) note that in rural Bangladesh a woman is compared to the land if a couple does not have offspring. "The land is blamed if it gives not a good harvest ... if a crop is not forthcoming it is because of the conditions of the land and its moisture rather than the seed."

7. It is noteworthy that a collaborative World Health Organization study on patterns and perceptions of menstruation (Snowden and Christian 1983) in ten countries (including India) does not address the issue of fertility in relation to popular perceptions of the

menstrual cycle. This is particularly striking because the study was largely oriented toward examining perceptions of menstruation in relation to family planning methods and issues.

8. The notion that conception would have the best chance of taking place immediately after a woman's period is well documented in English history from the 16—19th century (McLaren 1984: 71—72). In most references a woman's cycle is discussed in relation to her most fertile period, not her least fertile period as a means of birth control. A woman's least fertile period was perceived in relation to blood flow. Copulation just prior to or during menses was not thought to result in conception as the seed would not be able to "root" before being washed away.

9. Subsequent to the preparation of this paper two ethnographic studies were received which make reference to lay notions of times of fertility. Interestingly, they draw attention to the two folk models presented in this paper: the open uterus model and the wet-dry uterus model. The first study by Kay (1977) notes that among Mexican-Americans in Tucson, an idea exists that the week before menstruation is a time when a woman is fertile because her uterus is open. Likewise, a woman must be careful not to engage in coitus after a baby is born as her uterus is open at this time as well (the duration is not specified). The second study by Niehof (1985) describes the ideas of women living on the island of Madura in Indonesia:

    Most women do not regard their menstrual cycle as consisting of fertile and infertile days and those who do, unfortunately misunderstand it. They think that they have a greater chance to conceive on the days just before and just after menstruation, and consider the mid-period of the cycle to be sterile. The reversal of the actual pattern of fecundity is caused by the association of dry with sterile and moist with fertile. The womb is thought to be dried in the middle of the cycle. Just before menstruation it is thought to be moist and swollen with blood, providing an ideal host environment for the seed. After menstruation the womb is thought to be like an open wound, facilitating penetration and settling of the seed (Niehof 1985: 223—224).

10. Sixty-five key informant interviews with married women aged 25—38 having at least one child were initially carried out by the authors over a period of seven months in rural villages of Horana, Ratnapura, and Matara districts of low country Sri Lanka. All informants were literate and lower middle class. Twenty to twenty-two informants in each district were interviewed. An additional 35 interviews of women with similar socio-economic and age backgrounds were carried out by graduate students, all seasoned health workers from the Sri Lankan Bureau of Health Education. Data were collected from known informants in Galle, Colombo, Kalutara, and Kurenagala Districts. The range of ideas noted in this paper was further substantiated by focus group interviews carried out by research staff of the Family Planning Association of Sri Lanka (personal communication, Victor de Silva, June 1985).

11. McGilvray (1982: 52) notes that among Batticaloa Tamils the uterus is commonly referred to as a flower and fecundity a time when it is in bloom. In a recent (1986) field trip to South Kanara, the image of a woman's uterus opening and closing like a flower was recorded during an interview with an ayurvedic *vaidya* concerning his prescription practices for women having problems conceiving. A plant image-based fertility education program has been attempted in India. Thormann (1984) in a report on the promotion of natural family planning in India describes the successful use of fruit imagery in teaching about a woman's cycle in the Mother Teresa Missionary of Charity in Calcutta. The following image was used: "Just as a fruit on a tree grows to maturity, gets ripe, falls down and gets rotten, so on the first day of the ovulation cycle the woman knows her ovum (fruit) is starting to ripen. She is aware of dampness, her temperature is rising, her mucus

goes from being sticky to like egg white. After ovulation the mucus gets sticky and dries up. The ovum is dead, the woman feels dry." Note that this image overlaps with traditional ideas about heat, wetness, and dryness.

12. This is not say that in Sri Lanka menstruation is not associated with overheating, for it clearly is. For example. restrictions against bathing involve the idea that the coolness of a bath may interfere with the process of menstruation.

13. There is a popular belief among middle class women with little education that the need for a hysterectomy after menopause is related to engaging in sex too soon after delivery. This act is described as causing the intestines and uterus to "come down." We documented three separate cases where women feared pregnancy to the point of attempting to bring on their menses (see Note 21) after engaging in intercourse within three months following delivery.

14. Part of this perception may have some scientific validity. Muslim women in southwestern Sri Lanka do tend to wean their children early or to place them on formula soon after birth. Research has found that the frequency and intensity of infant suckling induces prolactin activity which inhibits ovulation (Delgado et al. 1978; Huffman et al. 1978).

15. Interestingly, a majority of women interviewed did not think that breastfeeding in itself reduced one's chances of becoming pregnant — it was only when breastfeeding was coupled with a time of non-menstruation.

16. In South Kanara the waxing and waning of the moon are likewise linked to fertility and infertility. For example, a central fertility ritual known as *kedvasa* is begun on a no moon (*amavase*) day when the earth is said to be menstruating. During the three day ritual, fields may not be plowed nor wild plants gathered. As in Sri Lanka, most crops are sown while the moon is waxing (*shukla paksha*). During the waning period (*krishna paksha*), trees are cut for timber as it is said they will be "hard." Trees cut in *shukla paksha* are thought to be "soft" and can rot more easily.

17. Traditional methods of birth control on the Contraceptive Prevalence Survey included rhythm and withdrawal. On the World Fertility Survey, traditional methods included abstinence in addition to rhythm and withdrawal. We choose to use the term "safe period" instead of rhythm method so as to present the practice as it is perceived by villagers (see Note 2).

18. On a methodological note, we would emphasize that the collection of accurate quantitative data about traditional practices of birth control is problematic. Our experience, corroborated by that of CPS and WFS survey interviewers, is that data collection on traditional practices is far more difficult than data collection on modern methods. Some degree of social distance is afforded by the technological status of modern methods. Indeed, the community has become somewhat desensitized to discussions of "methods" through the media, if not interactions with health/medical staff. Discussion of traditional fertility control entails the discussion of "practices" (as opposed to methods). One's practices are highly personal and individualistic and are rarely, if ever, discussed in Sinhala culture, even among friends.

19. Shedlin and Hollerbach (1981) propose a model for fertility decision making and stress that it is a process which may change with each successive birth. It seems that the Sri Lanka data concords with this model.

20   Efficacy would depend on the duration and regularity of a woman's cycle as well as ideas about fertility and safe days. There may be a notable difference in the efficacy of birth control practices among those believing the 15-day range beginning on the first day of menses and the range beginning on the fourth day of menses.

21. We might note that among couples where communication between husband and wife about safe period did exist, it was far more common for men to initate discussions of the topic than women.

22. A similar idea of "bringing down the period" through the use of traditional medicines has been noted by Shedlin (1982: 82) in Mexico. Shedlin makes the point that these women do not see this practice as abortion and speak of it comparatively freely. This idea has also been reported in Malaysia (Ngin 1985: 35), Afghanistan (Hunte 1985: 53), and Jamaica (Brody 1985: 168).

23. Dr. Nanda Ratnapala, personal communication, 1984.

24. Recent interest in natural family planning has been expressed by the Family Planning Association of Sri Lanka and international donor agencies. There is some evidence that natural planning programs elsewhere in South Asia have achieved notable degrees of success. Rao and Mathur (1970), for example, have documented an All India Insitute of Hygiene and Public Health program designed to teach Indian women to recognize times of fertility by the use of a wall calendar which calculated "baby days" from the time of a woman's menstrual bath. Baby days were denoted as the eight days falling between the 11—18th day after the onset of menstruation. According to a more recent study, the Billings ovulation method of natural family planning was successfully introduced on a trial basis in South India (Mascarenhas et al. 1979). This method is based on self recognition by women of their fertile and infertile period by the subjective sensation of wetness in the genital area. Given an idea as to when her fertile period occurred, illiterate women were able to calculate and mark on a color coded chart (available to their husbands) dry and wet, safe and at risk to pregnancy days. Limitations of the Billings method include the existence of widespread leucorrhoea and cervitis amongst the rural population, as well as a lack of privacy for the practice of sympto-thermal techniques. Moreover, the cost effectiveness of the method is questionable (Betts 1984). We are not advocating this technique in this paper. We have rather identified young married couples (age 25—35) as a focal group for fertility health education efforts which focus on combined safe period/ condom use as well as the need for contraceptive behavior during postpartum amenorrhea.

25. The kind of research process which we have in mind accords with a micro-approach to demographic research presented by Caldwell et al. (1984). With respect to the probable response of the Sinhalese population to the kind of education advocated, we may note the experience of Chullawathi (1985). As part of her study, this health educator found that 98% of the mothers whom she interviewed wanted information about the safe period. Indeed, she notes that many women visited her at her quarters attempting to acquire additional information. With respect to the form of information desired, 72% of her sample wanted to receive information interpersonally from health workers, with 52% of the sample requesting written materials along with or in lieu of interpersonal communication.

REFERENCES

Betts, K.
    1984 The Billings Method of Family Planning: An Assessment. *Studies in Family Planning* 15: 235—266.
Brody, E.
    1985 Everyday Knowledge of Jamaican Women. *In Women's Medicine: A Cross Cultural Study of Indigenous Fertility Regulation*. L. Newman, ed: Pp. 162—178. New Jersay: Rutgers University Press.
Buck, B., L. Kincaid, M. Nichter, and M. Nichter
    1983 Development Communication ith the Cultural Context: Convergence Theory and Community Participation. *In Communication Research and Cultural Values.*. W. Dissanayake and Abdhul Rahman Mohd Said, eds. Pp. 106—126. Singapore: Amic Press.
Caldwell, J.
    1980 The theory of wealth flow. *In Determinants of Fertility Trends: Theories Re-examined*. Chariotte Hohn and Rainer Macksen, eds. Pp. 75—98 Belgium: Ordina.

Caldwell, J., P. Reddy, and P. Caldwell
    1984   *The Micro Approach in Demographic Investigation: Toward a Methodology.* Paper
           presented at the Seminar on Micro Approaches to Demographic Research, Aus-
           tralian National University, Canberra, September 3—7.
Chullawathi, M. K.
    1985   *Lay Ideas on Fecundity During a Woman's Monthly Cycle and Post-partum till
           Twelve Months.* Master's Degree Project Report, Post Graduate Insitute of Medicine,
           University of Colombo, Sri Lanka.
Contraceptive Prevalence Survey
    1983   *Sri Lanka Contraceptive Prevalence Survey Report 1982.* Department of Census and
           Statistics of the Ministry of Plan Implementation and Westinghouse Health Systems.
           Colombo, Sri Lanka.
Das, V.
    1976   Masks and Faces: An Essay on Punjabi Kinship. Contributions to Indian Sociology,
           New Series 10 (1): 1—30.
Dash,Vd. Bhagavan
    1975   *Embryology and Maternity in Ayurveda.* New Delhi: Delhi Deary Publishers.
Delgado, H., R. Martorell, E. Brineman, and R. Klein
    1978   Nutrition, Lactation, and Post Partum Amenorrhea. *American Joural of Clinical
           Nutrition* 31: 322—327.
Douglas, M.
    1966   *Purity and Danger.* London: Routledge and Kegan Paul.
Dube, L.
    1978   *The Seed and the Earth: Symbolism of Human Reproduction in India.* Paper
           presented at the Tenth International Congress of Anthropological and Ethnological
           Sciences. New Delhi, India, December 12.
Finch, B. E. and H. Green
    1963   *Contraception through the Ages.* London: Peter Owen.
Fruzzetti, L. and A. Ostor
    1976   Seed and Earth: A Cultural Analysis of Kinship in a Bengali Town. Contributions to
           Indian Sociology, *New Series 10*(1): 97—132.
Gould, K.
    1969   Sexual Practices and Reproductive Decisions. *Journal of the Christan Medical
           Association of India 44*: 547—550.
Hansen, F. A.
    1975   *Meaning in Culture.* London: Routledge and Kegan Paul.
Harrel, B.
    1981   Lactation and Menstruation in Cultural Perspective. *American Anthropologist 83*:
           796—823.
Huffman, S. L., A. K. M. Chowdhury, and W. H. Mosley
    1978   Postpartum Amenorrhea: How is it Affected by Maternal Nutritional Stores?
           Science 200(43—46): 1155—1157.
Hunte, P.
    1985   Indigenous Methods of Fertility Regulation in Afghanistan. *In Women's Medicine:
           A Cross-Cultural Study of Indigenous Fertility Regulation.* L. Newman, ed. Pp. 45—
           74. New Jersey: Rutgers University Press.
Inden, R. and R. Nicholas
    1977   *Kinship in Bengali Culture.* Chicago: Chicago University Press.
Johnson, S. and L. Snow
    1982   Assessment of Reproductive Knowledge in an Inner-City Clinic. *Social Science and
           Medicine 16*: 1657—1662.
Johnson, S., L. Snow, and H. Mayhew
    1978   Limited Patient Knowledge as a Reproductive Risk Factor. *The Journal of Family
           Practice 6*(4): 855—862.

Jordan, B.
    1987 *Modes of Teaching and Learning: Questions Raised by the Training of Traditional Birth Attendants.* Institute for Research on Learning, Report No. IRL—0004. Palo Alto, Calif.
Kay, M.
    1977 Mexican-American Fertility Regulation. *Communicating Nursing Research 10*: 279—295.
Maloney, C., K. M. A. Aziz, and P. Sarker
    1981 *Beliefs and Fertility in Bangladesh.* International Center for Diarrhoeal Disease Research, Dacca, Bangladesh.
Mandelbaum, D.
    1970 *Human Fertility in India: Social Components and Policy Perspectives.* Berkeley: University of California Press.
Mascarenhas, M., A. Lobo, and A. Ramesh
    1979 Contraception and the Effectiveness of the Ovulation Method in India. *Tropical Doctor 9*:209—211.
Mayer, A. C.
    1960 *Caste and Kinship in Central India: A Village and Its Region.* Berkeley: University of Califormia Press.
McGilvray, D.
    1982 Sexual Power and Fertility in Sri Lanka: Batticaloa Tamils and Moors. *In Ethnography of Fertility and Birth.* Carol MacCormack, ed. Pp. 25—73. London: Academic Press.
McLaren, A.
    1984 *Reproductive Rituals: The Perception of Fertility in England from the Sixteenth Century to the Nineteenth Century.* London: Methuen Press.
Nag, M.
    1968 Factors Affecting Human Fertility in Non-Industrial Societies: A Cross-Cultural Study. *Yale University Publications in Anthropology*, No. 66. Reprinted by the Human Relations Area Files Press.
Ngin, C. S.
    1985 Indigenous Fertility Regulating Methods among Two Chinese Communities In Malaysia. *In Women's Medicine: A Cross Cultural Study of Indigenous Fertility Regulation.* L. Newman, ed. Pp. 26—40. New Jersey: Rutgers University Press.
Nichter, Mark
    1981a Negotiation of the Illness Experience: The Influence of Ayurvedic Therapy on the Psychosocial Dimensions of Illness. *Culure, Medicine and Psychiatry 5*: 5—24.
    1981b Idioms of Distress: Alternatives in the Expression of Psychosocial Distress: A Case Study from South India. *Culture, Medicine, and Psychiatry 5*: 5—24.
Nichter, Mimi
    1982 *The Use of Metaphor as a Communication Strategy.* M.A. Thesis, University of Hawaii, Department of Communication.
Niehof, A.
    1985 *Women and Fertility in Madura.* Ph.D. Dissertation, University of Leiden, Department of Social Anthrooplogy.
Pollack, M.
    1983 *Health Problems in Sri Lanka: An Analysis of Morbidity and Mortality Data.* American Public Health Association, Washington, D.C.
Rao, M. N. and K. K. Mathur
    1970 *Rural Field Study of Population Control (1957—1969).* All India Institue of Hygiene and Public Health, Calcutta.

Rubel, A., K. Weller-Fahy, and M. Trosdal
    1975 Conception, Gestation and Delivery According to Some Mananabang of Cebu. *Philippine Quarterly of Culture and Society 3*: 131—145.
Shedlin, Michele
    1982 *Anthropology and Family Planning: Culturally Appropriate Intervention in a Mexican Community*. Ph.D. Dissertation, Columbia University.
Shedlin, M. and P. Hollerbach
    1981 Modern and Traditional Fertility Regulation in a Mexican Community: The Process of Decision Making. *Studies in Family Planning 12*(67): 278—296.
Snowden, R. and B. Christian
    1983 *Patterns and Perceptions of Menstruation*. A World Health Organization International Collaborative Study. London: Croom Helm.
Thormann, M.
    1984 *Natural Family Planning in India: An Overview*. Consultant Report, USAID, New Delhi.
Trautmann, T.
    1981 *Dravidian Kinship*. Cambridge: Cambridge University Press.
World Fertility Survey
    1978 *First Report of the World Fertility Survey (1975)*. Department of Census and Statistics. Colombo, Sri Lanka.

2. THE ETHNOPHYSIOLOGY AND FOLK DIETETICS OF PREGNANCY: A CASE STUDY FROM SOUTH INDIA

A series of successive pregnancies subject most rural South Indian women to dietary restrictions for a significant part of their lives (Gopalan and Naidu 1972). While folk dietary restrictions have frequently been cited in Indian health sector reports (Voluntary Health Association 1985b; United States Department of Health, Eduction and Welfare 1979) as negatively affecting the health status of pregnant women among the rural poor, little attempt has been made to understand how and to what extent. Moreover, few studies have examined in any detail the contingency between popular notions of ethnophysiology, lay health concerns, preventive and promotive health behavior, and folk dietetics.[1] In this paper, we investigate these issues in southwest peninsular India. An initial topic explored is the relationship between lay ideas about appropriate baby size and food consumption behavior. Both the quantity and quality of foodstuffs deemed appropriate to consume during pregnancy are considered. Alternative patterns of food consumption associated with baby size preference and reasons for this preference are discussed in relation to folk health ideology. Concepts of ethnophysiology and pathology are highlighted in relation to specific dietary practices and folk medical behavior. Public health ramifications of the study are discussed and suggestions made toward enhancing nutrition education efforts by greater anthropological perspective.

Our suggestions of ways of enhancing nutrition education should not be taken to mean that we consider malnutrition in rural India to be primarily a problem of health education, for this is clearly not the case. Economic considerations far outweigh the conceptual. However, economic explanations for the food habits of rural poor pregnant women are insufficient.[2] Within the "continuum of poverty," resources are maximized to varying extents by those with similar economic capacities. Moreover, income increments among the low and lower middle class have not been strongly associated with substantial alterations in dietary behavior (Baroda Operations Research Group 1972; Thimmayamma et al. 1976). Issues affecting dietary behavior, in addition to purchasing capacity, are health ideology, competing felt needs, and the relative importance of converting limited funds into food once a perceived minimal requirement of staple food has been reached. Our conceptual analysis of the folk dietetics followed during pregnancy is meant to complement socioeconomic analysis of income investment and nutritional analysis of nutrient intake and absorption.

30

STUDY AREA AND METHODOLOGY

Our discussion of the folk dietetics and ethnophysiology of pregnancy draws from both personal fieldwork experience and the survey research efforts of a community diagnosis of health project conducted in rural areas of Puttur Taluk, South Kanara District, and Ankola Taluk, North Kanara District, Karnataka State (Nichter 1987). These regions are approximately 300 km apart and differ significantly in respect to regional language, folk traditions, patterns of settlement and residence, levels of overall economic development, and relative health status. South Kanara is more densely populated and relatively "developed" in comparison to North Kanara. The aggregate health status of South Kanara District is the highest in the state, while North Kanara is ranked 11th out of 19 districts in Karnataka (Population Centre 1978). Despite their differences, both regions share many of the same features of folk health culture.

Initial fieldwork was carried out in South Kanara. Participant-observation was used as a method for collecting data on general dietary patterns and special dietary practices followed during pregnancy. The dietary behavior of a cohort of ten pregnant women was periodically observed. Data on the ethnophysiology of pregnancy was obtained from both lay and specialist informants with care placed on distinguishing between specialist and lay knowledge bases.

The layperson in any society rarely turns attention to the body or its processes until one of these processes malfunctions of seems to have done so by cultural criteria (Fabrega and Manning 1973; Fisher 1974). When first interviewing villagers about notions of physiology, we found that they had difficulty in speaking about body processes abstractly, although they could provide names for most major body organs. We were best able to gather data about lay notions of general physiology and the physiology of pregnancy in the context of illness by being present when the ill described their symptoms to family members or to indigenous medical specialists. Descriptions were noted down and later discussed with a variety of other informants — laypersons as well as indigenous specialists, including midwives. The accounts presented here are descriptions of *lay* informants recorded during field interviews. In some cases, notions about physiological processes are discussed in relation to physical disorders. In other cases, analogies, a common means of description used by informants to explain body processes, are highlighted.

Following the collection of qualitative data, a data profile on the ethnophysiology and folk dietetics of pregnancy was constructed. Key ideas concerning the contingency of pregnancy, appropriate dietary behavior, and preferred baby size, identified on this profile, were surveyed to ascertain their pervasiveness in the general population. The survey was conducted during the participatory research exercises of a community diagnosis of health project facilitated by the authors in a later period of fieldwork. Survey data in turn generated additional issues for qualitative investigation.

Community diagnosis survey data on the perceived relationship between baby size and food consumption are presented from both North and South Kanara districts. The data are introduced to document a general preference for small babies by rural South Indian women and to raise questions about the nature of folk beliefs and dietary behavior associated with this prefer- ence. The cultural reasoning behind the folk dietetics of pregnancy is discussed in the remainder of this paper, which focuses on in-depth analysis of data from South Kanara.

BABY SIZE AND FOOD CONSUMPTION: THE BIG BABY/SMALL BABY DILEMMA

The diets of pregnant and lactating women of the low income groups are deficient in several respects. The major reason for the low intakes has been found to be the poor purchasing capacity. But an important additional reason is the practice of food taboos and food fads which prevented the intake of certain nutrient foods both during pregnancy and lactation. The fear of a difficult delivery as a consequence of a large infant also prevented some pregnant women from consuming adequate amounts of food (Voluntary Health Association 1975b).

A preference among rural Indian women for smaller babies and a tendency for pregnant women to consume less as opposed to more food has been noted in passing in both anthropological and public health reports (Brems and Berg 1988; Katona-Apte 1973; Mathews and Benjamin 1979; U.S. Department of Health, Education and Welfare 1979).[3] Common explanations as to why a small baby is desired and less food eaten during pregnancy have been ease in delivery and fear of pain associated with difficult delivery. These explanations, while relevant, tend to underestimate pregnant women's concern for the health of their babies. In reality there are several factors involved with baby size preference and food consumption habits during pregnancy. Single-answer or one-sided explanations tend to gloss over a complex of ideas associated with notions of ethnophysiology and preventive health.

A consideration of community diagnosis survey data focusing on three interrelated questions serves to facilitate discussion on this complex of ideas:

1. For the health of the baby, is it better for the baby to be relatively large or small at birth?

2. During pregnancy, is it better for a woman to eat a greater amount of the food, the same amount of food, or less food?

3. If less food is consumed during pregnancy will the baby be large or small?

The Community Diagnosis Survey

A purposive sample of 200 rural poor households in North Kanara and 82 households in South Kanara was selected for the survey. Women who had young children were interviewed. Sample selection reflected the social and demographic characteristics of the two field areas as well as assumptions entertained by health planners as to variables influencing the health behavior of the "rural poor." Informal discussions with health planners at a national, state, and regional level revealed implicit assumptions that health behavior (not just status) would be positively influenced by any or all of the following: increased access to government health facilities and trained medical practitioners, increased health education efforts by Primary Health Centre (PHC) staff, and rises in general education and economic status.

The terms "rural" and "poor" were defined contextually. A mapping of the social landscape revealed that a trajectory of rural settlements with varying access to transportation facilities and the services of medical practitioners existed in both field areas. Three types of settlements were chosen for study: interior villages with poor access to transportation and cosmopolitan medical practitioners, roadside villages with good access to transport and a resident medical practitioner, and small crossroads towns (population 5,000 to 12,000) in which government medical facilities coexisted with the offices of private medical practitioners. Including these three types of locales within a sampling frame provided a means of evaluating behavioral and attitudinal changes associated with increased access to a broad range of practitioners, government health facilities, and government health workers as well as greater varieties of food, medical resources, and the media. In order to select representative settlements for sampling, the general distribution of health resources was ascertained by making a crude spot map of all available practitioners (traditional, eclectic, and cosmopolitan). This endeavor was undertaken with the assistance of PHC field-workers, local chemists, herb merchants, and local practitioners.

Relative levels of poverty on the poverty continuum were defined by community advisors selected from the local population. For the purposes of this paper, economic status is discussed in relation to a higher and lower strata among the rural poor. Both samples were also stratified by educational status and caste culture. The educational status of women informants is discussed in relation to two levels: illiterate women and literate women who had attended school beyond third standard but not beyond ninth standard. In North Kanara, specific castes were the primary unit of study. Residence in North Kanara was primarily in single-caste nucleated settlement, making for caste-centered social networks. In South Kanara where multicaste nonnucleated settlements and social networks were prevalent, broader caste groups were surveyed (see Table I).

The following three questions were asked of participants in the survey.

TABLE I. Survey Sample Characteristics.

Variable	South Kanara (N = 82)	North Kanara (N = 200)
Locale		
Town	29 (35%)	58 (29%)
Progressive roadside village	28 (34%)	21 (11%)
Interior village	25 (30%)	121 (60%)
Economic status		
Very poor, family monthly income Rs. 100—300	52 (63%)	136 (68%)
Intermediate poor, family monthly income Rs. 301—600	30 (37%)	64 (32%)
Education		
Illiterate	65 (79%)	148 (74%)
Literate	17 (21%)	52 (26%)
Caste	Brahmin 6 (7%)	Karve 5 (3%)
	Christian 8 (10%)	Chamagara & Holeya 9 (5%)
	Muslim 10 (12%)	Kamapanths 10 (5%)
	Harijan 18 (22%)	Ambiga 13 (7%)
	Shudra 40 (49%)	Achari, Kalasi & Madivala 13 (7%)
		Sonagar & Vaisha 14 (7%)
		Harikant 20 (10%)
		Nadava 21 (11%)
		Ager 25 (13%)
		Namdhari 30 (15%)
		Halakki Gowda 40 (30%)

Chi-square tests in many cases reveal statistically significant differences (p < 0.05) between responses from North Kanara and from South Kanara, which is more densely populated, more economically "developed," and where the aggregate health status is relatively high.

Question 1: For the Health of the Baby, Is It Better for the Baby to Be Relatively Large or Small at Birth? A majority of informants from both regions expressed a preference for a relatively small baby. The preference for a small baby was significantly more common in North Kanara (see Table II). Chi-square tests revealed that within each region the frequency of people who prefer a relatively small or large baby did not differ significantly according to locale, economic class, literacy, or caste.

Question 2: During Pregnancy, Is It Better for a Woman to Eat A Greater Amount of Food, the Same Amount of Food, or Less Food? Interviewers met

TABLE II. Preferred Baby Size.

	Size of baby		
	Small	Large	Total
South Kanara (N = 82)	55 (67%)	27 (33%)	82
North Kanara (N = 200)	180 (90%)	20 (10%)	200
Total	235	47	282

$x^2 = 20.4; p < 0.001.$

with considerable ambivalence from informants when they tried to differ-entiate whether women thought it better to eat less food during pregnancy or to eat a normal staple diet. Response to the question most often contrasted "less food and the same amount of food with more food." Discussion revealed that intervening variables, related to the amount of work the pregnant woman was doing at any given time, the season, or her general state of health made it difficult to differentiate less from the usual diet in a precise manner.

A majority of informants from both regions thought it advisable to eat less or the same amount of food as opposed to increasing food intake. Signif-icantly fewer women in North Kanara believed in restricting the quantity of food eaten (see Table III).

Chi-square tests revealed that within each region, the quantity of food regarded as appropriate did not differ significantly with respect to locale, literacy or caste.

In South Kanara, a greater number of the very poor thought it appropriate to restrict food intake during pregnancy. A significantly greater percentage, but not a majority, of the relatively better off deemed it better to eat more food during pregnancy (see Table IV).

Also, in South Kanara a significantly greater proportion of those who

TABLE III. Appropriate Amount of Food Consumed During Pregnancy.

Region	Quantity of foods eaten		
	Less or the same	Greater quantity	Total
South Kanara (N = 82)	61 (74%)	21 (26%)	82
North Kanara (N = 200)	120 (60%)	80 (40%)	200
Total	181 (64%)	101 (36%)	282

$\chi^2 = 4.63; p < 0.05.$

TABLE IV. South Kanara: Appropriate Amount of Food Consumed During Pregnancy.

| | Quantity of staple foods eaten | | |
Economic status	Less/Same	Greater	Total
Very poor (N = 52)	42 (83%)	9 (17%)	52
Intermediate poor (N = 30)	18 (60%)	12 (40%)	30
Total	61 (74%)	21 (26%)	82

$\chi^2 = 4.02; p < 0.05.$

preferred a small baby regarded it appropriate to restrict food intake during pregnancy. Of those who wanted a large baby, a significantly greater proportion said they ate more food during pregnancy (see Table V).

In North Kanara, almost all women preferred a small baby. Appropriate food quantity did not differ significantly according to baby size preference (see Table VI). Of the total sample population, 33% of the women who stated a preference for a small baby also deemed it appropriate to consume more food. A question arose as to whether the association of more food with smaller baby size revealed a mode of reasoning or whether chance or error had determined the responses of the 78 women (Tables V and VI).

To query the possibility that women might think that eating more food resulted in a smaller baby, the following question was posed: "If a pregnant woman eats less food while carrying on a normal work routine, will the baby be relatively large or small?"

Question 3: If Less Food Is Consumed During Pregnancy, Will the Baby Be Large or Small? More than 50% of respondents in each region associated eating less with having a large baby. Between locales, the proportions of women giving this response was not significantly different (see Table VII). In North Kanara, chi-square tests revealed no significant differences according to locale, economic status, literacy, or caste.

TABLE V. South Kanara: Preferred Baby Size in Relation to Appropriate Food Consumption.

| | Preferred baby size | | |
Appropriate amount of food to eat	Small	Large	Total
Same or less food	50 (82%)	11 (18%)	61
More food	6 (29%)	15 (71%)	21
Total	56 (68%)	26 (32%)	82

$\chi^2 = 17.8; p < 0.001.$

TABLE VI. North Kanara: Preferred Baby Size in Relation to Appropriate Food Consumption.

| | Preferred baby size | | |
Appropriate amount of food to eat	Small	Large	Total
Same or less food	108 (90%)	12 (10%)	120
More food	72 (90%)	8 (10%)	80
Total	180 (90%)	20 (10%)	200

$\chi^2 = 0.06$; N.S.

TABLE VII. Baby Size When Less Food is Consumed.

Region	Small	Large	Total
South Kanara (N = 82)	36 (44%)	46 (56%)	82
North Kanara (N = 200)	82 (41%)	118 (59%)	200
Total	118 (42%)	164 (58%)	282

$\chi^2 = 0.34$; N.S.

TABLE VIII. South Kanara: Baby Size When Less Food is Consumed (Breakdown by Locale).

| | Baby size when eating less | | |
Locale	Small	Large	Total
Town	8 (28%)	21 (72%)	29
Roadside Village	10 (36%)	18 (64%)	28
Interior village	18 (72%)	7 (28%)	25
Total	36 (44%)	46 (56%)	82

$\chi^2 = 11.86$; $p < 0.001$.

In South Kanara, chi-square tests revealed that baby size thought to result from restricted food intake varies significantly according to locale and economic class. A greater proportion of women from interior villages associate eating less with having a small baby, and a greater proportion of roadside villagers and townspeople associate eating less with having a larger baby (see Table VIII). A greater proportion of the very poor associate eating less with having a larger baby and the greater proportion of the intermediate poor associate eating less with having a small baby (see Table IX).

TABLE IX. South Kanara: Baby Size When Less Food is Consumed (Break-down by Economic Class).

Economic class	Baby size when eating less		Total
	Small	Large	
Very poor	18 (34.6%)	34 (65.4%)	52
Intermediate poor	18 (60%)	12 (40%)	30
Total	36 (43.9%)	46 (56.1%)	82

$\chi^2 = 4.0; p < 0.05.$

GENERAL IMPLICATIONS OF THE SURVEY

A majority of rural poor women in both field areas expressed the opinion that for the health of the baby, a relatively small baby at birth was preferable to a large baby. Differences in responses of rural poor women within each region were not significantly related to differences in economic strata (of the poor), locale (in the rural continuum), educational backgrounds (literacy), or caste communities.

In general, more women deemed it appropriate to eat less or the same amount of food during pregancy as opposed to more food. Differences in the distribution of this opinion among rural poor women respondents within each region was not significantly related to locale, educational backgrounds, or caste community. Data suggest that relative economic status may influence opinion on this issue. In South Kanara, but not in North Kanara, economic status was significantly related to ideas about appropriate food intake during pregnancy. A greater percentage of the very poor think it advisable to eat less or the same amount of food during pregnancy than the relatively better off. In North Kanara, however, no such association was made.

Mixed ideas exist as to whether eating less will produce a larger or smaller baby. Three questions warranting qualitative investigation were generated by the survey data: (1) What kinds of ideas exist as to how food consumption affects baby size? (2) How is a large baby viewed? (3) What are the conceptual and behavioral factors that influence whether a woman eats more or less or the same during pregnancy?

Qualitative Research on South Kanarese Folk Dietetics During Pregnancy: Food Consumption and Baby Size

From our own perspective, it is understandable why some informants associated the eating of less food with small baby size. But what reasoning underlies an alternative association of less food intake with larger baby size?

An understanding of this association requires a consideration of the ethnophysiology of pregnancy, most notably the concept of *baby space*.

While South Kanarese women distinguish between the womb and belly, this distinction is blurred during pregnancy in respect to the location where a baby "grows." In Tuḷu, the term *banji* may be used to refer to the stomach or womb during pregnancy. A pregnant woman is referred to as a *banjinalu* (Manners 1886).[6] The custom of stomach binding after delivery practiced by some women reflects the association of baby space and stomach space. If the stomach is not bound it is thought that after the delivery a lot of room will remain in the stomach requiring much rice to fill it. The fetus is viewed as growing in a space occupied by food, wind (gas from gaseous foods), and according to some villagers, urine. Many women noted that the *more space* occupied by other substances, the *less space* the baby would have in which to grow. Accordingly, these women deemed the eating of more food to result in a smaller baby. This notion, in conjunction with a general preference for a relatively small baby provides the rationale for a number of folk dietetic patterns. A few dietary restrictions and lay medical practices followed during pregnancy may further illustrate this point.

While a preference exists for smaller babies at birth, a notion exists that a baby must have enough space for movement during pregnancy if a baby's proper development is to occur. For this reason, pregnant women avoid the consumption of gaseous (*vayu*) foods such as sweet potato, jackfruit, bengal gram, and dhal. These foods are believed to cramp the living space of the fetus, making the baby roll in the stomach and causing, in extreme cases, the umbilical cord to get wrapped around the fetus' neck. Pregnant women commonly link breathlessness to cramped body space — the cramping of the body space shared by baby, food, air, and urine.[7] When breathlessness occurs, women may opt to eat less or attempt to urinate more as a means of reducing this symptom. Some women remove liquid from their stomachs by consuming decoctions such as cumin and aniseed to increase the frequency of urination. Women believe that more frequent urination will increase "baby space" and decrease the risk of a baby consuming urine, a factor linked to the bloated "large" appearance of some stillborn babies.

How is a Large Baby Viewed?

The latter reference to sickly babies having a bloated appearance introduces an important dimension to the small baby preference issue. *A big baby is not necessarily viewed as a healthy baby.* A popular distinction drawn by villagers in discussing body image is between a muscular (*pushti*) body associated with vitality and strength (*dhatu*) and a body characterized by "loose watery flesh." One's *dhatu* is often spoken of both in reference to strength and the capacity to maintain positive health (Nichter 1983). Villagers speak of wanting a strong *pushti* baby and not a large "puffy" baby. It is not simply that South Indian women want a small baby for ease in delivery; they want a baby having strength and positive survival characteristics.

A better understanding of attitudes toward size and strength may be gained by considering analogies posed by villagers when discussing this topic. Villagers noted, for example, that despite the small grain size of indigenous rice in comparison to larger hybrid varieties, indigenous rice was rich in *dhatu*, required less fertilizer and nutrients for growth, and was more durable than hybrid grain varieties. In a similar manner, villagers noted that while a large baby of a landlord fed solely on prestigious tinned formula might have a large impressive body (like the fat landlord), such a body had little strength or capacity for hard work. This type of body was compared to a jackfruit, which is large in size but from which one derives little strength or sustenance, or a *chevu* plant, which if manured grows quickly but is of no practical use or benefit to anyone.

Another association between large babies and ill health centers on what villagers describe as a "puffy" baby; a baby who, though large in appearance, is bloated. We did not personally have the opportunity to see the type of puffy baby described by informants as large and unhealthy, nor were we able to collect reliable data on the incidence of such babies. Some of the symptoms of puffy babies suggest the possibility of a child born to a diabetic mother, an infant with tetany, a child born of a mother subjected to extensive sulfur medication, or some malfunction of a fetus' ability to take in nutrients and expel wastes. The incidence rate is perhaps not as important as the publicity that would result from the birth and subsequent death of a bloated baby. It may furthermore be noted that infants who exhibit swelling as a sign of protein calorie malnutrition are often described by parents as being "like that from birth" or having a "constitution" predisposed to this body condition. By constitutional rationale, swelling during infancy may be associated post facto with actual or attributed puffiness at birth.

Factors Influencing the Dietary Behavior of Pregnant Women

In addition to a concern about baby size, a number of other factors influence the dietary behavior of pregnant women. We may consider these factors in two groups: factors influencing the quantity of food consumed and factors influencing the quality of foods consumed.

Three factors in addition to baby size influence the dietary behavior of pregnant women, or at least are employed as explanations for dietary behavior: bodily movement, constitution, and morning sickness. Some pregnant women eat less food due to a decreased felt need for food concordant with the notion that food need and digestive power are relative to body movement. Digestive power as well as food need are associated with body activity. For example, a young infant who has not yet begun to crawl vigorously is not thought to require as much food and water as is needed when the child begins to move actively about. When the work load of a pregnant woman is decreased during a slack work season her diet during that trimester of pregnancy may also be reduced. Slack work seasons are also times of economic difficulty so the rationale cited may be a justification for scarce resources not being more favorably allocated to pregnant women. On the other hand, two cases were recorded where women opted to reduce their food consumption due to decreased movement although they had the resources to maintain, if not increase, their food consumption.

A second factor used to explain the quantity of food eaten during pregnancy is body constitution. Many informants emphasized that appropriate food consumption for pregnant women varied in accord with their body constitution (*prakṛti*). Poor appetite and limited digestive capacity engendered by long-term malnutrition were observed by the researchers to be interpreted as constitutional attributes related to food need. For example, one woman with a long-standing riboflavin deficiency manifested as angular stomatitis was compelled by folk health ideology to eat a rather bland, tasteless (unchillied) diet for several months, a diet that exacerbated her existing state of malnutrition. Concordant with her restricted diet came appetite loss measured by the amount of the rice she consumed. Over time, the family spoke of her angular stomatitis as constitutional, as indicative of a predisposition toward heat also revealed by dry skin and brittle hair. The woman's diminished appetite came to be interpreted as a normal state rather than a state that had developed. During her pregnancy the woman consumed a meager diet even by local standards. Her food intake did not attract attention, however, because it was seen as "constitutional." An observation cited by informants in support of an association between constitution, appetite, and food need was that some people who are continually hungry eat a lot but remain thin, while others eat less and appear to gain weight.

A third factor influencing both the quantity of food eaten during pregnancy and the interpretation of pregnancy desires is morning sickness. Morning sickness is an important factor limiting the amount of food a woman will eat regardless of her ideas about the optimum quantity of food to eat for the health of the fetus. A number of explanatory models of morning sickness coexist. Some women view dizziness and nausea during pregnancy as hereditary, others as a toxic reaction, and still others as caused by an increase in *pitta* and bodily heat.

Pitta, an *ayurvedic* term generally translated as bile, is for the layperson a symptom complex associated with dizziness and nausea, yellow excretions from the body, a bitter taste in the mouth, and overheat in the body. Some informants viewed nausea and vomiting as signs that a pregnant woman's desires had not been satiated and postulated a causal relationship between increased desire, heat, and *pitta*. Others linked *pitta* to an increase in bodily heat resulting from the process of pregnancy. According to folk medical tradition (no doubt influenced by *ayurveda*) sour is a taste identified with reducing *pitta* symptoms. For this reason, pregnancy cravings for sour fruits such as unripe mango or lemon were interpreted by informants as the body seeking to reduce *pitta*.

The discussion of morning sickness introduces two important health concerns that influence the quality of foods eaten during pregnancy: heat and toxicity. Pregnancy is considered by villagers to be a time of increased body heat. An analogy is sometimes drawn between a woman's body being heated in the same way as a fruit during the process of ripening. Most fruits are deemed by villagers to be hot in their unripe state and relatively cool when ripe. As in the ripening process, pregnancy is a time of rapid transformation and development. A woman's body is naturally hot during this process. Her body becomes cool when the baby is fully ripened, when she delivers.

While increased heat is deemed natural during pregnancy, villagers believe that overheat is dangerous. Minor swelling of the hands and feet are seen as ubiquitous signs of increased heat in the body during pregnancy and are not paid much concern. Burning sensation during urination, scanty urine, or white discharge are taken more seriously as signs of significant overheat. These conditions are generally treated by herbal medicines or diet as opposed to cosmopolitan medicines, because the latter are generally ascribed to be heating for the body and thus contraindicated during pregnancy.

Abortion is commonly attributed to overheat in the body, as is the delivery of a child deemed premature. The very classification of a premature baby is linked to ideas involving the effect of overheat. One way to determine whether or not a baby is premature is by the absence of head hair. Baldness is attributed to an excess of heat in the body. Premature babies are treated by lay therapy that places emphasis on cooling the baby. One method of cooling the baby included smearing the baby with "cooling" algae from the bottom of a well.

The eating of foods classified as heating are decreased if not restricted during pregnancy in order that a pregnant woman's already heated body not become excessively hot, resulting in abortion. For this reason, fruits considered heating, such as papaya and pineapple, heating vegetables such as pumpkin (*Curcurbita maxima*), bitter gourd (*Momordica charantia*), and bamboo shoots, and heating grains such as wheat are avoided. The intake of salt, a heating substance, is likewise reduced. The eating of foods classified as cooling is advocated, including such items as tender coconut water, greengram, millet, amaranth, and cumin.

A second health concern during pregnancy that accords with notions of ethnophysiology is toxicity. During pregnancy a woman's body is considered to be prone to toxicity (*nanju*). An excess of toxins accumulates during pregnancy due to the retention of impure blood usually expelled during menstruation. Several informants noted a propensity for pregnant women to develop wound infections and linked this to blood impurity. If a woman becomes pregnant during lactation and has not yet resumed her menstrual cycle, especially high levels of retained toxins are thought to exist in the body. Concern is expressed that the developing fetus will suffer problems, linked to *nanju*, such as skin infections. A man's sperm, a foreign substance retained inside a woman during pregnancy is also spoken of as *nanju*. In the first trimester of pregnancy, if a woman experiences discomfort or morning sickness, others may describe this as the effect of the husband's *nanji* growing inside her, *nanji bulenaga seeksankada jasti.*

During pregnancy the eating of foods classified as *nanju* producing or *nanju* aggravating are contraindicated. These foods include jackfruit and unctuous vegetables such as brinjal, vine spinach, and drumstick. They also include some of the most commonly eaten and valuable sources of protein, including popular varieties of fish (most notably Indian mackerel, prawns, shellfish, and crab) and blackgram. Herbal decoctions prepared from the bark of *benga* (*Pterocarpus marsupium*) and *pongare* (*Erythinia indica*) are consumed, as they are considered to both purify and cool the blood. These decoctions are deemed warranted when signs of *nanju* and overheat, such as swelling in the hands or feet, appear. Aside from the possibility of a baby being harmed by the *nanju* present in a mother's blood, the baby can be affected by gulping *nanju* food (or urine) while in utero. Folk medicines, such as aniseed and cumin decoctions, are consumed by pregnant women to increase urination as a means of purification. In some families newborn babies will be force-fed water to make them vomit out impurities or will be given the juice of *kepala* (*Ixorea coccina*) flowers to prevent "bad" water from entering the baby's system. In other areas of South India, babies are fed a spoonful of castor oil for similar reasons (Katona-Apte 1973).

The appearance of vernix on newborn babies is taken as a sign that the mother did not follow a proper diet during pregnancy. Foods such as jackfruit and beaten rice are attributed to cause this pastiness on the skin of the newborn — a condition concordant with the physical properties of these foods. To avoid the formation of the vernix on the baby, some pregnant women in the second trimester of pregnancy regularly eat a handful of rice chaff followed by a spoonful of hot oil mixed with water as a means of ensuring a "clean" baby at delivery. This mixture is somewhat like the materials a woman uses to cleanse her body while taking an oil bath. Poor women noted that the wealthy who can afford to consume clarified butter (*ghee*) during pregnancy do not have babies with vernix, as the *ghee* cleanses the baby's skin. One popular midwife in South Kanara encouraged her clients to consume a raw egg mixed with hot water once a week as its slippery consistency was thought to reduce vernix formation.

FOLK DIETETICS AND INDIGENOUS HEALTH CONCERNS: RAMIFICATIONS FOR PUBLIC HEALTH

Folk dietary patterns followed during pregnancy by rural South Kanarese women have public health ramifications. As a means of highlighting nutritional aspects of these dietary patterns, we may consider how women qualitatively and quantitatively alter their diet when pregnant in accord with health ideology. In respect to the quantitative intake of food we may consider the probable caloric and protein intake of rural women who do and do not increase their diet during the second trimester of pregnancy.

Our computations are only estimates based largely on impressionistic self-report data, cross-checked when possible by spot observational visits. Inasmuch as the correspondence between dietary reports and actual behavior is known to vary significantly among some groups, additional observational and food quantification research is indicated.[8] Our interview data from ten pregnant women who stated they consumed on an average slightly less than their normal diet was cross-checked four times a month (at different meal times) by local interviewers known to informant families and of similar economic status. By and large, periodic spot visits during food consumption substantiated informant accounts. The variety of foods consumed was checked by seven-day food variety studies conducted during each trimester of pregnancy requiring daily self-reports to local interviewers.

Ten women were also interviewed who stated they consumed more food during their last pregnancy. Unfortunately, pregnant women who considered increased food intake appropriate and within their means were not identified for observation during the project. Our data on these women is therefore entirely impressionistic and based on self and family reports.

One of the factors instrumental in our studying the folk dietetics of pregnancy was the relationship between maternal dietary habits, infant birth weight, and child mortality.[9] As a means of emphasizing the practical implications of this study and the need for additional research on food intake, we present as background a brief nutritional profile of rural South India, with special attention directed toward pregnant women as a group at risk.

Based on studies carried out by the National Institute of Nutrition, Gopalan et al. (1971) estimated that women of childbearing age (15—45 years) represented 21.2% of India's population and that at any given time 20 million women were pregnant. More recent estimates[10] suggest that 3.1% of the rural population are pregnant at any given time.

It has been estimated that between half and 69% of the rural population of South India has protein-calorie malnutrition (Dandekar and Rath 1971; Cantor Associates 1973).[11] If the data on maternal food intake during pregnancy presented in this paper is at all representative of rural South India, there is good reason to believe that pregnant women are significantly under-represented in the general estimates of those malnourished.[12] In addition to protein-calorie malnutrition, 30—50% of South Indian pregnant women suffer from anemia (hemoglobin below 10 g per 100 ml).[13] The nutrient stores of those having successive pregnancies are continually depleted.

Malnutrition among pregnant women contributes significantly to high rates of pregnancy wastage, maternal mortality, low birth weight babies, infant mortality, and low nutrient stores in infants as well as mothers during lactation.[14] Pregnancy wastage among those consuming less than 1,850 Kcal and 44 g protein daily has been estimated at 30% (Gopalan and Naidu 1972).[15] Anemia has been directly responsible for 10—20% of maternal deaths and in another 20% it has been cited as a contributing factor (Gopalan et al. 1971; Indian Council of Medical Research 1975). The livers of infants born to mothers of low socioeconomic groups contain only 60% of expected iron, folate, and vitamin B_{12} stores (Indian Council of Medical Research 1975). Such children are at greater risk of developing anemia in early infancy.

Forty-six percent of all deaths in India occur among children 0—4 years of age. A closer consideration of the age distribution of these deaths reveals that 60% occur between the ages of 1 day and 12 months. Nineteen percent of infant deaths occur in the first week of life, 14% between 8 and 28 days after birth, and 17% occur between 1 to 6 months after birth (USAID 1980; Prema 1978). While the infant mortality rate of India is approximately 129/1,000, studies have found that infant mortality rates for babies weighing 2,000 g is approximately 350/1,000, for babies weighing 2,001—2,501 g, 250/1,000, and for babies weighing 2,501 g or greater, 85/1,000 (USAID 1980).[16] It is estimated that a contributing cause of 44% of infant deaths (0—6 months) is low birth weight.

Qualitative Patterns of Dietary Prescriptions and Restrictions

When a male member of a family is ill it is not uncommon for the diet of the family to be altered in accord with indigenous dietary prescriptions, or for the individual to be offered special foods. Males receive preferential treatment in the allocation of staple food resources in health, and preferential treatment during illness when special foods for health needs are secured on their behalf. When a woman is ill or pregnant, provisions for securing special foods are rarely made. As in the case of the woman with angular stomatitis cited earlier, many women avoid eating foodstuffs prepared for the family which are contraindicated during illness or pregnancy. They rarely alter the family diet for their own accord or purchase special foods. Observation of pregnant women among the poor revealed that dietary *restrictions* influence dietary behavior far more than the dietary *prescriptions* reported to us. For example, during pregnancy, the commonly eaten nutrient-rich low-cost foods listed in Table 10 are either consumed less or not at all by women when available to other family members. The consumption of nutrient-rich prescriptive foods, such as greengram (B complex, protein), millet (protein, calcium), and coriander and cumin (iron) were not observed to increase significantly unless frank symptoms of overheat were prominent.

Quantitative Patterns of Food Consumption During Pregnancy

Deferring to the survey data initially presented, we find that 180 of the 282 women surveyed stated that it was best to consume the same if not less rice when pregnant. A cohort of 10 South Kanarese women who reported they were eating less or the same amount of rice (parboiled) during and before pregnancy were periodically observed. A liberal median estimate as to midterm pregnancy rice intake for these women was 430 g of rice per day during a season of more plentiful food. This would yield approximately 1,500 Kcal and 36.6 g of protein a day. From limited field observations of actual dietary practices we would estimate another 300 Kcal and 8 g of protein intake a day by way of other foodstuffs. Taking 2,500 Kcal and 55 g of protein as the nutrient requirement for the second trimester of pregnancy,[17] we would estimate that the aforementioned group of rural women meet, at best, 72% of their caloric requirement. While 80% of their crude protein requirements appears to be met, protein is not maximized for growth until basic calorie requirements are fulfilled, so protein is expended for calories.

One hundred and two informants favored an increase in the consumption of rice during pregnancy. Most of these informants stated that they were in no position to satisfy their present needs let alone increase their intake. Ten women who stated greater consumption was appropriate were in a position to consume rice adequate to felt needs. These women were interviewed regarding the approximate amount of rice they consumed daily during the second trimester of their last pregnancy. From an analysis of impressionistic data, an estimated mean of 600 g of rice was consumed per day by these women. This would yield 2,634 Kcal and 51 g of protein. Add to this another 300 Kcal and 8 g of protein from other foods and both a pregnant woman's calorie and crude (not amino-specific) protein requirements are met.

Economics aside, it would appear that notions of ethnophysiology and

TABLE X. Example of Nutrient-Rich Foods Restricted During Pregnancy

Food	Reason for restrictions	Otherwise scarce nutrient in this food
vine spinach	consistency	vitamin A, Calcium, iron
drumstick	toxic, heating	iron, calcium
bengal gram	gaseous	B complex, protein
blackgram	gaseous, toxic	B complex, protein
groundnuts	toxic	B complex, protein
beaten rice	fear of vernix	calcium, iron
soy-enriched wheat bulgar	heating	protein
Indian mackerel, prawns, shellfish	toxic	protein, calcium

preferred baby size bring about dietary behavior that significantly affects nutritional status. This is true in a complex of ways, for increased or decreased food consumption may be related to either having a large or small baby. It is assumed by some health planners that changes in attitude toward baby size and dietary behavior will come with increased primary education, contact with health personnel, and contact with the media. Field observation and survey data did not substantiate this view among the rural low-class continuum. Economic stratum was associated with a greater preference for increased consumption of food (but not a large baby) in South Kanara (but not in North Kanara). Education and locale (access to the media) did not significantly affect baby size preference or notions of appropriate dietary behavior.

We would suggest that one reason education has had little impact on ideas about maternal food consumption and baby size is because indigenous health concerns and notions of ethnophysiology have not been appreciated or addressed. Nonappreciation has led to such ethnocentricity as health messages that emphasize baby size rather than baby strength, a more appropriate indigenous health concern. The ramifications of this oversight are highlighted by a brief consideration of the reactions of some villagers to preventive medicines promoted by Government Primary Health Centre field staff in accord with the large-baby theme.

Health Concerns and Medicine-Taking Behavior During Pregnancy

Notions of ethnophysiology affect medicine-taking behavior as well as folk dietetics during pregnancy. This has already been noted in a discussion of the health concern "overheat" and women's reluctance to consume medicines perceived as heating. We now consider the theme of baby size and the rural population's response to three important preventive medicines offered to pregnant women free of charge: ferrous sulfate, tetanus toxoid, and multi-vitamin tablets.

During a survey focusing on the lay population's maximization of existing health resources, we noted a reluctance by pregnant women to receive these preventive medications from Primary Health Centre staff in both field areas. This was true even among those women who had already been assisted, or were planning on being assisted, during delivery by a government nurse-midwife. Interviews with pregnant women revealed that these three medica-tions were highly suspect. They were not suspected of being family planning medications, as we first imagined, but were rejected because of their attributed characteristics. Black ferrous sulfate tables, for example, were perceived by many villagers as weakening the blood or interfering with the digestive process, as opposed to producing blood (Nichter 1980). Pregnant women perceive a tablet as an inappropriate form of medication because a hard pill is believed to be difficult to digest and is thought to share the same body space as the fetus. In a medicine preference survey, 100 informants were nearly unanimous in their opinion that a liquid tonic — and not tablets — constituted an appropriate medication form for use during pregnancy and postpartum. This is one reason that liquid *ayurvedic* tonics are so popular during these times. These tonics are perceived as easily digestible, blood producing, and *dhatu* promoting.

Another reason for not taking ferrous sulfate — omitting it entirely or taking only one pill instead of the recommended three — involved the manner in which PHC staff promoted the supplement. Health staff commonly stated that the tablets were "good for health" and a "tonic to produce a big baby."[18] While this explanation might be appropriate in a Western context or for those with a cosmopolitan orientation, it is quite inappropriate for the lay population in rural South India. Our interviews revealed that many village women perceived ferrous sulfate tablets as a powerful and heating medicine capable of producing a large, but not necessarily healthy, baby.

An unfortunate association was drawn between ferrous sulfate and tetanus toxoid. The latter was considered an "injection tonic." Tetanus toxoid was rarely named or explained to villagers in relation to tetanus, a disease for which an indigenous term (*dhanurvata*) exists. It was rather ambiguously described in the same manner as ferrous sulfate — "good for health — a tonic for a big baby." What is unfortunate about this representation of ferrous sulfate and tetanus toxoid as tonics causing large bodies is that folk health concerns could have been employed judiciously to explain these medications more accurately and in a more culturally sensitive manner. Ferrous sulfate could just as easily have been presented as a medicine for increasing blood and strength in the mother and baby. Tetanus toxoid could have been presented as a medicine that decreased a particular toxicity to which pregnant women are prone.

In a related manner, multivitamin tables are rejected by village women. For a rice eater, a state of normality and good health is measured against a set of routine body signs: food transit time, routine defecation patterns, urine color, urine frequency, and so forth (Nicher 1983). One normal body sign for South Indian rice eaters is clear urine. Yellow urine is deemed a sign of *pitta* and overheat, a condition for which medication is sought and a condition deemed particularly dangerous during pregnancy. On three separate occasions we observed woman consulting a traditional practitioner about *pitta*-related symptoms (yellow urine, dizziness, nausea, burning sensation) after having been given "pills" by PHC staff for one reason or another. In one case, the pills given by the PHC staff had been taken two weeks previously, resulting in yellow urine. The other symptoms that concerned the women (nausea and vomiting) were post facto linked to the pills and the incidence of yellow urine; the pills had been discontinued after one day of use.

One last case dramatically illustrates how notions of ethnophysiology affect medicine-taking behavior during pregnancy. During a PHC deworming campaign a pregnant woman whose feces were tested was found to be infected with common roundworm, *ascaris lumbricoides.* When it was suggested by a young PHC field-worker that she take piperzine citrate to rid herself of worms, the woman and, in fact, her entire neighborhood were shocked at what they considered most harmful advice. In fact, a few villagers mumbled about how this was further evidence of the government's plot to reduce population. Within local conceptualization, any medicine heating enough to rid one of worms was certainly heating enough to cause an abortion.

CONCLUSION

There are many ways of approaching the study of folk dietary behavior. In the South Kanara study, it was found to be more advantageous to focus on what a pregnant woman does to enhance her chances of delivering a healthy baby than to dwell on either what she does not do or on her fears of a difficult delivery. Our reason for this focus was to generate information useful to health educators in their efforts to reduce infant mortality by increasing maternal weight gain. From our own experiences, we considered it doubtful that village women could easily be convinced to eat more (even where resources permitted this) by stressing that a large baby was good for health. An alternative approach was to generate information on coexisting health concerns and notions of ethnophysiology that could better be used as themes for culturally appropriate nutrition education programs.

The paper suggests that increased awareness of the contingency between ethnophysiology, folk health concerns, and folk dietetics could do much to generate alternative approaches to nutrition education that are culturally appropriate (Nichter and Nichter 1981). For example, data on the folk dietetics of pregnancy suggest culturally appropriate themes for nutrition education efforts, such as baby space, baby strength, blood purity, health as full bloodedness, and *dhatu* as an indigenous concept of promotive health. Lack of sensitivity to such themes may indeed prove detrimental to public health efforts. The poor response of pregnant South Kanarese women to ferrous sulfate and tetanus toxoid is a case in point. Attempting to alter diet without giving credence to folk dietetics is like attempting to fix a roof (nutrition program) without paying attention to the cultural foundations (notions of ethnophysiology) or pillars (health concerns, felt needs) of the house.

NOTES

1. For example, numerous studies have discussed dietary restrictions and prescriptions during illness, pregnancy, confinement, lactation, and weaning with reference to the

hot-cold conceptual framework. While some of these studies have made reference to notions of physiology found within the classical humoral doctrines of great traditions, a paucity of data exists on lay concepts of physiology as they relate to notions of hot and cold. It is noteworthy that one does not find a single reference to a study of lay notions of physiology in relation to diet in Christine Wilson's annotated bibliographies (1973, 1979) on studies of culture and diet.

2. On the limitations of economic explanations for dietary behavior see Taylor et al. (1987b). Several studies have shown that birth weights follow a socioeconomic gradient (Prema 1978). While this may reflect better dietary habits during pregnancy associated with greater purchasing power, this is not necessarily the case. Economic strength in relation to access and use of health care facilities, and a consideration of the number of young pregnant women in different economic strata are two major factors that need be considered in assessing birth weight data.

3. In a survey conducted by Matthews and Benjamin (1979) in Tamil Nadu, few if any women were found to eat anything extra during pregnancy and many did not feel that lack of food would harm the baby. In survey areas not influenced by a health education project between 38% and 93% of women did not feel less food would harm their baby and between 76% and 88% did not eat more during pregnancy. In a more recent survey commisioned by the Indian Ministry of Health and Family Welfare (1985), it was found that a significant percentage of private practitioners and indigenous midwives, in addition to mothers, disapproved of increasing food consumption during pregnancy. In Gujarat, for example, 45% of mothers and 78% of private practitioners deemed it unwise to increase food consumption. Preference for a small baby has been noted in several other areas of the world from East Africa to Latin and South America, the Philippines, and Burma (Cruz 1970; Foll 1959; Gonzales and Behar 1966; Harfouche 1970; Katona Apte 1977; Todhunter 1973; Sharma 1955; Trant 1954; Wellin 1955; Good 1980; Kay 1980; Fuglesang 1982.) Brems and Berg (1988) provide an updated list.

4. All women informants had at least one living child under 7 years of age and two-thirds had a child under 4 years of age. Roughly two-thirds of informants were under 40 years of age and one-third were above 40 years of age (by crude reckoning).

5. From an observation of villagers at PHCs, a relatively large baby was considered to weigh over 2.8 kg. More rigorous research is required to determine lay perceptions of what constitutes a normal-size baby. The term "large baby" irrespective of weight was often used to describe a baby who appeared bloated.

6. Alternatively, a pregnant woman may be called a *garbhini*, a term referring to the *garbha kosha*, a more general term for womb (Manners 1886). An idea expressed by one midwife was that there were many *garbha kosha* in the stomach. During each pregnancy, one *garbha kosha* was utilized to contain the baby within the stomach.

7. Katona-Apte (1971) has noted that among women in Tamil Nad it is believed that extra food consumed during pregnancy would lead to irregularity of breathing and choking.

8. A review of methods useful in the collection of data on food consumption and a discussion of differences between self-reported and observed nutrient intake may be found in Krantzler et al. (1980, 1982).

9. It is recognized that several factors other than pregnancy weight and pregnancy weight gain influence birth weight. These factors include length of gestation, emotional stress during pregnancy, and the mother's rate of infections during pregnancy. The latter (incidence of diarrhea, respiratory illness, urinary tract infections) may well interfere with placental function and the maternal-fetal transfer of nutrients. On the variety of factors that may influence birth weight see Margen (1982). On the relevance of seasonal infection rates as a factor influencing neonatal mortality see Taylor et al. (1978b).

10. Personal correspondence from Marianne Anderson, Office of Health, Nutrition, and Population, USAID, New Delhi, India.

11. Using national sample survey data from 1961, Dandekar and Rath (1971) estimated that about a third of the rural population diets are inadequate in calories. This estimate is based on conservative international standards of basis caloric requirements (2,250 Kcal) and a drop in the mean available calories per capita in the last 20 years. We view these figures as impressionistic and only suggestive of the magnitude of malnutrition in rural India. An important limitation of this kind of data is that nutritional norms for a reference man (65 kg) and woman 55 kg) age 20—39 are misleading when used to examine the nutritional status of a population. The Food and Agricultural Organization (FAO 1978) has pointed out that figures for recommended nutrient intakes should not in themselves be used to justify statements that undernutrition, malnutrition, or overnutrition is present in a community or group, as such conclusions must always be supported by clinical or biochemical evidence. The FAO also notes that the methodological basis for estimating energy and protein requirements are weak inasmuch as they are based on studies of healthy young men. The reference figures do not take into account inter-individual variability. Studies such as those by Dandekar and Rath (1971) have used average energy requirements of a population to determine levels of malnutrition and the poverty line. On the issue of measurement of malnutrition, see Srinivasan (1980). Other studies such as the Tamil Nadu Nutrition Study (Cantor Associates 1973) suggest that approximately one-half of Tamil Nadu meet less than 80% of caloric needs.

12. In reference to surveys that have actually tried to assess the nutritional status of pregnant women, Gopalan and Naidu (1972) have noted that one survey carried out in cosmopolitan South India found 43% of pregnant women with frank signs of malnutrition. Another survey (Rao and Gopalan 1969) revealed that the incidence of nutritional deficiency signs was significantly higher (51%) in pregnant women who had had more than three pregnancies than among those who had three or fewer pregnancies (28%).

13. Gopalan et al. (1971) and a WHO (1973) report on nutrition programs and health in India estimated that 30% of pregnant women have hemoglobin below 10 g per 100 ml. The Tamil Nadu Nutrition Study (Cantor Associates 1973) estimated that anemia affected 50% of pregnant women. The Voluntary Health Association (VHA 1975b) estimated that 15—20% of Indian women are anemic at the onset of pregnancy and that 60—70% have hemoglobin levels less than 11 g per 100 ml. Research suggests that in mild and moderate degrees of anemia in pregnancy, iron deficiency was the main factor while in severe forms folate deficiency is clearly evident (VHA 1975a). The net iron loss during pregnancy in Indian women is around 350 mg. To meet this demand, a woman needs to absorb 2—3 mg of additional iron daily. Iron absorption from food during pregnancy ranges from 10% in the first trimester to 25—30% at term. On this basis, the iron requirement during pregnancy is computed to be around 40 mg per day — or greater for women with poor iron stores and low hemoglobin levels at the onset of pregnancy. According to a VHA report (1975a), the mean iron intake of low-income groups is around 18 mg iron per day, 45% of the recommended allowance. Other hemopoietic factors such as vitamin C, folic acid, and vitamin B_{12} are also deficient.

14. Shah and Shah (1979) identified weight during pregnancy and amount of weight gain during pregnancy in underweight women as important factors influencing birth weight. If a 38-kg woman gained 6 kg rather than 2 kg, the average weight of the infant increased from 2.27 kg to 2.50 kg.

15. Gopalan and Naidu (1972) mention a study by P. S. S. Sunder Rao who systematically followed 2,537 rural and 2,021 urban women belonging to the lower socioeconomic groups subsisting on diets providing less than 1,850 Kcal and 44 g protein daily. The pregnancy wastage observed was about 30%.

16. Based on a retrospective study of 10,000 perinatal deaths and 20,000 health controls, Mehta (1980) found that 75% of the perinatal deaths weighed less than 2,500 gms.

17. We have used FAO/WHO (1973) nutrient requirement guidelines for caloric needs

during the later half of pregnancy (2,500 Kcal). Additional energy requirements are assessed at 100 Kcal during the first trimester and 300 Kcal during the first trimester and 300 Kcal during the latter stages of pregnancy. For protein requirements, we have followed the guidelines suggested by the Voluntary Health Association of India. Protein requirements based on a diet of cereals and tubers was estimated to be 55 g by VHA and 63 g by FAO/WHO. The VHA (1975a) compiled a table of mean nutrient intake levels of Indian pregnant and lactating women in low-income groups based on dietary surveys carried out in various regions of India. The average energy intake during pregnancy was 1,400 Kcal (to our 1,800 Kcal) and protein intake was 43 g (to our 44.6 g). Our estimates were made on the basis of a season of more plentiful food. For estimates of another survey of nutrient intakes of pregnant and lactating women see Pasricha (1958).

18. Kay (1980) notes that foods like milk are avoided during pregnancy among Mexican Americans because mothers are afraid they will make the baby large and difficult to deliver. However, vitamin and iron preparations are popular and taken in preference to herbal remedies as a means of "enriching blood." The importance of explaining dietary supplements such as ferrous sulfate, folic acid, and vitamin A to lay populations in accord with emic as opposed to etic health concerns is evident. Good (1980) notes that in Iran doctor's advice is suspect because it does not accord with culturally constituted common sense:

I pay my doctor twenty tomans for each visit. I didn't buy any of the medicines he said to buy so the baby wouldn't be so large I'd have to have a caesarian ... some of those doctors want babies to be so large that they will have to perform caesarians to get them out! (1980: 148)

REFERENCES

Baroda Operations Research Group
    1972 *Food Habits Survey Conducted in Southern India* (Vols 1 and 2). Protein Foods Association of India.
Brems, S. and A. Berg
    1988 Eating Down During Pregnancy. Unpublished Discussion Paper. UN Advisory Group on Nutrition, September. Population and Human Resources Department, The World Bank.
Bonfil-Bantalla, G.
    1970 Conservative Thought in Applied Anthropology: A Critique. *In Applied Anthropology*, A. A. Clifton (ed.) pp. 246—53. Boston: Houghton Mifflin.
Cantor Associates
    1973 *Tamil Nad Nutrition Study: An Operations Oriented Study of Nutrition as an Integrated System in the State of Tamil Nadu*. Washington, D.C.: United States Agency for International Development.
Cruz, P. S.
    1970 Maternal and Infant Nutritional Practices in the Rural Areas. *Journal of the Philippino Medical Association 46*: 668—682.
Dandekar, V. M., and N. Rath
    1971 *Poverty in India*. Bombay: Indian School of Political Economy.
Fabrega, H., and P. Manning
    1973 The Experience of Self and Body: Health and Illness in the Chiapas Highlands. *In Phenomenological Sociology: Issues and Applications*. George Psalkas, ed. New York: J. Witz and Sons.
Fisher, S.
    1974 *Body Consciousness*. New York: Jason Aronson.

Foll, C. V.
  1959 An Account of Some of the Beliefs and Superstitions about Pregnancy, Parturition, and Infant Health in Burma. *Journal of Tropical Pediatrics 5*: 51—59.
Food and Agricultural Organization (FAO)
  1973 *Energy and Protein Requirements: Report of a Joint FAO/WHO Ad Hoc Expert Committee.* Rome: Food and Agricultural Organization.
  1978 *Report of the First Joint FAO/WHO Expert Consultation on Energy Intake and Requirements (Danish Fund in Trust, TF/INF 297).* Rome: Food and Agricultural Organization.
Fuglesang, A.
  1982 *About Understanding.* Uppsala, Sweden: Dag Hammarskjold Foundation.
Gonzalez, N. S., and M. Behar
  1966 Child Rearing Practices, Nutrition, and Health Status. *Milbank Memorial Fund Quarterly 94*: 77—95.
Good, Mary Jo Delvecchio
  1980 Of Blood and Babies: The Relationship of Popular Islamic Physiology to Fertility. *Social Science and Medicine 14b*, 147—156.
Gopalan, C.
  1974 The Nutritional Problems of India. Journal of the Indian *Medical Association 62*: 224—227.
Gopalan, C., S. C. Balasubramanian, B. V. Ramasastri, and K. Rao
  1971 *Nutrition Atlas of Asia.* Hyderabad: National Institute of Nutrition.
Gopalan, C., and N. Naidu
  1972 Nutrition and Fertility. *The Lancet,* November 18, pp. 1077—1079.
Harfouche, J. K.
  1970 The Importance of Breastfeeding. *Journal of Tropical Pediatrics 16*(3) (Monograph No. 10).
Indian Council of Medical Research
  1975 Report on Nutritional Status and Pregnancy. *Cited in Nutrition in Pregnancy and Lactation, Fact Sheet M-3.* New Delhi: Voluntary Health Association of India.
Jyothi, K. K., and R. Dhakshayani
  1963 A Study of Socioeconomics, Diet, and Nutritional Status of a Rural Community near Hyderabad. *Tropical Geographical Medicine 15*: 403—410.
Katona-Apte, J.
  1973 Food Behavior in Two Districts. *In Cultural Anthropology and Nutrition 2B, Tamilnadu Nutrition Study.* Report to USAID Mission, New Delhi, India.
  1977 The Sociocultural Aspects of Food Accordance in a Low Income Population in Tamilnadu, South India. *Environmental Child Health (April)*: 83—90.
Kay, M.
  1980 Mexican, Mexican American and Chicana childbirth. *In Twice A Minority: Mexican American Women,* M. Melville (ed.). St. Louis: C. V. Mosby.
Krantzler, N., and B. Mullen
  1980 *Measuring Food Intake Patterns.* Paper presented at the 4th Annual Meeting of the West Coast Nutritional Anthropology Society.
Krantzler, N., B. Mullen, E. Comstock, C. Holden, H. Schutz, L. Grivetti, and H. Meiselman
  1982 An Annotated Indexed Bibliography on Methods of Measuring Food Intake. *Journal of Nutrition Education 14*(3): 108—119.
Manners, A.
  1886 *Tulu-English Dictionary.* Bangalore: Basil Mission Press.
Margen, S.
  1982 Studies of Maternal Nutrition and Infant Outcome: Statistical Versus Biological Significance. *Birth 9*(3): 197—200.
Matthews, C. and Benjamin, V.
  1979 Health Education Evaluation of Beliefs and Practices in Rural Tamil Nadu: Family Planning and Antenatal Care. *Social Action 29,* 377—392.

Mehta, A.
  1980 *Perinatal Mortality Survey in India.* Paper presented at the 3rd International
        Seminar on Maternal and Perinatal Mortality, New Delhi, India.
Ministry of Health and Family Welfare
  1985 *Monitoring Communication Needs for Health and Family Welfare.* Unpublished
        series of six state reports.
Mitra, A., and S. Mukherji
  1980 *Population, Food, and Land Equality in India, 1971: A Geography of Hunger and
        Insecurity.* Bombay: Allied Publishers.
Nichter, M.
  1980 The Layperson's Perception of Medicine as Perspective into the Utilization of
        Multiple Therapy Systems in the Indian Context. *Social Science and Medicine
        14*(B): 225—233.
  1984 Project Community Diagnosis: Participatory Research as a First Step toward
        Community Participation in Primary Care. *Soc. Sci. Med. 19*: 3 237—252.
  1986 Modes of Food Classification and the Diet-Health Contingency: A South Indian
        Case Study. *In Modes of Food Classification in South Asia.* R. Khare and K.
        Ishvaran, eds.
Nichter, Mark, and Mimi Nichter
  1981 *An Anthropological Approach to Nutrition Education.* Newton, Mass.: International
        Nutrition Communication Service Publications, Education Development Center.
Pasricha, S.
  1958 A Survey of Dietary Intake in a Group of Poor Pregnant and Lactating Women.
        Indian Journal of Medical Research 46: 605—610.
Population Centre
  1978 Classification of Districts in Karnataka State by Health Status. *Population Centre
        Newsletter 4*(3). Bangalore.
Prema, K.
  1978 Pregnancy and Lactation: Some Nutritional Aspects. Indian Journal of Medical
        Research 68 (Supplement), October, pp. 70—79.
Rao, V. K., and C. Gopalan
  1969 Nutrition and Family Size. *Journal of Nutrition and Dietetics 6*: 248—266.
Shah, K. P., and P. M. Shah
  1979 Relation of Maternal Nutrition and Low Birth Weight. *Indian Pediatrics 14*(11):
        961—966.
Sharma, D. C.
  1955 Mother, Child, and Nutrition. *Journal of Tropical Pediatrics 1*: 47—53.
Srinivasan, T. N.
  1980 *Malnutrition: Some Measurement and Policy Issues.* World Bank Staff Working
        Paper No. 373. Washington, D.C: World Bank Publications.
Spradley, J.
  1979 *The Ethnographic Interview.* New York: Holt, Rinehart & Winston.
Taylor, A., I. Emanuel, L. Morris, and R. Prosterman
  1978a Child Nutrition and Mortality in the Rural Philippines: "Is Socioeconomic Status
        Important?" *Tropical Pediatrics and Environmental Child Health* (April): 80—86.
Taylor, C., A. Kielmann, and C. LeSweemer
  1978b Nutrition and Infection. *In Nutrition and the World Food Problem.* M. Recheigl, ed.
        Pp. 218—243. Basel, Switzerland: Kaiger.
Thimmayamma, B. V. S., P. Rau, V. K. Desai, and B. N. Jayaprakash
  1976 A Study of Changes in Socioeconomic Conditions, Dietary Intake and Nutritional
        Status of Indian Rural Families Over a Decade. *Ecology of Food and Nutrition 5*:
        235—243.

Todhunter, N. E.
  1973   Food Habits, Food Faddism, and Nutrition. *World Review of Nutrition and Dietetics 16*: 286.
Trant, H.
  1954   Food Taboos in East Africa. *Lancet* (October): 703—705.
United States Agency for International Development (USAID)
  1980   Paper presented by Cathy LeSar at a Title Two Workshop on Malnutrition and Mortality, March 25—27, New Delhi, India.
United States Department of Health, Education, and Welfare
  1979   *Background Paper on India's Health Sector.* Washington, D.C.: Office of International Health.
Voluntary Health Association
  1975a *Anemia in Pregnancy.* Fact Sheet M-7. New Delhi, India.
  1975b *Nutrition in Pregnancy and Lactation.* Fact Sheet M-3. New Delhi, India.
Wellin, E.
  1955   Maternal and Infant Feeding Practices in a Peruvian Village. *Journal of the American Dietary Association 31*: 889—894.
Wilson, C. S.
  1973   Food Habits: A Selected Annotated Bibiography. *Journal of Nutrition Education 5*(1): Supplement 1.
  1979   Food Custom and Nurture: An Annotated Bibliography on Sociocultural and Biocultural Aspects of Nutrition. *Journal of Nutrition Education 2*(4): Supplement 1.
World Health Organization
  1976   *Nutrition Programs and Health Report of the Regional Office for Southeast Asia.* November, New Delhi.

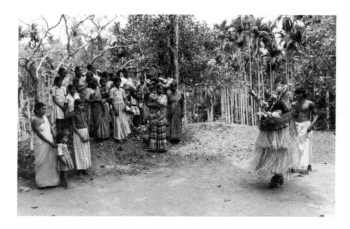

Women attend a spirit possession ritual, *bhuta kola,* as a means of receiving the blessing of
fertility for themselves and their land as well as protection against illness for their children.

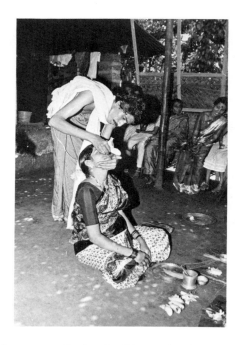

Fertility is a cultural construct. During the 7th month of pregnancy, a ritual medicine is
inhaled through the woman's right nostril to enhance the chances of her having a male child.

3. MODERN METHODS OF FERTILITY REGULATION: WHEN AND FOR WHOM ARE THEY APPROPRIATE?

According to the 1982 Sri Lanka Contraceptive Prevalence Survey (CPS), 99 percent of ever-married women interviewed had knowledge of at least one contraceptive method, and 97 percent knew of a supply source or service point for this method. Fifty-five percent of currently married women interviewed during the survey had engaged in some form of contraception related behavior. This figure represents a significant increase over the findings of the 1975 World Fertility Survey (WFS) in Sri Lanka which found that 32 percent of married women interviewed had engaged in some contraceptive practice. The most popular method of contraception reported by the CPS was female sterilization, the method having been adopted by 17 percent of all women surveyed. Prevalence rates for other means of birth control were: rhythm, 13 percent; withdrawal, 5 percent; other traditional methods, 7 percent; male sterilization, 4 percent; condom, 3 percent; pill, 3 percent; and IUD, 3 percent. Between the 1975 WFS and the 1982 CPS surveys, reported prevalence of female sterilization and traditional contraceptive practices nearly doubled, while pill and condom use increased slightly and IUD use declined significantly.

What is noteworthy about this survey data is that the reported increase in method use in the seven year period between the two surveys was largely due to an increase in the use of traditional contraceptive practices rather than modern methods (CPS 1982; Nichter and Nichter 1987). Two thirds of CPS respondents stated that they did not want more children. Of these women, 40 percent reported using traditional practices, 24 percent reported using modern methods and 40 percent reported no birth control related behavior. An issue raised by this data is why modern methods of family planning have not been more widely adopted by a largely literate population expressing a clear need to limit their family size.[1] Sri Lanka has one of the highest literacy rates in the developing world (males 90%; females 82%) and family planning services are widely available throughout the country. What is more, those Sri Lankans who use traditional practices rather than modern methods tend to be the most educated and are just as likely to reside in urban as in rural areas.[2]

An assumption maintained by many health planners is called into question by the Sri Lankan data: The assumption is that literacy, access to modern contraceptive methods and deployment of an increased number of family planning workers will add to a steady rise in modern contraceptive method use given a situation where economic decision making favors birth control.[3] This reasoning assumes that 1) couples will adopt family planning methods because they are available and have been sanctioned by doctors and 2) that users will be satisfied with the effectiveness of the contraceptive services offered. In the Sri Lankan context, these assumptions beg reconsideration by both health care service research focusing on quality of service and medical anthropological research focusing on users' perceptions of effectiveness — by what means and at what cost.

In Sri Lanka and throughout the third world many women have tried temporary methods of family planning and have opted to discontinue their use. Explanations by professionals for dropouts and non-compliance center on "rumors involving fear of side effects". Often such explanations reflect a blaming of the victim posture, particularly in circumstances where screening or follow-up care services are not available and the primary focus of family planning workers is meeting target quotas. These are issues requiring health service research. Our interest at present is to explore predisposing cultural factors which enter into a household's decisionmaking about 1) the adoption of alternative modern family planning methods and 2) at what point to adopt such methods in a woman's reproductive career. This requires sensitivity to the health concerns associated with modern contraceptive methods from the users' perspective. We will endeavor to move beyond the rhetoric of non-compliance which simplistically links nonadoption of modern contraceptive methods to "fear of side effects," "the spread of unscientific rumors", and the impact of culture as "superstition impeding progress." Our approach will be to investigate nonadoption and discontinued use in relation to tacit cultural knowledge about ethnophysiology, popular understanding of how modern methods function, and lay cost benefit analysis based upon cultural perceptions of health, food availability and work load. We will highlight popular Sinhalese interpretations of how family planning methods work and health concerns associated with these methods. We will consider reasons why the poor find particular contraceptive methods unsuitable for their use despite the fact that they desire to space or limit their number of childern. Drawing upon cross-cultural literature, we will document similar concerns about family planning methods in other countries in order to emphasize that the concerns of our Sinhalese informants are not unique. Rather than being portrayed as groundless from an etic biomedical perspective, these concerns will be shown to be reasonable given *different sets* of premises about health, body physiology and pathology.

THE RHETORIC OF RUMORS AND SIDE EFFECTS

Considerable mention of rumors about side effects exists in the cross-cultural family planning literature. Typically, such literature (e.g. Population Reports 1984; Bogue 1975) identifies rumors about side effects and then proceeds to demonstrate why these claims are unscientific from a biomedical perspective. Family planning workers are asked to develop effective communication strategies to "dispel" these false rumors by providing accurate information in a convincing way. In some countries, workers have been asked to "develop rumor registries, trace rumors to their sources and provide persuasive rebuttals" (Population Reports 1984). Tracing rumors to their source is no small task if one takes source to mean the source of their appeal and credibility, not just source as a rumor grapevine to be traced to individuals. Identifying an individual as a source is much a case of moving the target to score a bullseye. Rumors about contraceptive methods would not appeal to the public if they did not resonate with some already existing tacit knowledge about the body — knowledge embedded in and reproduced through popular health practices and discourse about health.

Before we embark on a search for the source of popular health concerns associated with family planning methods, it is prudent to scrutinize the very use of the terms "rumor" and "side effects". Rumor denotes second hand information and connotes information which is groundless, made up, and secretive. The way the term is often employed in family planning literature, one is led to believe that rumor is part of a covert conspiracy against the dominant biomedical culture. Such thinking is clearly unproductive. One rarely comes across people who have rejected modern medicines for both themselves and their families. It is useful to consider both the production of knowledge about modern contraception and the production of knowledge about rumors, side effects and noncompliance as the aforementioned are influenced by explicit and implicit agenda. What is identified as "rumors" by outsiders often constitutes popular health knowledge counter to that of a dominant medical culture. In such contexts, the term "rumor" is pejorative and indexes power relations between a dominant knowledge system and popular health culture. For our purposes it is necessary to differentiate between 1) popular discourse about family planning methods, including the experience of users, which is well grounded in popular health culture and which invokes common health concerns, 2) popular discourse about family planning methods which tends to be value laden commentary on modernity and the deterioration of traditional values and 3) discourse reflecting idiosyncratic opinion about family planning methods underlay by personal agenda such as discrediting a doctor, power brokerage, etc. While these kinds of discourse often merge, we will focus on the first and will not use the term rumor for what appears to us to be popular interpretive understanding of experience and potential experience.[4]

The term "side effects" must likewise be scrutinized for it infers at least two distinct meanings. In its most general use, the term denotes an effect other than that directly intended. A differentiation need be made between 1) a side effect which occurs and is unrelated to the effectiveness of the method and 2) a negative effect which although undesired is deemed to be functionally related to the way in which the method works. We will refer to the latter as a "negative primary effect" of a method and the former as an unintended side effect. A point we will emphasize is that what some health workers flippantly term "side effects" may be interpreted by the lay population as a symptom set primary to the functional effectiveness of a contraceptive method.

METHODOLOGY

Before discussing lay perceptions of modern contraceptive methods a few words are in order regarding our own methods of data collection and the characteristics of our informants. Unstructured ethnographic interviews were carried out with sixty married couples aged 25—40 having at least one child. All informants were lower middle class and literate. Most informants had at least a sixth standard education. Twenty couples were selected from each of three districts (Horana, Galle and Ratnapura districts) in low country Sri Lanka. The researchers established rapport with informants prior to an investigation of family planning methods through interviews on children's health. After seeking permission to discuss family life, each informant was asked to describe what they had heard about family planning methods from health professionals, family members and friends. Informants were next asked what relative health benefits and concerns were associated with various methods. Those health concerns voiced were followed up upon by questions relating to ethnophysiology, pathology, and how various methods functioned in the body. Informants' own experiences with modern methods were elicited only after an opportunity had been provided for them to voluntarily discuss these experiences.

ORAL CONTRACEPTIVES: HOW THEY FUNCTION

As a category, modern English "*ingrisi*" medicine is spoken of in general discourse as heating and powerful. While *ingrisi* medicine is praised for fast action, it is commonly referred to as having "uncontrolled" side effects. The English term "side effects" has been incorporated into popular discourse from the media. Informants tended to interpret "side effects" as inherent toxicity and heatiness, the effects of which are unpredictable and emergent over time. In contrast, traditional herbal medicine (*Sinhala behet*) is perceived as rendering control and balance. Indigenous interpretations of birth control pills incorporate preexisting ideas about powerful western medicine. Sri Lankans are leery, in general, of any western medicine which has to be taken for a long period of time because of a sense of increasing toxicity and heat. While short term benefits of western medicine are appreciated, long term complications are suspect.

A pervasive notion among informants was that the pill worked because of its heating effect in the body. Several explanations were offered in this regard. Some informants noted that taking these pills every day raised the heat level of the body to such an extent that male and female *dhatu,* a substance associated with vitality and strength, was burned up. This was expressed in Sinhala by the phrase, *dhatu pichenava,* literally *dhatu* burns. Others informants explained that the extreme heat in the body caused by taking the pill diluted the *dhatu, dhatu direvenava,* to the point where it was no longer strong enough to create a fetus.

Similar ideas have been reported by Shedlin (1977) who states the following from her fieldwork amongst Mexican women:

Oral contraceptives or the 'pill' seem to have generated the most variations in beliefs about how it works. It is seen as a medicine which affects the blood or liquid of the woman, man or both, either to make one or both liquids too weak to join together to begin the formation of the baby. It was also said to enter the uterus and force everything out, or to dissolve the joined liquids and cause them to 'bajar' (go down). Thus it is seen as functioning before conception to prevent it, or after conception to destroy it and cause everything involved to leave the body. (p. 13)

Another health concern noted by rural Sinhalese women informants was that the excess heat in a woman's body caused by taking the pill rendered the womb dry. Over time, a dry womb became incapable of accepting male seed. As one informant explained, "A dry womb is like a dry field. If you plant seeds in a field which is not moist, the seed will not take to the soil. A womb which has become totally dry through continued use of birth control pills becomes useless." Long term dryness leads to decaying and deterioration of the womb. In the words of another informant: "The womb deteriorates just like a piece of wood left in the sun for many months. It becomes brittle and finally turns to powder."

A concern about drying of the uterus rendering a woman infertile has been noted elsewhere. Good (1980) has noted that Iranian women believe the pill prevents pregnancy "through some action on the uterus, making conception at a later time unlikely" (p. 152). Specifically, Good notes that Iranian women believed that the pill dries the uterus. For this reason, many of her young, educated informants opted for abortion as a birth control method rather than risk loss of fertility and a drying of the uterus by taking the contraceptive pill. The condom was also viewed as having adverse effects on the uterus by depriving it of moisture. Many Iranian women complained that the pill caused one's entire body to "dry up" and thus hastened the onset of memopause and old age. Premature drying is a serious matter for Iranian women, as it is believed "that the uterus becomes dry and less strong as a woman gets older and thus less receptive to the male seed."(1980: 152). The Iranian concern that dryness leads to infertility appears to be quite similar to ideas expressed by some of our Sri Lankan informants.

While birth control pills are promoted as a temporary method by health educators, many Sinhalese believe they cause permanent damage to the body and are, in effect, a permanent method. A concern voiced by many young women wanting to space their children was that after taking the pill for some time, their chance of conceiving when they once again wished to was diminished. The fear that temporary family planning methods such as oral contraceptives will make women permanently infertile has been reported worldwide: El Salvador (Bertrand et al. 1982); Iran (Good 1980); India (Rogers 1973); Philippines (Mercado 1973). This concern was found to have influenced the timing of when some of our informants choose to utilize the pill. Of twenty informants using the pill (from a separate sample of birth control pill users) almost one third spoke of choosing this "temporary" modern method: 1 after a minimum optimum number of children (in most cases two) had been born, 2) where a final decision was pending with respect to having one more child. Their use of the pill appeared to be related to the delaying of a final decision about family size, or use of a permanent method more than child spacing per se.

THE PILL: SIDE EFFECTS AS PRIMARY NEGATIVE EFFECTS

Several symptoms were commonly noted by informants when they described how birth control pills negatively affected health.[5] The symptoms listed below were deemed by at least one third of our informants to be primary negative effects of the pill — symptoms manifesting from the way the method functioned to diminish fertility. The following symptoms were cited:

TABLE I. The Pill.

Symptom	Caused by pill through:
Weight reduction	Heatiness
Burning sensation in urinary tract, digestive tract, hands and feet	Heatiness
Headaches	Heatiness
Nausea and vomiting	Heatiness; toxicity
General body pain	Heatiness
Stomach pain	Heatiness (causes wounds to erupt in the stomach)
Joint pains	Heatiness (causes blood to dry up interfering with body movement)
Drying up of breastmilk	Heatiness
Rashes, diarrhea in nursing baby, general failure to thrive of nursing baby when mother is taking the pill	Heatiness of breastmilk

The most commonly reported negative effect of the pill worldwide is general weakness and leanness: Iran (Good 1980); Botswana (Liskin 1984), Egypt (DeClerque et al. 1986; Krieger 1984; Morsy 1980) and Morocco (Mernissi 1975). In addition to possible physiological effects of the pill on appetite and the absorption of nutrients among a population at risk to malnutrition,[6] it is necessary to consider cultural dimensions of weakness and leanness discourse. Here it is important to pay credence to both referential and indexical aspects of this discourse: notions of ethnophysiological process and physical feelings people referred to when they speak of weakness or leanness as well as what they are attempting to do by communication to others (as well as themselves) feelings of weakness. In many cases, talk of weakness may refer to the physical while indexing social relations, the social body.[7] In a similar manner, leanness may refer to actual body size as well as index relations of power and substance in one's psychosocial lifeworld.

Birth control pills are not only considered heating and drying but are in other ways deemed harsh, *sarai*, for the body. As discussed elsewhere (Chapter 7), the heatiness and harshness of modern medicine is commonly linked to concerns about blood quantity/quality and flow, digestive capacity and in turn general strength and vitality. Concern about *igrisi* medicine being heating and toxic and capable of effecting blood and digestive capacity increases user's sensitivity to a wide range of symptoms. The presence of diffuse symptoms may be interpreted in relation to the pill especially in a context where psychosocial distress associated with fertility and sexuality are involved. Similarly, discourse about the pill and loss of weight while taking the pill may refer not only to heatiness, but may index problematic social relations of which pill discourse is itself symptomatic. In Iran, for example, Good (1980) notes that the pill is thought to cause a set of complaints — heart palpitations, weakened nerves, hand tremors, shortened tempers and loss of weight. Good notes that such symptoms comprise a language of somatization for feelings of anxiety and ambivalence associated with contraception and sexual intercourse, fertility and infertility, and the stresses of a woman's life linked to being a wife and a mother.

Discourse about the pill in Sri Lanka, as in Iran, is multivocal. The following example exemplifies this point. One informant, a neighbor, complained to us that she was becoming lean, *kettuyi*, since taking the pill but actually she appeared rather plump. The term *kettuyi* was used referentially to imply a lack of strength and body weakness. What became apparent overtime was that the woman was using a somatic idiom of distress to indirectly communicate to us problems she was having with her husband which entailed a weakening of their social relationship and growing psychosocial distance. These problems preceded her taking the pill and involved her husband's use of alcohol (arrack), itself a heaty substance. Interestingly, her husband had lost weight due to his drinking, but did not complain of this. He plunged the family into debt and argued against his wife having a second child. Indeed, he tried to convice her to undergo a sterilization for which she would received a cash bonus from the government. The woman's anxiety was articulated vis à vis the weakness-thinness idiom, an idiom which allowed her to indirectly communicate that she was feeling powerless in her situation as well as her body. This informant used the pill as a convenient marker in her health discourse to relate to concerned others ambivalent feelings she was having about her husband and her own identity, feelings associated with a loss of her sense of person defined in relation to her husband. The similarity of this case to the case material described by Good in Iran is striking.

Another problem related to heatiness as a "primary negative effect" of birth control pills is their impact on breastmilk. Birth control pills are associated with both a reduction in the quantity of breastmilk produced, and the quality of breastmilk which becomes heaty. The latter was associated with *mandama dosha*, an illness marked by a failure to thrive (often protein calorie malnutrition), diarrhea, and skin rashes. We came across few women in our interviewing who had actually taken birth control pills while breast-feeding. However, the idea that heating birth control pills would reduce breastmilk made intuitive sense to a large majority of our informants.

The case of one of our more modern informants from Colombo city gave us the impression that the taking of birth control pills might constitute a strategy some women use to stop breastfeeding in a context where it is culturally supported. The woman began taking the pill after five months of breastfeeding while expressing a desire to return to work, against the wishes of her mother-in-law. The informant brought to her husband's attention family planning advice offered to her by a health educator which emphasized the need for contraception six months after delivery as a means of birth spacing. Complaining of condoms, she began taking oral contraceptives on her own initiative, much to the disappointment of her mother-in-law. Speaking to her mother-in-law, we were told that taking any heaty medicine constituted a valid reason to stop breastfeeding. In this case, which we do not believe is common, the use of a contraceptive was negatively related to breastfeeding and strategic, associated with a woman's work opportunities. The negative relationship between contraceptive use and breastfeeding duration has been more widely reported in Africa than Asia (Knodel and Debavalya 1980; Jain and Bongaarts 1981; Lesthaeghe, Page and Adegbola 1981; Zurayk 1981; Oni 1986). It raises an important policy dilemma for developing countries committed to child survival, family planning, and increasing employment opportunities for women.

In a study of side effects experienced by users of oral contraceptives in Sri Lanka, Basnayake et al (1984) reported nausea, vomiting, headaches and dizziness as widespread. The authors conclude that Sri Lankan women report similar side effects to women of other cultures and that these reduce as the body becomes accustomed to the pill. The study is a good example of the limitations of biomedical studies of "side effects" which strictly rely on surveys; seek to provide biomedical reasons for symptom occurrence; and offer psychosomatic explanations for their commonality without cultural depth. Surveys are as often revealing of the mentality and gaze of their designers as of the people to whom they are administered. Indeed, survey data is often an artifact of the survey instrument itself. It is striking that in the Baanayake study no complaint of heatiness was noted. This is surprising when one considers that in our interviews the most common health concern associated with the pill was heatiness. Baanayake structured interviews around a prepared questionnaire untilizing symptoms most commonly noted in the West. Interviewers conducting the survey asked about side effects, but failed to investigate relationships between symptoms cited and the processes underlying their occurrence. The user's health culture was overlooked.[8]

The Basnayake report places emphasis on habituation to the pill with respect to the prevalence and severity of physical symptoms. Habituation is an important Sinhalese as well as biomedical health concept (Nichter, Chapter 7). What Basnayake fails to appreciate is that habituation is a process that entails becoming "accustomed" to something, not just physically accommodating it. A cultural dimension to habituation exists. Sinhalese informants made it clear that becoming habituated to the harshness of *ingrisi* medicine and contraceptive methods in the short run does not guarantee that one will not suffer long term consequences from continued use. Long term habituation requires more than just the body accommodating to the "fix" in the sense of not being "shocked" by its presence, manifest as physical-symptoms. It entails provisions for conterbalancing and removing negative primary effects of fixes.

Many of our informants noted that taking harsh birth control pills over time would be detrimental not only for a woman's future fertility, but also for her general health. Taking a brith control pill everyday is seen as doing something daily to weaken one's health. A concern existed that since pills were bad for helath, they should only be taken when absolutely necessary. For some informants this meant that they would take a pill only on those days when it was likely they would "mis" (have coitus) with their husbands, or after they had had coitus. For others, this meant taking the pill during days perceived to be times of peak fertility. As noted in Chapter 1, cultural perceptions of peak fertility do not always coincide with biological fact. Researchers working in other cultures have found that pill use is mediated by ideas about its negative effects. Krieger (1984), for example, found that amongst Egyptian women, the misuse of the pill was associated with beliefs about the method: the pill was perceived as a potent, toxic substance that should not be ingested daily. Moreover, its potency was regarded to have sustained action, making daily consumption unnecessary to achieve protec-tion.[9] Among our Sir Lankan informants, we found that it was not uncommon for a woman to discontinue taking the pill when she felt ill, not only from symptoms overtly associated with heat — such as diarrhea and fever — but from more general symptoms such as weakness and giddiness. Tucker has noted similar contraceptive behavior in Peru:

Pills are given with minimal explanation so that most respondents do not understand the proper way to use them. Women often start taking their pills on the wrong date, forget to take them for a few days or quit in the middle of the cycle because "they do not feel good." (1986: 312)

SURVEYS ON PILL USE : A CAUTIONARY NOTE

Two issues remain to be discussed with respect to lay knowledge of the pill. The first involves use of the pill as an abortive as well as a "temporary" method; the second, the manner in which informants answered survey-type questions about their knowledge of the pill. A common notion we encountered is that if contraceptive pills were powerful enough to weaken the *dhatu* or in some other way prevent conception from occurring, then taking several pills at once should effect the body sufficiently to heat, dry, or push out the fetus. One of our informants was in the process of obtaining birth control pills from the Government Health Worker for this purpose when we interviewed her, and four other informants voluntarily told us without prompting that they had taken multiple tablets as a means of menstrual regulation when their period was overdue. In a study of twenty mothers who had used self treatment for abortion in Galle District (Chullawathi 1985), it was found that 25% had utilized birth control pills for this purpose. Good (1980) has likewise noted the use of the pill in Iran to induce abortion. It was not uncommon for Iranian women to take a month's supply in a day to bring on menstruation when they suspected they were pregnant with an unwanted child. Another use of the pill observed by us in South India and reported by Campbell and Stone (1984) in Nepal involved the management of menstruation in relation to ritual regulations involving states of pollution. Some women used the pill not for contraception, but rather with the purpose of delaying their menstrual period so they could participate in a religious festival, wedding, etc.

Bearing in mind that the misuse of birth control pills as an abortive is commonplace in Sri Lanka, we may suggest that the findings of the CPS may be less than accurate. According to the CPS, 82% of the woman surveyed "had knowledge" of the pill. The question that arises is what kind of knowledge did they have? From discussions with CPS interviewers, we found that misinterpretation of survey questions by laypersons was quite common. Campbell and Stone (1984) among others (Marshall 1972; Smith and Radel 1972) have pointed out the problems of knowledge, attitude and practice studies in their validation study of family planning survey research in Nepal.

In addition to language problems (e.g. the use of high language), they found that "problems arise when the concepts embedded in a question evoke special meanings and associations for respondents. People respond not to the formal content of a question, but to associations the questions have for them (1984: 31)". Campbell and Stone cite data about abortion as a case in point. They note that all villagers interviewed by their research team knew of abortives, but less than half claimed knowledge of abortion on a national KAP type survey. Dominant cultural values casting negative associations on abortion led informants to immediately focus on threatening and gossipy associations which the word carried "causing them to reinterpret straightforward questions put to them in personal terms."[11] Similarly, Marshall (1972) found in India that although every man in the village where he worked knew of vasectomy, one half of the 53 respondents on a KAP survey said they had not. Similarly, informants who had adopted contraception (vasectomy, loop) did not mention their adoption.

In our research on birth control pills, the dynamics of interviewing proved complex for related, but somewhat distinct reasons. When asked if they had heard of the pill, all of our respondents answered that they had. We then asked if they knew how the pill was used, and the majority answered affirmatively. When probed for details, however, it was found that many women had very vague ideas as to the use of the pill and some regarded the pill to be an abortive, not a means of temporary contraception. We suspect that "knowledge of method" as reported in the CPS needs to be interpreted with considerable latitiude. Knowledge of "what" remains the question. With the high valus placed on literacy in Sinhalese society, we found that informants did not want to appear "uneducated" by not "knowing" about the pill.

STERILIZATION: HOW IT WORKS

Tubectomy is the most popular family planning method in Sri Lanka and according to the CPS, 17 percent of all married women in Sri Lanka have undergone sterilization. Several different ideas were noted as to how this method works. One common idea was that the operation was a turning of the womb, *bukka harenava*, causing the entrance to the womb to be blocked so that male *dhatu* could not enter and mix with female *dhatu*.[12] Another idea was that the mouth of the womb is stitched closed to prevent conception. Other informants described the operation as a tying of a woman's tubes, *nara*, to prevent *dhatu* from coming into the womb. Informants working on a tea plantation near Kandy interviewed as part of a separate study[13], perceived that the operation was a cutting and tying of the *nara* with a piece of plastic fishing line, *tangoose*. Practical everyday experience with fishing line led them to question the permanence of the operation. They conceived of possible slippage in the tying between times of tautness and slackness. It

was feared, for example, that if a woman climbed steep hills or did considerable bending and lifting work, this line might loosen or break off rendering
the operation ineffective. Some informants expressed the opinion that an
operation was not a reliable method — i.e. that one could become pregnant
either because the stitches were not tight — allowing *dhatu* to leak inside —
or because the stitches could come out altogether. Informants in two of our
field sites related stories about a woman who had become pregnant after
having an operation. In each area we were told that the local doctor and
family health worker had explained that "the stitches had loosened", providing a prototype for method failure which supported popular imagery of
method function. With regard to this data, it is interesting to note that in a
study conducted in the U. S. (Johnson, Snow and Mayhew 1978: 859),
women informants noted that sterilization was reversible and that "the tubes
would spontaneously untie in seven years."

A less common idea which emerged during the study was that a woman's
body was cooled by the operation, due to significant blood loss. This cooling
of the body created an environment in which it was not possible to conceive.
This reasoning followed the indigenous notion that a woman must maintain
an optimum level of heat in order to conceive. The idea here is the reverse of
that articulated about birth control pills in which overheat in the body
rendered the method effective.

With respect to vasectomy, the most common explanation for how the
method worked was that the tube, *nara* which carries the *dhatu* was cut and
tied, so that *dhatu* could no longer come out. As a result, semen, which is
composed of *dhatu* and other fluids becomes thin and watery. Some men
emphasized that when aroused the *dhatu* continues to want to burst out but
is blocked. This creates a pressure comparable to the feeling of hemorrhoids.
Various male informants stated that this blocking effect could either heighten
or inhibit sexual capacity, in either case resulting in frustration. Significantly
less data was collected on user understanding of vasectomy, in part because
fewer informants had either personal experience with the method or knowledge of others who did. Interestingly, among those who did discuss vasectomy, the Sinhalese phrase "*shakti ena nahara kapala*" was commonly used,
literally the vein that brings *shakti* is cut. The use of the word *shakti*, life
energy, as opposed to *dhatu* in this phrase is important because it notes how
a vasectomy is not just seen as effecting a man's semen but rather is
conceived of as weakening one's vigor, vitality, and most critically, one's life
energy.

SIDE EFFECTS OF STERILIZATION

The most common negative symptoms noted in discourse about sterilization
were weakness and the inability to do heavy work.[14] Also mentioned by

females was a set of symptoms commonly including: leanness, decreased digestive capacity, less appetite, heavy bleeding during menses, painful menses (blockage of a normal flow of substance); and decreased sexual desire. Males additionally mentioned pain during urination and pain during intercourse due to a blockage and pressure. Once again it may be emphasized that these symptoms must be considered in their own right as well as being part of a somatic idiom of distress having symbolic and indexical meanings. This became very clear to us while following a forty year old middle class woman complaining of appetite loss and weakness one year following a tubectomy. Discussions with an ayurvedic practitioner who had been treating the woman for well over twenty years, revealed that these complaints were at once caused by deranged humors and constituted a means by which she withdrew from an unsatisfactory sexual relationship with her husband. He had treated the couple for this problem nine years before the operation. Following each sexual contact the woman would complain to her husband of multiple somatic complaints and would visit the practitioner at significant cost to the family. She would additionally state that she was unable to engage in strenuous work for some days.

CONDOM USE

According to CPS data, the reported use of condoms in Sri Lanka is limited to less than 3 percent of the population, representing an increase of just under one percent in the seven year period between the WFS and the CPS surveys. Notably, a significantly lower percentage of women reported knowledge of the condom than all other methods of contraception, with the exception of withdrawal. This data is surprising when one considers that the Preethi condom social marketing campaign has been described as a landmark in the fertility reduction efforts of Sri Lanka (Goonasekera 1976).[15]

Why is reported knowledge and use of condoms so low in Sri Lanka? A number of possibilities exist. First, it is possible that women respondents on the WFS and CPS (neither survey had male respondents) were embarrassed to claim knowledge of a method utilized strictly by men. A second possibility is that other cultural factors — beyond gender — mitigate against reporting condom use. Research revealed that when first introduced by the Government Family Planning Association, condoms were most commonly used by men who were visiting prostitutes. Such an association of the condom with illicit sexual activity has also been reported in Peru (Tucker 1986), the Middle East (Sukkary-Stolba and Mossavar-Rahmani 1982), and India (Marshall 1973). In India the condom was traditionally used only with prostitutes. Marshall notes that "because of the resulting guilt by association, it would have been especially embarrassing to both men and women for a person to purchase or be known to use a condom" (1973: 129). In Sri Lanka, an association still remains between condom use and elicit sex. Moreover, condom use is looked down upon by the middle class who consider them a low class contraceptive method and associate them with "uncultured" sexual relationships engaged in by the "uneducated."[16] Government dispensary personnel and private pharmacists reported that many men in the rural areas who do use condoms prefer to take a bus trip to the next town to purchase condoms to preserve their anonymity. They preferred a trip which would cost at least a rupee plus the price of a condom to obtaining a condom at a local clinic for the low cost of five paise (1/20 of a rupee).

All of our informants had knowledge of the condom and how it was used. Two health concerns were associated with their use. Condoms were described as heating and burning (*ushnayi* and *darelayi*) for both the male and female partner. This "side effect" was linked to friction and the heatiness of rubber. Several informants noted that this effect could be counterbalanced by drinking cooling tender coconut water the morning following intercourse. A similar belief has been noted by the researchers in India. A second health concern was that condoms interfere with the natural flow and exchange of *dhatu* between men and women. In both Sri Lanka and South India it is believed that women derive a source of vitality and health during intercourse when they receive male *dhatu*. Men, on the other hand, are generally thought to be weakened by sexual intercourse. This idea underlies the popular Sinhalese practice of a newly married wife serving her husband egg coffee on mornings following intercourse as a means of replenishing his *dhatu* supply. According to village lore, a man will become lean following marriage while the new bride becomes fat from the supply of *dhatu* she absorbs from their lovemaking.[17] This notion is offset by a health concern about lovemaking when one is weak or in ill health. Intercourse at this time is thought to increase weakness and render one more vulnerable to debilitating illness.

Condom use interferes with what may be thought of as *dhatu* economics — a concern taken more seriously by the poor maximizing scarce resources than by those having abundant food resources and more capable of replenishing *dhatu* supply. For the poor, *dhatu* represents a penultimate form of vitality produced by the body through a chain of transformations from food to blood to *dhatu*. To discard such a valued source of vitality is considered wasteful. There is a balance as well as supply side to *dhatu* economics. Informants referred to a balancing which occurs from an exchange of substance between partners. Five of our male informants spoke of loosing "something" of benefit from a woman when a condom was worn. Three of these informants used the hot-cold idiom to express a sense of imbalance following condom use while two described themselves as being "unsettled" after intercourse. One informant during a small group discussion over a vintage bottle of arrack alcohol aptly summarized his feeling to the approval of his four companions: "When we use the condom it is something like drinking sweet toddy, but not drinking fermented toddy! The fermented toddy gives you a kick, but the sweet toddy doesn't!"

IUD: HOW IT WORKS

The IUD or "loop" is not a popular method of contraception in Sri Lanka. According to CPS data, only 2.5 percent of married women respondents reported using this method, one percent lower than the findings of the WFS in 1975. While most of our informants had heard the name "loop", few could describe this method beyond stating that it was some kind of barrier which prevented male *dhatu* from entering into a woman. Notably, some women discussed the IUD referring to it as an operation. Indeed, in one case where a woman had stated to us that she had had an operation, it turned out that she had not had a tubal ligation as we imagined, but an IUD insertion. For this woman, any procedure which involved lying down in a clinic where a doctor used long instruments inside her body constituted an operation!

A very vague sense of ethnoanatomy emerged from discussions about the loop. Few women, even users, had an understanding of where the loop was placed inside of them. Lack of a clear idea as to placement was reflected in a popular health concern involving migration of the loop within the body. Informants spoke of the loop being gradually pushed up toward the stomach and beyond. Many conceptualized no clear separation between the womb and stomach or imagined one opening into the other. A fear was expressed that if the loop was pushed into the stomach, an operation would be required to remove it. If this was not done the loop could move up to the lungs and kill the woman. Women at greatest risk were deemed to be those who engaged in sex more frequently for the loop was imagined to "move up" during more vigorous sexual activity.

The idea that an IUD can travel in the body and lodge in the head or lungs had been noted in Botswana (Larson 1983), Kenya (Huston 1979), India (Population Reports 1984), Mexico (Shedlin 1977), and Tunisia (Sukkary-Stolba and Mossavar-Rahmani 1982). In Peru, Tucker notes that "some women thought that the IUD floats in the body and can perforate the lungs or brain and eventually kill them" (1986: 312). Respondents there reported that the IUD attacks the head and the nerves. Another common idea in Sri Lanka was that the loop could fall out after it was inserted. At the time of insertion, women are advised by health personnel to "feel for the string" when they urinate. When they fail to find it they suspect it has fallen out, or that it has been pushed up. Some women noted that heavy work could cause an IUD to fall out. Shedlin (1977: 14) has noted similar concerns about the IUD in Mexico: "They were concerned it would fall out, get lost, appear in various orifices of the body, cause them to become stuck together with their husbands, be felt by their husbands, etc." Other informants in Sri Lanka stated that if a woman had sex with more than one partner, her vagina might become larger causing the loop to fall out. Therefore, if a loop did fall out, it created suspicion that the woman had been having extramarital affairs.

Misconceptions about the IUD are common worldwide. Marshall notes in India (1973: 128):

The IUD was believed by the villagers to operate by increasing the heat in a woman's genital region above the threshold at which conception could occur. Under normal circumstance this would not be considered physically dangerous to a woman, but if she were afflicted with certain ailments that were thought to be "hot" — such as smallpox, diarrhea, or venereal disease — then the additional heat from an IUD could kill her. Since a woman could not be assured of escaping such a disease after she had adopted a loop, the method was best avoided.

A lack of understanding about the loop has also been noted by Johnson, Snow and Mayhew (1978) in a study in the U.S. Among their informants, 53% had incorrect information on the IUD's mode of action. The IUD was seem by many women as a plug that kept the sperm and egg from getting together. This notion of something "plugging" the female was reported by 39% of these women to be dangerous to health (1978: 858).

NEGATIVE EFFECTS

In Sri Lanka, as in Egypt (Morsy 1980: 82), one of the main health concerns underscoring resistance to the IUD is a loss of blood following insertion. Users attributed weakness from the IUD to an increase in menstrual blood loss, which a majority of women were not informed might occur. Some informants assumed that this loss of blood was in some way involved with the functioning of the method itself constituting a primary negative effect. In one instance, an informant stated that she had suffered from continuous bleeding for one month following her loop insertion, but had not sought follow-up care. When we asked her why she thought this bleeding had occurred, she remarked:

The loop is something made of plastic so it creates a lot of heat. It is like wearing rubber slippers — when you wear them, your feet feel hot and you get heating side effects. The bleeding is caused by this heatiness. Heatiness and bleeding are to be expected. This is how the method works.

Another idea reported was that the loop could cause "cancer." Probing the meaning of cancer we found that the term was taken from the media and incorporated in everyday speech to denote chronic ill health caused by a foreign body inside the body. Informants associated the presence of a foreign body with heatiness, toxicity, and wounds within the body resulting in rough (scar like) tissue — cancer.

Ideas circulating about the IUD may in large part be due to the lack of explanation offered to women about possible side effects. In India, for example, Cassen (1978) has noted ". . . it was felt that it was sufficiently hard to persuade women to use the IUD at all and would be harder if they had to be told that they might experience pain or bleeding" (1978: 158). This strategy was not successful in India and rumors, in part based on ethnoanatomical knowledge, spread that the IUD could migrate within the body to the heart and lungs, could cause penile injury or even death to the husband during intercourse. IUD adoption rates dropped dramatically.[18] Side effects of the IUD are now explained and taken more seriously by program personnel (Ainsworth 1985).

An ethical problem related to health service may well contribute to the unpopularity of the loop in Sri Lanka. In rural Ratnapura, the loop was widely adopted when it was first introduced, but within a few years many women discontinued its use. A number of informants in this region spoke of the loop being unreliable and falling out. When we interviewed family health workers about this, we were told that there was little if any screening before loop insertion.[19] Upon investigation we found one reason decreasing the reliabiltiy of the loop involved women who had had a loop inserted after they found out they were pregnant, thinking this would result in an abortion.[20] When their pregnancy became visible, it gave rise to the notion that a woman could get pregnant, even when having a loop. When confronted with a pregnant woman following an IUD insertion, clinicians commonly acted "kindly" suggesting the possibility that the IUD may not have been positioned correctly. In so doing, they alleviated suspicion that the woman might have engaged in extra marital sexual affairs should her husband have been away prior to loop insertion.

SOCIAL CLASS AND PERCEPTIONS OF CONTRACEPTIVE METHOD APPROPRIATENESS

We asked a lower middle class informant who was a long term satisfied user of both a loop and sterilization why some women complained of bleeding and weakness after these procedures while others, like herself, did not have such problems. She replied that each person's body was different so it responds differently to family planning methods. When we asked in what way people's bodies were different, she remarked that some were more heaty than others. She further explained that the pill and loop were very heaty and harsh so they were not good for women with heaty bodies who could not afford to eat cooling foods. "If a woman doesn't eat cooling foods while taking the pill, she looses the ability to conceive — she dries up. If she can eat cooling food while taking the pill, she may still be fertile when she stops."

Three important inpressions emerged during this interview: 1) that people with different bodies repond differently to modern methods, 2) if one uses a method which has a negative primary effect or an unintended side effect, it is possible to counterbalance this effect thereby reducing harm to the body, and 3) a chief means of reducing negative effects especially blood loss was by consuming cooling and strength producing foods. Following this interview we spoke to serveral lower middle class and poor informants. What emerged was a widespread impression that modern methods of contraception were appropriate for those who could afford to consume milk, eggs, meat and particular varieties of fish.

Important lessons can be learned from considering distinct social class perceptions of contraceptive appropriateness evaluated in relation to the parameters of resources and risk. According to the poor, the diet of the wealthy enabled them to cope more effectively with the primary negative effects of contraceptive methods. While birth control pills might be appropriate for the middle class, they were not an appropriate method for the poor because they could not afford to routinely balance the heating side effects of pills with the consumption of tender coconut water and cow's milk. Of the six lower middle class women whom we interviewed who were presently using the pill, all went into elaborate detail about their strategies for cooling their bodies. Not having enough resources to routinely consume special foods, one resorted to bathing frequently with well water and drinking large quantities of cold water. Four of these women noted that they restricted the intake of heating foods such as dry fish, thus reducing their dietary resources, in an effort to counter balance excess heatiness in their body.

The idea that nutritious food can offset harmful effects of fertility regulation methods has been noted cross-culturally. For example, in Morocco it was reported that although pills can cause heart palpitations, they can be used safely by women rich enough to afford a balanced diet (Mernissi 1975). As one of her informants noted:

If you eat only starch and you can never afford milk, meat or bananas . . . you are already weak and the pill is therefore dangerous for you because it affects the heart. A weak body cannot take the pill. The day I can afford to have a banana and a glass of milk I will start using the pill again. Until then I have to find another method which is less dangerous (1975:422)

Writing about Egypt, Morsy notes that:

The ingestion of powerful medications is also believed to require the consumption of large amounts of nourishing food. This belief illuminates a rationalization by women for their refusal to consume birth control pills. Women who have used these pills complain that they cause weakness . . . strong medicine like this needs good eating and we are poor peasants. (1980:93)

Similar ideas abut the need for "good food" while taking the pill have been noted by Sukkary-Stolba and Mossavar-Rahmani (1982) in their five country study in the Middle East.

It is not only the negative primary effects of the pill which are believed to be offset by optimum food resources. Many Sri Lankan informants expressed the view that if a woman could afford to eat eggs, milk, meat, and fish, and refrain from hard work for three months following sterilization, weakness and general malaise could be mitigated. By following this regimen, a woman's body would be allowed to replenish its supply of *dhatu* which had been lost.[21]

Two points need to be highlighted. First, decisions as to whether or not to adopt various family planning methods/practices are made bearing economic and social constraints as well as perceptions of health risk in mind.[22] Second, contraception is associated with an increased vulnerability to ill health, which may be mitigated by folk dietetic prescriptions and restrictions. Among the poor, dietary prescriptions are often unaffordable. The result is that those already in a debilitated state tend to interpret past health problems as exacerbated, if not caused by, a contraceptive method. Medical staff commonly interpret complaints of "side effects" as being psychosomatic. They fail to comprehend the way in which family planning methods are thought to function and impact on bodily processes as basic as digestion and blood production and as subtle as *dhatu* production and all it entails.

SECRECY AND THE IDEAL OF CONTROL: THE IMPORTANCE OF RUMOR

Let us now consider the phenomena of rumor as distinct from cultural knowledge, or what may more aptly be considered culture based common sense. Although the Sinhalese are more open to discuss modern methods of birth control than traditional practices (Chapter 1), there is some reticence especially among the low-middle class, to publicly admit that one is using a family planning method. Within the dominant Sinhalese Buddhist culture, control is a highly regarded social value associated with doing or wanting nothing in excess. As Amarasingham (1981) has noted, Sinhalese Buddhist ideology proscribes moderation as an ideal. Anything in excess is believed to lead to unhappiness and ultimately to suffering. Applied to birth control, this cultural value manifests in public secrecy about contraceptive method adoption. Control of one's sexuality is a source of respect and social status. Admitting to using a method amounts to "telling that you are unable to control your sexual urge and that you are uncultured". Our middle class informants commonly spoke of the uneducated having more children because "they cannot control themselves". These same informants were often the first to emphasize secrecy about method use "so neighbors will not come to know and spread rumors."

The importance of secrecy varies by ethnic group, social class and residence pattern. For example, among lower middle class informants in rural Horana and Ratnapura districts, great effort was expended on bypassing the normal methods of condom distribution to maintain secrecy.[23] The desire for secrecy was further found to effect women's willingness to contact family health workers about IUD related problems. Some informants expressed a reluctance against frequent visits by the family health worker fearing that this would suggest to neighbors that they were using a family planning method. This kind of behavior points out the weakness of the assumption that greater geographic accessibility to family planning resources necessarily leads to greater use.

An emphasis on control of one's sexuality has given rise to social seclusion as well as secrecy. A widespread concern among males is that methods of family planning adopted by women afford them license to engage in extra-marital sexual relations. A few informants in Sri Lanka and many more infor-mants encountered during fieldwork in South India reported altered forms of social behavior following contraceptive adoption, particularly tubectomy. In cases reported by women, husbands were described as acting more protec-tive of them, monitoring their coming and going and questioning their participation in social activities. As a means of reducing a husband's suspicions, some women who had actively participated in community affairs and social activities decreased their participation following sterilization. These informants described a deep sense of loss over their forced with-drawal from social interaction. Family planning methods had removed them from being victims of unplanned families, but they were now victims of suspicion — confining them once again.

A sensitivity to cultural values and the devastating impact of rumor also influences the way in which doctors explain pregnancy when a husband has a vasectomy or when a woman claims she is practicing birth control, but becomes pregnant-especially after her husband has left for migrant work elsewhere. In this situation, health care providers are faced with discrediting either the woman or the method. Given the grave situation which may result from accusing the woman of infidelity in a country with a high suicide rate, health care providers consistently stated that when faced with such a situation they usually stated that the pregnancy might be the result of a method failure. Of eight doctors questioned, six stated they had faced such a situation at least once in the past three years. Although these doctors behaved in a culturally tactful and kind manner, they served to reduce confidence about family planning methods.

CONCLUSION

One of the biggest problems with contraceptive use survey data is that the terms "knowledge" and "familiarity" have been confounded. "Knowledge" of a family planning method as reported on the CPS, the WFS and similar surveys can mean anything from recall of the name of a method to experi-ence with or familiarity with someone who has tried the method, to knowledge as an objectified construct of how the method actually functions. Different forms of contraceptive knowledge exist ranging from tacit knowledge and prototype experience to explanatory models developed in relation to popular health concerns, interpretations of information from biomedical and/or traditional medical tradition and rumors as heresay. A greater appreciation of the range of knowledge people have of contraceptive methods will help to broaden an understanding of contraceptive use and non-use among particular groups. A better understanding of the production of knowledge about contraception by practitioners and laypersons alike will provide insights into the ideologies and motivations underlying the generation of discourse about family planning as a subject in context, not isolation.

It would appear obvious that there is a significant need to prepare a population conceptually when introducing preventive health technical fixes such as immunization (Nichter 1989) and family planning. Additionally, there is an ongoing need for understanding how local populations are interpreting the way in which such fixes work in the short run and effect health in the long run. To neglect popular health culture or classify it as marginal, misinformation, rumor or whatever is to be medicocentric and to blame the victim for poorly thought out health programs. The physical and cultural experience of biotechnical fixes can not be neatly separated in terms of mind and body. It is necessary to consider public reponse to fixes both in relation to how they are delivered (physically and conceptually) and experienced bioculturally. Fertility regulation is an emotionally charged area of biotechnology where there is much contention among practitioners as well as the public. Real risks exist and there is a need for ongoing monitoring among peoples having different physical, nutritional, health and cultural characteristics. The tendency to hastely label biocultural experience as untruth or rumor needs to be studied in its own right.

We have recast the issue of "rumors about side effects" in this paper, calling attention to the need for greater sophistication in the analysis of why there is concern — not simply resistance — about contraceptive use. A focus on side effects instead of health concerns as embedded in health culture is as limited a focus of analysis as a consideration of "barriers to demand" instead of "opportunities for demand." The former assumes one knows what another should want and demand. It begins with what is being offered. The latter considers what another wants or feels is necessary and puts available technology to work maximizing opportunities and expanding consciousness to meet demand.

It is prudent to bear in mind that:

The consequence of modern science and technology has not been to overwhelm common sense views and render them insignificant, but to modify them somewhat and increase their cultural significance. (Holzner and Marx, 1979)

NOTES

1. CPS data indicates that the percentage using traditional methods was positively associated with education. This is not the case in the use of modern methods (Sri Lanka 1983: 77) cited in Gendell (1985). For example, 21% of women who had completed primary school used traditional methods compared to 29% of secondary school (and over) educated women — both groups averaging 30—31% utilization of modern methods.

2. Several government health education officers told us that the group who had the most questions and the most doubts about modern methods of family planning were the educated — particularly teachers. Often these doubts were associated with information printed in local newspapers wherein large headlines announced news such as "Oral Contraceptives Cause Cancer." We found that the statistics that often followed these headlines established that cancer was relatively rare. Informants, however, tended to remember headlines not supporting data.

3. The Matlab Project in Bangladesh indicated that while access to contraceptives is a necessary precondition for the adoption of family planning, contraceptive prevalence rates are not always high when contraceptives are simply physically available (Phillips et al 1982). There is a real need to understand the user's perspective when designing and modifying family planning programs. KAP surveys are an insufficient mode of research. Qualitative information is required not only on how decisions about reproduction and contraception are made, but more elementary, about the rationale behind these decisions — i.e. the meaning of modern methods. Such an approach has been advocated by Marshall and Polgar (1976) who have called for a phenomenological approach — "one that demands an understanding of existing and potential fertility regulation methods from the perspective of the client population."

4. In this regard, we concur with DeClerque et al (1986) that the origin and transmission of rumor should be considered in the wider context of social dynamics. Festinger et al. (1948) have noted that the need for external control often underlies the occurrence of rumor. Of concern in this paper is what to label as a "rumor" and what the ramifications of label use are when applied to indigenous knowledge. We propose that the word not be broadly used by professionals to denote the emic form of an etic vantage point.

   On another note, we would point out that rumor may also reflect a cultural style of communication. Rumor, as talk about others and their experience, may provide an opportunity for discussion of one's feelings in a culture where more direct communication is inappropriate. Speaking through rumors may allow one to discuss an issue with a culturally appropriate degree of social distance.

5. In Sri Lanka the drying, heating effect of the pill on one bodily process is generalized to other processes. A drying of the breastmilk is associated with the drying of the womb — an idea also reported in Iran (Good 1980). The drying-reducing effect of the pill is also associated with weight, an overdetermined symbol of well being in South Asia.

6. DeClerque et al. (1986) suggest that in relation to the ubiquitous complaint of weakness there maybe unique side effects generated through the combined use of high dose pills and endemic health problems (such as anemia) among Egyptian women.

7. Ethnographic research relating to the issue of weakness may be found in Morsy 1980, Good 1980, Nichter 1981 and DeClerque et al. 1986.

8. Margarita Kay (1985) has raised a related point in her work with the Mexican-American community. She has noted that Mexican American women do not accord the same attributes to birth control pills and other forms of contraception as are found in the scientific educational materials they are given. She suggests that contraceptive providers have a poor understanding of what properties are salient to their users. The Basnayake report exemplifies this point.

9. In another study in Egypt, Khattab (1978) found that among 70 pill users in a rural village, 24 (35%) were using the pill incorrectly. Many were using the same brand of a 28 day pill cycle where vitamin tablets were intended for the seven days of the menstrual flow. She noted that women started with the supplementary pills while others alternated pills with vitamins to counteract side effects.

10. Seaton (1985) has also stressed that "In less developed countries, the problem of ensuring client compliance in family planning programs are aggravated by educational and cultural environments that do little or nothing to promote an understanding of the perceptions and practices of contraception" (p.52).

11. In addition to problems relating to cultural styles of communication and the dynamics of knowledge production is the limited capability of a structured interview to create an environment fostering the articulation of tacit knowledge. While structured surveys may prove reliable for collecting certain types of microdemographic data, they are an insufficient way of researching the meaning of health related behavior, the production of knowledge about health and family planning, and the interpretation of lived experience.

12. In South Kanara District, Karnataka, India, a tubectomy is referred to as turning the pregnancy bag over, *garbha chila madistare*. Mathews and Benjamin (1979) have similarly reported that a tubectomy in Tamil Nad is described as "twisting the uterus" or "turning it upside down." A vasectomy in both areas is described as cutting a nerve, *nara*, by many people.

13. This study was carried out in conjunction with the Department of Census and Statistics in 1984.

14. Informants noted that since the operation caused weakness it was more economically viable for the wife to be sterilized than the husband. If a wife could no longer do hard work outside of the home after the operation, she could at least continue with the housework.

15. Preethi, a term which means happiness in Sinhala and Tamil, was chosen as the name for the condom and a hand signal was designed so it could be obtained from shops by demonstrating a non-verbal cue thus reducing embarrassment. Although we found that the product was widely known, the hand signal was much less recognized than we had expected from its popularity as described in the literature. In fact, the hand signal approximates another commonly used non-verbal cue meaning excellent, *niame*.

16. As used by the middle class, the words uneducated and uncultured are often used interchangeably as markers of inclusion/non-inclusion. They do not refer so much to one's literacy or formal education but rather to their knowledge and public adherence to Buddhist precepts and practice.

17. A variant idea is that the *dhatu* of a young woman is particularly rejuvenating for an old man — one reason why old men like to marry young girls (Harrison 1976).

18. People speak of the slow progress of family planning programs in India prior to 1976 as if it demonstrated the absence of any widespread desire to limit one's family. What may in fact have been demonstrated by the low adoption levels was the low level of acceptability of the IUD and vasectomy as offered within the government programs.

19. Loops were inserted once a month during a special clinic day. All women interested in loop insertion therefore had to appear at that time, irregardless of when they had had their last menses. Loop insertion is ideally performed during menses. Many women, however, had insertions at other times of the month.

20. Some women had loops inserted to induce abortion. After loop insertion bleeding is heavy leading these women to believe that "everything inside would be pushed out." If the loop failed to abort pregnancy, some women would return to the clinic the following month and have it removed.

21. The type of food that a person can afford is a factor which also impacts on sexual

behavior. As one Tamil informant explained, "With our present food situation, we can afford to have sex only one to three times a month. This is not because we don't enjoy sex but because when we lose *dhatu* and don't take proper foods to replace it we become weak." Times of high sexuality were often pay day, a time when alcohol consumption was also greatest.

22. Ainsworth (1985) has provided a useful review of the literature on perceived social and health related costs of practicing contraception and strategies developed to reduce the costs and satisfy unmet needs related to quality of service and access to information method and follow up service.

23. Coastal Muslims preferred birth control pills delivered directly to the home for the same reason. The need for secrecy was not found among Tamils working on tea estates who preferred to go to sterilization camps in a group. Truckloads of women working on the plantations were driven to the Government Hospital for these camps. When we inquired if this did not make women shy (i.e. that everyone could plainly see what they were doing) we were told by several informants that they felt shy to go alone.

REFERENCES

Ainsworth, M.
  1985 *Family planning programs: The clients' perspective.* World Bank Staff Working Papers Number 676. Population and Development Series Number 1. The World Bank, Washington D.C.
Basnayake, S., Higgins, J. E., Miller, P., Rogers, S., and Kelley, S. E.
  1984 Early symptoms and discontinuation among users of oral contraceptives in Sri Lanka. *Studies in Family Planning Volume 15*, Number 6. Nov./Dec., 285—290.
Bertrand, J. T., Araya, J. d., Cisneros, R. J., and L. Morris
  1982 Evaluation of family planning, communication in El Salvador. *International Journal of Health Education 24*(3): 183—194.
Bogue, D. J.
  1975 *Twenty-five Communciation Obstacles to the Success of Family Planning Programs.* Media Monograph 2. Communication Laboratory, Community and Family Study Center, University of Chicago, Chicago, Illinois.
Campbell, J. and Stone, L.
  1984 The use and misuse of surveys in international development: An experiment from Nepal. *Human Organization Vol. 43*, No. 1: 27—37.
Cassen, R. H.
  1978 *India: Population, Economy, Society.* New York: Holmes and Meier.
Chullawathie, M. K.
  1984 *Lay Ideas on Fecundity During Women's Monthly Cycle and Post-Partum until Twelve Months.* M. Sc. Field Project, Post Graduate Institute of Medicine, Colombo, Sri Lanka.
DeClerque, J., Tsu, A. O., Abul-Ata, M. F., and Barcelona, D.
  1986 Rumor, misinformation and oral contraceptive use in Egypt. *Soc. Sci. Med., Vol. 23* (1), pp. 83—93.
Department of Census and Statistics
  1978 *World Fertility Survey, Sri Lanka, 1975: First Report* (Colombo: Ministry of Plan Implementation).
Festinger, L., Cartwright, D., Barber, K., Fleischel, J., Gottsdarker, J., Keyer, A., and Leavitt, G.
  1948 A study of rumor: its origin and spread. *Human Relations 1*, 464—486.
Gendell, M.
  1985 Stalls in the fertility decline in Costa Rica, Korea, and Sri Lanka. World Bank Staff

Working Papers: Number 693. *Population and Development Series* Number 18, Washington, D.C.

Good, M. J. D.
  1980 Of blood and babies: The relationship of popular Islamic physiology to fertility. *Soc. Sci. Med., Vol. 14B*, pp. 147—156.

Goonasekera, A.
  1976 *Commercial Distribution of contraceptives in Sri Lanka: The Preethi Experience.* (mimeo)

Government of Sri Lanka, Department of Census and Statistics, Ministry of Plan Implementation and Westinghouse Health Systems
  1983 *Sri Lanka Contraceptive Prevalence Survey Report: 1982.* (Colombo: Dept. of Census and Statistics, Ministry of Plan Implementation)

Harrison, P.
  1976 Marketing Preethi in a small package. *Human Behavior*, March.

Holzner, B. and Marx, J.
  1979 *Knowledge Application: The Knowledge System in Society.* Boston: Allyn and Bacon.

Huston, P.
  1979 *Third World Women Speak Out.* New York: Praeger.

Johnson, S. M., Snow, L., and Mayhew, H.
  1978 Limited patient knowledge as a reproductive risk factor. *The Journal of Family Practice, Vol. 6*, no. 4.

Kay, M.
  1985 Mexican American fertility regulation. *Communicating Nursing Research Vol. 10*, pp. 279—295.

Khattab, M.
  1978 Practice and non-practice of family planning in Egypt. *In* A. Molnos (ed.) *Social Science in Family Planning*, pp. 22—29. International Planned Parenthood Federation, London.

Krieger, L.
  1984 *Body notions, gender roles, and fertility regulating methods used in Imbaba, Cairo.* Doctoral dissertation, Dept. of Anthropology, University of North Carolina, Chapel Hill.

Larson, M. K.
  1983 *Botswana: family planning myths and beliefs.* Cited in Population Reports No. 28, 1984.

Liskin, L.
  1984 *After contraception: dispelling rumors about later childbearing.* Population Reports No. 28. Population Information Program, Johns Hopkins University, Baltimore.

Marshall, J. F.
  1972 *Culture and contraception: Response determinants to a family planning program in a North Indian village.* Ph.D. dissertation, University of Hawaii.
  1973 Fertility regulating methods: cultural acceptability for potential adopters. *In* G. W. Duncan, E. J. Hilton, P. Kreager and A. A. Lumsdaine (eds) *Fertility Control Methods: Strategies for Introduction.* New York: Academic Press.

Marshall, J. F. and Polgar, S. (eds.)
  1976 *Culture, Natality, and Family Planning*, Monograph 21, Chapel Hill, North Carolina: Carolina Population Center, pp. 204—218.

Matthews, C. and Benjamin, V.
  1979 Health education evaluation and belief and practices in rural Tamil Nad: Family planning and antenatal care. *Social Action 29*: 377—392.

Mercado, C. M.
  1973 Application of social science methodologies to information and education. In IPPF-

SEAOR. Presented at the Eighth Meeting of the Regional Information & Education Committee. Singapore, May 9—11.

Mernissi, F.
  1975 Obstacles to family planning practice in urban Morocco. *Studies in Family Planning* *6*(12): 418—425, Dec.

Morsy, S.A.
  1980 Body concepts and health care: Illustrations from an Egyptian village. *Human Organization Vol. 39*, No. 1, Spring, 92—97.

Rogers, E. M.
  1973 *Communication Strategies for Family Planning.* New York: Free Press.

Seaton, Brian
  1985 Non compliance among oral contraceptive acceptors in rural Bangladesh. *Studies in Family Planning 16*: 1, 52—58.

Shedlin, M.
  1977 *Body image and contraceptive acceptability in a Mexican community.* Paper presented at the Symposium on Body Concepts and Implications for Health Care, Annual Meeting of the American Anthropological Association, Houston, Nov. 29— Dec. 3.

Smith, S. E. and Radel, D.
         The KAP in Kenya: A critical look at KAP Survey Methodology. *In* Marshall & Polgar (eds), *Culture, Natality and Family Planning.* Chapel Hill, North Carolina: Carolina Population Center.

Sukkary-Stolba, S. and Mossavar-Rahmani, Y.
  1982 The cultural context of fertility in five middle eastern countries. Unpublished manuscript.

Tucker, G. M.
  1986 Barriers to modern contraceptive use in rural Peru. *Studies in Family Planning Vol. 17*, No. 6/Pt. 1., Nov./Dec, 308—317.

SECTION TWO

ILLNESS ETHNOGRAPHIES

INTRODUCTION

In this section I focus attention on illness classification, the manner in which different illnesses are and are not spoken about, perceptions of illness causality and patterns of health care seeking. Several features of illness related discourse are discussed in Chapter Four followed by an ethnographic investigation of states of malnutrition in South India and diarrheal illness in Sri Lanka. The latter two chapters include data on notions of etiology and patterns of curative resort. I may briefly note the importance and limitations of such data.

To understand how illness is perceived in South Asia it is necessary to appreciate the wide range of factors thought to predispose, cause, confound, and aggravate illness. This is a complex subject because one symptom (or a set of symptoms) may be caused by a number of different factors influencing the body alone or in conjunction with other factors. Very few types of illness or symptom states are thought to be caused by one and only one etiological factor. In most instances of ill health, several factors are implicated by the afflicted and/or significant others.

Often different members of a household or extended therapy managment group will have varying opinions about the cause or course of an illness. Their ideas are emergent with multiple forms of knowledge being produced in context. These forms of knowledge range from the knowledge of prototype illness experiences and illness narratives to knowledge negotiated between people. They include explanatory models constructed around popular metaphors as well as labels which imply sociomoral relations.

Knowing how actors describe illness, perceive etiology and evaluate courses of treatment is important to an understanding of popular health culture. It is not, however, sufficient to explain why households or individuals respond in particular ways to illness episodes. Health behavior is complex and based upon contingencies of social and economic as well as cultural significance. When studying health care decision making, predisposing, enabling and service related factors need to be considered in relation to household dynamics, time and resource demands, the impact of education etc. Just as important, it needs to be recognized that sickness is viewed as

83

more than a set of disvalued symptoms. Symptoms are often interpreted as signs of misfortune and vulnerability within the overlapping domains of one's lifeworld.

In South Asia, correspondences are drawn between poor health and events in other areas of life. For example, the infertility of a woman or the poor growth of a child may be linked to failed crops or poor yield and associated with stars, spirits, witchcraft or one's fate. In life, an opposition is broadly perceived between:

labba (profit): *dosha* (trouble)
       health: illness

Recognizing that ascriptions of etiology are often emergent, negotiated and context specific, it is valuable to identify popular ideas about illness causality, characteristics and appropriate treatment. While of limited predictive value, this data provides descriptive generalizations against which actual behavior patterns may be studied. In chapters five and six, which examine states of malnutrition and diarrhea, I employ a mix of case study and survey data to provide a thick description of these health problems and a sense of cultural heterogeneity in the way they are interpreted. Health care practices are highlighted to emphasize the ramifications of interpreting illness in various ways.

4. THE LANGUAGE OF ILLNESS, CONTAGION AND SYMPTOM REPORTING

I spent the morning observing a rural clinic attended by a Harijan caste doctor hailing from the next district who had practiced in this district for the past two years as a government medical officer. I was particularly curious to see how he would interact with both Harijan and higher caste Shudra patients. While I was busy taking notes on the doctor's meticulous display of purity, to the point of folding a white handkerchief on his chair before sitting, an agricultural laborer hobbled into the clinic and complained of having *meenu kannu*, literally fish eye. The doctor peered into his eyes which were inflamed, and pressed his index finger checking routine signs of anemia. Without an exchange of words, he then proceeded to write a prescription for eye drops. A B_{12} injection was administered and a packet of black ferrous sulfate tablets was given to the man with instructions as to dose, but no mention of the need to take them following meals. The patient thanked him, placed a few rupees on the table which was whisked away automatically, and proceeded to leave. There was something in the patient's gait, the way he stumbled out of the office, which led me to strike up a conversation with him outside a chemist shop an hour later. *Meenu kannu*, it turned out, was a deep abscess (pitted keratolysis) in the sole of the foot caused by stepping on sharp rocks while carrying a heavy headload of wood or other material. Why the name *meenu kannu*? The abscess looked like a fish eye and vis à vis the doctrine of signature, villagers believed it to be caused by stepping on or over a fish eye. The man had been given medicine for inflamed eyes and anemia yet he seemed satisfied. I couldn't help but wonder why. Upon investigation, I found that an indigenous means of treating red inflamed eyes was to rub cooling oil on the sole of the foot so as to draw the heat downward. The man thought the eye medicine he purchased was a cooling medicine which would draw the heat upward from his foot. He recognized the black ferrous sulfate tablets given to him at the clinic as the pills doled out by the village auxiliary nurse midwife. He decided not to take them, at least not now. After having an injection one had to be careful about heatiness and these pills were viewed as heaty.

I talked to the doctor later about *meenu kannu* and he expressed minor embarrassment but genuine interest in the incident, blaming the ignorant villager for not speaking up and believing in folk superstitions.

INTRODUCTION

I introduce this chapter on the language of illness with a fieldnote vignette to emphasize the practical importance of this subject in addition to its inherent anthropological significance. The language of illness is a multifacted field of inquiry for which there is a very limited cross-cultural literature. In the present study I focus on the language of illness in South Kanara.* The chapter is divided into four sections. In the first section, a brief critical review of broad approaches to the study of the language of illness will be provided as a means of placing the current study in context. In subsequent sections I turn to nine aspects of the language of illness in South Kanara. Considered in section two are illness nomenclature, the social dynamics of illness discourse, knowledge of illness categories, the negotiation of illness identities, and power relations as a feature of illness labeling. Section three is directed toward three issues pertinent to international health: the language of contagion, strategic symptom reporting, and the medicalization of ambigiously defined symptom states. Section four moves from interactional to more structural aspects of the language of illness. Considered is the way in which verbs and tenses implicity designate contrasting features of illness onset and course. Further illustrations of why it is important for those engaged in international health to appreciate native illness classification will be provided in chapters five and six.

SECTION ONE

THEORETICAL APPROACHES TO ILLNESS SEMANTICS AND THE LANGUAGE OF ILLNESS: AN OVERVIEW

Ethnoscience

Over the last twenty five years, two major approaches to the study of illness conceptualization and the language of illness have emerged in the literature. The first, of whom Frake (1961) is an exemplar, is an ethnoscience approach. Emphasis is placed on a taxonomic analysis of illness classification and the distinctive features which constitute the boundaries of illness categories. The underlying premise of this type of ethnosemantic analysis is that the disease universe is exhaustively subdivided in each culture into conceptually distinct mutually exclusive illness categories. These emic categories reflect culturally meaningful parameters of difference, patterns of contrast defining class inclusion and exclusion at various levels of specificity. Two kinds of data are essential to this approach to the language of illness. First, through observation of illness discourse and/or the deployment of such

---

* For the purposes of this chapter I will restrict myself to a consideration of Kannada language and not consider the Tulu language spoken in this region.

methods as sentence frame questionnaires which probe inclusion/exclusion by responses to posed statements (D'Andrade 1976), the principles by which natives classify their universe are identified in relation to levels of specificity. Second, and less explicit in existing ethnosemantic studies, is the study of the dynamics of discourse which engage a particular level of specificity. In other words, the issue is raised as to why an illness is identified and spoken about in a more general or specific manner in different contexts. For example, when is an upset stomach referred to rather than a "touch of the flu", a slight case of diarrhea or salmonella? Important here is the issue of social relations which crosscut diagnostic specificity.[1] Entailed, but not discussed in the ethnoscience literature, is a recognition of both the "referential" pointing feature of language and the "indexical" dimension of communication which involves the negotiation of knowledge and the constitution of social relations (Silverstein 1976, 1979).

The referential function of language lies in its ability to point to persons, objects, events and processes. Reference rests ultimately on a perceived correspondence between "content" of expressions and some state in "the real world". Contrastively, indexical meaning is dependent on the same feature(s) of the context in which the expression is uttered. It is not simply the case that some signs are indexical or that indexical meanings are simply "added on" to referential ones. Interview discourse (and I would add diagnostic discourse) is highly indexical, because the meaning of responses is contingent on the questions that precede them, previous questions-answer pairs, the social situation, the relationship between the interviewer and interviewee and host of other factors. (Briggs 1986: 42)

Frake has been criticized for subscribing to a static view of illness classification. Often overlooked is the attention he placed on the contextual use of language in describing illness and the production of knowledge at levels of contrast responsive to social role contingencies:

Diagnosis is not an automatic response to pathological stimuli; it is a social activity whose results hinge in part on role-playing strategies. Do the patients and his consultants wish to emphasize the former's disability, which prevents him from discharging an expected obligation? Or do they wish to communicate that the person's lesion is not serious enough to interfere with his duties? (Frake 1961)

Recognized by Frake, but little explored, is a strategic dimension of the language of illness. Ethnosemantic studies in general and Frake's study of the language of illness among the Subanese (Mindanao, Philippines) have been criticized for their insensitivity to intracultural variation and the fallacy of cultural consensus. An identical cognitive code, a diagnostic template, is assumed to be shared by all inhabitants of a common culture. Frake describes the Subanese as having a health culture where there are no specialist healers and all people are diagnosticians:

Subanese operating with identical diagnostic concepts may disagree about the application of these concepts in a particular case, but rarely disagree on their verbal definitions of the concepts themselves (1961: 125).

Prototype theorists such as Rosch and Mervis (1975) have presented data which suggests that percepts belong to a category to the extent that they share attributes with a best example prototype, not each other. Classification occurs through a process of 'family resemblance' centered around prototypes. While the Subanese may share prototypical knowledge of the best example of a named illness category, their criteria for categorization may not be as straightforward as Frake suggests. Categorization entails more than inclusion/exclusion by concrete properties (overt symptoms). Prototypes often reflect clusters of interactional properties and metaphors (Kövecses 1986), not unitary immutable images. As Lakoff (1987) has argued, conceptual systems are not disembodied abstractions, but exist by virtue of being embodied by people who use them in thinking and doing. Classification is a process responsive to human experience, imagination, deep-seated and changing perceptions of the body, and social relations.[2]

Frake's approach to studying the language of illness through the construction of an illness taxonomy is a valuable first step for anthropologists studying the language of illness. It is much like a mapping exercise where major reference points are located and common patterns of movement are charted. However, the map is not the territory, all people do not know the territory in the same way, and general patterns of movement (classification, standard reference) tell as little about individual behavior, the forging of new paths, the taking of shortcuts, and the movement from one path to another. As Malinowski warned some time ago, ethnographers need beware of over systematizing conceptual organization for "this represents neither the natives mind nor any other form of reality" (1961: 229).

Semantic Illness Networks and Cognitive Models

The cognitive unity which Frake proposed in the 1960's has been superseded by more elaborate cognitive models. These cognitive models recognize a plurality of forms of knowledge and means of knowing (Holland and Quinn 1987) as well as the human capacity to maintain multiple perspectives about the same concept (MacLaury 1987).

It is one thing to say that villagers think within an indigenous health culture which encompasses locally known health phenomena, that the illnesses they experience fall within their system of classification or possible classification. It is quite another thing to say that the categories of illness within this culture are unambiguous and constitute an identical cognitive code shared by all members of a society. This places too much emphasis on the denotative features of illness and discounts the importance of evocative connotative meanings.[3] As Good (1977: 26) has noted, failure to take stock of the connotative dimensions of illness discourse is to "reify the conception of disease and reduce medical semantics to the ostensive or naming function of language."

Good (1977) argues that Frake has too closely modeled his approach to the language of illness on diagnosis as a medical activity. Moreover, his perception of diagnosis is ethnocentric. Too much attention is paid to symptomatology and etiology of illness to the exclusion of coexisting concerns and meanings contextually associated with illness and embedded in culture. Bibeau (1981) criticizes the ethnoscience approach as being too "grid oriented". He suggests that illness semantics may better be conceptualized "in the round" with each illness constituting a roundabout from which several points of arrival and departure exist as avenues of thought and feeling. Bibeau's depiction of illness semantics accords with MacLaury's (1987) formulation of 'vantage theory' which includes a notion of cognitive "coextensivity". This theory accounts for the indexicality of classification choice in context. A person does not merely name what he sees, but indexes his point of view. He mentally positions himself in relation to a choice of attending to either a construct's similarity with other constructs or its distinctiveness from them. Category (e.g. illness) and observer are inseperable.

The limitations of a strictly denotative referential approach to illness semantics and discourse were first discussed by D'Andrade (1972; 1976) following an exhaustive study of the denotative features of illness in the U.S. He found that illness is often conceived of in terms of its connotative features — its consequences and preconditions, relative seriousness, painfulness or curability — and less in terms of its distinctive features of category inclusion. It was Good's analysis of "semantic illness networks" in Iran, however, that provided an exemplar for a "connotative approach" to the study of illness conceptualization and discourse.

This second approach to comprehending illness categories posits them as sets (clusters, congeries) of words, metaphors, images, features, experiences, scenarios, and feelings (etc.) which come together in context. Illnesses are known vis à vis multiple forms of knowledge ranging from physiological symptoms (as they are culturally interpreted and individually experienced) and notions of causality to social interactions set into motion by assuming particular sickness labels (e.g. sick role, social stigma) and explanatory models fashioned out of previous illness experiences. This knowledge flows from semantic networks, pools of associations embedded in culture and enriched through personal experience. It is drawn upon episodically to produce fields of knowledge condensed around core cultural symbols/ metaphors which are polysemous (broadly connotative, widely symbolic, multivocal). Those employing the semantic illness approach, study the meaning of illness contextually in relation to emergent core symbols, health concerns and tacit knowledge emphasizing the fluidity as opposed to the rigidity of illness categories.

This second largely "connotative" approach to the study of illness is more sensitive than the first largely "denotative" approach in recognizing the negotiation of illness identities, a process which entails relations of power and status. Noted, but litte developed by either approach is a recognition that conceptual organization and the process of negotiating an illness identity are task responsive. Elaborating on the importance of tasks to conceptual thinking, Dougherty and Keller (1982: 769) have noted:

Named classes are inadequate as the sole guide to the conceptual units relevant to everyday behavior. The members of named classes can be described by numerous features relatively few of which are crucial to class distinctions. In the course of performance, attention will be focused differentially on specific features appropriate to the strategies for action, regardless of the importance of these features for category definition. The nature of the task then determines the nature of relevant features.

These researchers contrast a "taskonomy" with a taxonomy approach to the study of conceptual organization (they do not explicitly concern themselves with illness). Key to this approach is a recognition that knowledge production is episodic and often ephemeral. Constellations of information arise in context. Dougherty and Keller go on to suggest that:

Named distinctions reflect classes of broad contextual relevance. As such they must be sidestepped or further specified . . . for the task oriented project at hand. What leads to highly effective means of any (cultural activity) is flexibility in classification.

Flexibility is built into classificatory systems through ambiguity. As noted by Dougherty and Fernandez (1982: 827):

A social science anchored in the natural sciences, where the task is to untangle puzzles and defeat ambiguities, is likely to be neglectful of the centrality of ambiguity in the human experience . . . Ambiguity is not simply something to be denied or explained away; it is not simply an error in method.

Ambiguity and Specificity

Little recognized in the language of illness literature is the role of ambiguity in rendering flexibility.[4] Not only may illness categories be far less precise than Frake suggested, but specific ambiguity may be an important feature of illness classification and health care systems. For example, in our own culture "stress" exists as a catch-all for any number of symptoms and feelings.[5] It is a term which is denotatively problematic but connotatively rich.[6] "Stress", technically a response, has been objectified, conventionalized, and medicalized. It is given credibility by products advertised to reduce "it" and we treat "it" with cure as well as care. In everyday discourse we refer to stress knowingly and the legitimacy of this newly emergent illness category is measured by the fact that we may engage the sick role when having "it". What ever "it" is, we have a sense of knowing what another is talking about when they say they are experiencing stress. Stress is a culturally constituted final common pathway

(Carr 1978) for a whole range of feelings.[5] At other times, reference to stress or "just stress" constitutes a generalized end point in discourse beyond which personal information is not offered or requested. On this point, Last (1981) has noted that among the Hausa, certain stereotyped illnesses tend to be used not so much to describe a complaint as to pre-empt further discussion or diagnosis.

Ambiguity, like silence is multivocal in the sense of metacommunication. Reference to an ambiguious state may be used indexically to increase or decrease social distance. Named (specified) ambiguity also serves to reduce anxiety through a process of naming a state one has little control over as a means of gaining control over the unknown, what Fuller Torry (1973) has aptly termed "the principle of rumpleskilskin". Naming as mystification and a means of gaining control over a phenomenon is well recognized in the anthropological literature. Of particular public health importance, once an ambiguous state has been named, medicines are often marketed to cloak it, if not transform it. Behold the emperor's new clothes. These specifically ambiguous categories are a window of opportunity for a proliferation of "health" products which create or stretch the meaning of an illness category beyond the pale of previous imagination. Textually transmitted diseases are spread through the media and advertising.[6] A reservoir of consumers harbor the 'disease', having become infected by the product which bears its name.

Lack of precision in illness categorization has "coping value" in that it complements secondary elaboration when a treatment fails to prove effacious (in curing or healing). When a medicine slated to cure X does not prove effective then one of five possibilities exist: 1) it was the wrong medicine 2) the medicine was not suitable for the patient, 3) the illness is being compounded by some unknown factors preventing cure 4) the illness was improperly identified and treated — it is an illness of a different type, or 5) the illness has transformed to another illness requiring different treatment. Given these five possibilities there are numerous options for treatment, rendering hope and explaining failure. Ambiguity plays a major role in the latter two interpretive modes.

Social Labeling

A third approach to the study of illness conceptualization may briefly be noted as it will figure in the presentation of data on the language of illness in South India. This approach complements critical studies of medical systems and the social and historical contexts underlying the construction and distribution of illness categories (e.g. Foucault 1970, 1973). The social labeling approach to illness categorization focuses attention on the social construction and internalization of illness identities. The process of taking on an illness identity is "self constituting" in the same sense that engaging in familiar patterns of social relations entails the embodiment of tacit ideology (Bourdieu 1978). Social labeling theorists such as Waxler (1977, 1981) have pointed out that illness labels are internalized along with complexes of connotative meaning. One takes on an illness label and conforms to cultural expectations of what it is to be the bearer of the label. Person, illness identity, and performance merge in a social interactional field.[7] This approach reminds us that illness labels are not neutral, they impact and constitute social relations.

SECTION TWO

Illness Nomenclature in South Kanara

We may begin our examination of the language of illness in South Kanara by a consideration of illness names. This brief presentation will make it clear that a broad range of features of sickness underlay illness classification. These same features are taken into account when classifying individual illness episodes.

Illnesses are named in a variety of different ways. Bibeau (1981) has identified six modes of naming illnesses in Africa which have general relevance in South Kanara. These patterns are listed below followed by examples in Kannaḍa language as spoken in South Kanara:

1. Localization: Referring to the part of the body. In South Kanara, examples of this category abound:
   kivi soruvudu: ear dripping, discharge

   sandhu novu: joint pain

   karalu bene: intestinal pain

2. Resemblance: Referring to likeness of symptom, organic spatialization, resemblance as iconicity.
   gaja karna: literally elephant skin. Skin becoming tough hard like that of an elephant, excema.

   anekalu: literally elephant's leg, filariasis.

3. Representation: Similarity is posited by abstraction.
   Muttu: literally, touched. A term used by Brahmans to describe a menstruating woman. It signals the need for social distance.

   Sarpa suttu: literally, snake circling. This term is used to describe the progression of herpes, which follows a circular snake-like pattern.

   Faringi roga: foreigner's illness. This reference to venereal disease indexes a belief that it was brought to India by foreigners. Evoked is a set of connotations about the habits and behaviors of outsiders.

4. Etiological reference: Reference to causal agent or factor.
    Kallothu: stone step. This refers to stepping on a stone where a serpent has spit. This causes an abscess on the bottom of the foot. Much like *meenu kannu* described earlier.

    Ushna horakadde: literally heat coming out. Refers to bloody diarrhea caused by overheat in the body.

    pakki kadapu: literally, bird crossing. Refers to children's fits caused by a bird crossing over a sleeping child.

    bala graha: literally, child's planets. Fits caused by the influence of stars and planets.

5. Therapeutic reference: Cure is indexed by name.
    Kappe roga: literally, frog illness. This illness encompasses the disease whooping cough which is also called *nayi kemmu*, dog cough. Whereas the term dog cough is descriptive of the sound of the cough itself, frog illness is associated with both the rhythm of the cough and the use of frog meat as a folk cure. This cure is inspired by doctrine of signature type reasoning.

    Chinne dosha: literally in Tuḷu, sign illness. This is another name for *bala graha* which is associated with the effect of spirits or the stars. Some Kannaḍa speakers interpret *chinne*, sign, as *cinna*, which in their language means gold. This association may be fostered by the fact that ayurvedic medicine containing a small amount of gold ash is a popular cure for the illness.

6. Sociocultural imperative: A cultural value is indexed by an illness name.
    Mailige roga: literally impurity disease. Reference to impurity as cultural value indexes social distance during pox diseases. The house of the afflicted is marked by neem leaves and is socially isolated.

    Naga dosha: Trouble of cobra. Reference to a curse of cobra causing infertility. Indexed are imperatives about taboos to sacred animals of deities.

Most illness names in South Kanara refer to an outstanding feature of an illness (such as a predominant symptom) compare a symptom to a correlate in nature, or suggest an ascribed cause. The following examples illustrate the range of names which coexist:

A. States of illness named with reference to bodily experience:

    1) *chali jwara*   cold fever. This term is used to describe a state

	of sickness where the body experiences fever and chills.
2) *apasmara*	*apa*: no, *smara*: memory, i.e. a loss of memory, falling unconsciousness. This may refer to epilepsy as well as sudden fits not associated with spirit possession.
3) *kai-kalu naduka*	hand-foot shaking. This condition refers to general body weakness and/or nervousness.
4) *mai-kai novu*	body hand pain. This refers to general malaise as well as pain. Kannaḍa uses rhyme as a common feature when describing body feelings. For examle, *gudu-gudu* refers to the sound of the stomach grumbling.
5) *sihi muthra;* *sakre roga*	sweet urine or sugar illness. Ayurvedic *vaidya* further classify this illness into several stages of sweetness. "Honey sweetness", *janu muthra*, denotes the most serious stage.
6) *iruve hariyuvudu*	ants grazing or crawling. The sensation of dumbness, of pins and needles.

B. Illnesses named by external appearance

Shape and Size

1) *keppataraya*	king of chins. Mumps.
2) *gadde jwara*	tuber fever. A reference to malaria where there is a protrusion in the stomach region resembling a tuberous plant growth.
3) *raja kuru*	kingly abscess. A large abscess which appears on the spinal column having three heads. People say that each head of the boil is an eye of Shiva, to whom the ailment is attributed.
4) *rupayi hunnu*	*rupayi* boil. A boil as large and round in size as a coin.

Color

| 1) *kempu* | redness. This refers to cellulitis and a wide range of skin conditions accompanied by visible red rashes. |
| 2) *kempu kannu* | red eye. Another term for conjunctivitis. |

3) *arasina mundige*   turmeric sickness. A reference to jaundice.

4) *glani*   faded, that which has been discolored. This refers to the emotional state of depression.

C. States of illness/distress which suggest internal disorders with reference to hot/cold; notions of ethnophysiology; body humors.

1) *tale bisi*   hot head. A term used to describe anxiety as a state of uncontrolled heat rising to the head.

2) *nare nitrana*   nerve weakness. The term *nare* refers to channels in the body inclusive of nerves, veins, and arteries. People often use this term to refer to general feelings of instability, lack of well being, and lassitude. Physical weakness is often used as an expression of mental weakness.

3) *pitta*   reference to the humor *pitta*. Symptoms associated with the derangement of this humor include yellow excretions, bitterness in the mouth and dizziness as well as sudden rage. The name of the humor has become synonymous with an illness state.

D. Illness names which reflect a similarity between the illness and the appearance or behavior of an animal.

1) *dengi bapu*   crab swelling. This refers to an infection of the hand in which the fingers become bent, crusty and swollen taking on the appearance of crab's legs.

2) *nayi kemmu*   dog's cough. Whooping cough, because of the similarity in sound.

3) *koli kannu*   chicken's eye. Conjunctivits.

4) *hula tinnuvudu*   worms eating. Athlete's foot, caused by "worms chewing at one's feet".

E. Illnesses which have the names of goods and index divine intervention in etiology

1) *Devi*   The goddess *Devi* is believed to be the cause of smallpox and by extension the disease has taken on her name. As I will note shortly, the name is not used during an epidemic.

2) *sarpa sutu*	literally, cobra circling. Herpes which follows a circular pattern around the body. Because of its resemblance to a snake, villagers say that this disease is a curse of the serpent god, *Naga*.
3) *naga dosha*	literally, trouble of cobra. The common usage of this term is to denote childlessness. The cobra deity is associated with fertility. The curse of this deity is linked to a range of illnesses from skin rashes and leprosy to childlessness. Although other illnesses are believed to be caused by *naga*, they are not generally given this term.
4) *sanni patha*	High fevers of long duration such as typhoid are believed to be caused by the wrath of Sanni, a variety of malevolent spirit.

Talking about Illness

Speaking about illness is not a neutral event, nor is it merely referential. It is indexical of sociomoral relations and a means of establishing metonymic associations through the magical power of words (Tambiah 1968). Examination of a few features of illness discourse will highlight the importance of the connotative dimension of illness naming in context.

Several terms exist for the general category sickness. *Kayile* is used in cases of serious non-contagious illnesses such as asthma which linger, seem to get better, but recur. By contrast, *roga* is used to designate serious illnesses such as TB or leprosy, etc. which may or may not be contagious and/or curable. Sicknesses which are "*roga*" carry some measure of social stigma and fear. For this reason, the term *roga* is never used in the first person. Rather, the term *kayile* is employed. For example, if I was to inquire of a villager how his treatment for leprosy or herpes zoster was progressing, I would say *nimma kayile heg untu* and not *nimma roga heg untu*. Both literally mean "how is your illness?". The *roga* reference would only be used in discussing the sickness with someone other than the afflicted. *Sicku*, a neutral term adapted from the English word sick, has been adopted as a general all-purpose term for illness used in public discourse.

Conventions govern discourse about illness in the presence of the afflicted and in the company of others. For example the names of illnesses associated with divine punishment are not spoken of in the first person or in the presence of the afflicted because of connotations of responsibility or sin (*pappa*). To state directly that someone has leprosy would be to publicly imply that they, or some member of their lineage segment, has violated a serious taboo, such as killing a cobra. The same is true of conditions such as infertility or insanity which are associated with divine punishments.

Other illnesses are viewed as shameful and this in turn influences their description. Men are generally more straightforward about discussing their bodies and bodily sensations than women, especially higher caste or younger women. Women are described as *nachike*, a term indicating both shyness and shame. A woman's shyness becomes particularly evident during illness and pregnancy. When a woman experiences unusual bodily sensations she may speak of these symptoms to others, even health care providers, vaguely. In some cases she will refer to parts of her anatomy which are more general and less private than that actually affected, particularly if these parts call attention to her femaleness. For example, it was observed that women consulting an ayurvedic *vaidya* or doctor about a menstrual complaint often referred to this complaint indirectly. A patient often said *mai inda hogutade* "it goes from my body" rather than explicate the problem further. Menstruation is indirectly referred to in everyday speech as *muttu*, touched, or among Brahmans, *madi*, pure. These terms index social distance and convey to others indirectly that a woman should not be touched in her impure state.

Likewise, a woman who is pregnant for the first time may not mention this fact to other family members or outsiders, until they notice visible signs and confront her with their observation. On several occasions, Lady Medical Officers working in village Primary Health Centers mentioned to me that women consulted them about general weakness, when in fact they were pregnant. It was left to the doctor to observe their condition during the course of an examination.[8]

Spirit linked diseases are not referred to directly for reasons beyond etiquette. The names of serious, spirit-linked illnesses are considered powerful in themselves. Saying the name of a disease such as leprosy is thought to invite the illness to come into one's body.[9] The significance of this belief is that villagers will not mention without qualification the spirit linked names of serious illnesses. Some villagers will refer to a disease such as leprosy, *kushta*, by using a different name entirely. Brahmans, for example, call leprosy "elder pain", *hire bene*, as the disease is considered the most serious and thus, by analogy, the eldest of diseases. Likewise, many villagers were reluctant to refer to pox illnesses (encompassing chickenpox) as *devi* or *amma*, two names of the mother goddess commonly associated with these diseases. They preferred to speak of the diseases as *mailige roge*, illnesses of pollution or filth. This reference indexed the perception that heat and impurity leave the body when pustulates open, a reason medicine is not taken during these illnesses to retard what amounts to a natural purification process. There is little doubt that villagers associate pox illnesses, measles and rubella with spirit contact. However, when I surveyed 80 households about what they thought caused these illnesses, few would mention *devi* or *bhuta* spirits or allude to the wind, *sonku*, of *bhuta*. A response of "don't know" or a naturalistic "efficient cause" (Glick 1967) like heat would be cited.

Villagers will not openly say they are suffering from any "big" illness, *dodda roga* or *maha roga*. They describe these illnesses indirectly often referring to how the illness, or its symptoms "have happened." For example, a villager with measles or chickenpox might simply say, *mai alli bittide* "it fell on my body" when asked which illness they were recuperating from. As a general rule, if an illness is of a serious nature, villagers will not speak of it when the sick person is within their proximity. When the sick person leaves the area, however, the illness may be referred to with qualification. A speaker may say *avarige kushta agide* "to him leprosy has happened", but the speaker will quickly emphasize his or her distance from the disease by adding *nanage illa avarige untu* "to me it isn't, for him it is."

Although not as explicit as reported by Kay (1979) for Mexican American bilinguals, code switching between English and native terms for illness states was observed to take place among the educated in South Kanara. Kay found that English or Spanish scientific terms would be used for grave diseases while local Spanish terms would be used for mild ailments and "cultural diseases" for which there was no conceptual translation. Observed in South Kanara was strategic code switching in both directions. For example, T.B. was at times preferred to the local term *kashaya roga* as the latter term indexed notions of excess (eg. sex, tea, tobacco, liquor) while the former was associated with a public health problem and public health activities. On the other hand, mental illness diagnosed by clinicians (eg. schizophrenia) was often described in local more ambiguous terms such as nerve weakness (*nara dosha*).[10] Choice of terms was influenced by social relations and evaluation of a term's connotations for those addressed. I noted occasions where a scientific term for mental illness was employed in discourse which linked the illness to a cause unrelated to the family. In other instances an ayurvedic or astrological term would be used which drew attention to the humors or the stars. In each case, the indexical, more than the referential, guided discourse while non-verbal communication played a prominent role in how far conversations would proceed.

Illness Identities: Consensus and Variability

To what extent do community members share common or fixed ideas and images of attributes which constitute illness categories? For familiar illnesses with prominent symptoms, a fair degree of consensus was found to exist with respect to prototypical symptoms. The characteristics of native illness categories which correspond to filiarisis, jaundice, mumps and whooping cough, were known and agreed upon by most people I interviewed in South Kanara. In the case of many other illness categories, however, consensus as to what constituted the criteria for class membership was poor. Informants often knew only one prototypical characteristic of an illness category and were unclear as to what characteristics distinguished different types of illness sharing this feature. Concordant with semantic illness network theory, discussions about an illness identity often entailed a wide range of factors-a person's past illness history, their age, the season, possible causes, individual body constitution, food etc. An idea was expressed by some informants that one type of illness might take on different characteristics depending on the age, constitution, or gender of the person.

The ambiguity of some diagnostic categories may be illustrated. Both the terms *sanni patha* and *vayide jwara* are used to describe the protypical symptom of high fever of long duration. When I asked 20 informants living within 8 miles of each other to cite other characteristics of these illnesses, 40% of the informants stated that the two illnesses were synonymous whereas 60% distinguished them as different types of illness, not simply illnesses at different levels of contrast. In depth interviews were held with members of two households who stated they had experienced one of the two illnesses within the last year. The members of the first household claimed that *vayide jwara* designated fevers which became higher at night and were accompanied by fits, excessive thirst, red eyes, body pains, head pains, and reddish yellow urine. They described cases of illness called "typhoid" by doctors as *sanni*. According to these informants, *sanni patha* was a term used for body pain and fever which would rise and fall on alternating days, but which did not specifically increase at night.

This distinction was not accepted by the second household-members of the same village, caste group, and economic class having a similar educational status. They described the symptoms of "gastroenteritis" (fever, nausea, painful muscle cramps, diarrhoea) as *vayide jwara*.[11] They did not propose nor recognize a rising night fever criteria of inclusion for this illness. *Sanni patha* they stated, was an illness much like "typhoid" or "pneumonia", but which doctors could not cure with injections. "Pneumonia" was demarcated by high fever with a mucus laden cough and "typhoid" as a high fever with fits. They stated that when vomiting occurred, *vayide jwara* transformed into *vanti bhedi*, a term associated with "cholera". The informant's use of the terms "cholera" and "gastroenteritis" was influenced by the media. It ambiguously designated acute, watery and bloody diarrhea.

Considerable ambiguity was also discovered with respect to the labeling of respiratory illnesses. Informants often communicated to each other about the characteristics of a respiratory illness by mimicking breathing sounds not specifying names per se. Observations at three clinics in the same town revealed that various informants utilized the term "chali jvara", cold fever, to describe the symptoms of malaria, acute bronchitis and pneumonia. When asked to compare and contrast the symptoms of this and other local terms for respiratory illnesses such as "shita jwara" and "pneumonia', widespread ambiguity was revealed.

Ambiguity and variance in the use of local illness terms can have serious public health repercussions. Members of households who would directly request medicines from chemists for a proxy patient often received medicine for the name of the illness they specified based on a chemist's translation of the term into English.[12] For example, in one instance I found that anti-malaria tablets were distributed to a person suffering from pneumonia because the complaint cited, *chali jwara*, was translated into English as malaria. The family member visiting the chemist shop used the term to refer to 'fever with chills' and was asked no further questions.

Moving from a single patient to an entire community, I was informed by a primary health center doctor in 1975 that in his service area Chloromycin was no longer responding to cases of typhoid. Upon investigation I found that Chloromycin marketed under the brand name Reclor was commonly being used in non-typhoid cases. Research found that 1) several local practitioners flippantly used the term typhoid for all high fevers, 2) chloromycin was liberally prescribed for high fevers, and 3) a chemist shop was selling this drug over-the-counter to all clients citing *sanni patha* or *vayide jwara* as their ailment. These terms were considered by the shopkeeper to be synonymous with typhoid. Carl Taylor (1976) has noted the occurrence of a related phenomena in the Punjab. He found that indigenous practitioners who could not read the English label on allopathic medicine they purchased, requested pharmacists who supplied them with drugs to label the bottles with Punjabi illness terminology in local script.

Sutaka vayu may be cited as an example of a specific ambiguous diagnostic category used to describe a wide variety of conditions rarely specified in discourse. *Sutaka vayu* is generally recognized as an ailment which follows delivery. It was characterized by various informants as caused by 1) the retention of impure menstrual blood, 2) gases which should be expelled from the body during delivery but which are retained and go to the head, 3) the eating of toxic (*nanju*) food prior to delivery or during confine-ment causing impure blood and bad gases. The most common symptom associated with *sutaka vayu* is fits following delivery. The meaning of "fits" is very broad and the term is used very loosely.

Observations of instances when the term, *sutaka vayu*, was applied revealed that it could be used to refer to a wide range of deviant behaviors or unusual physical symptoms emergent during confinement. In one case, a married woman began scolding her husband, laughing loudly and being argumentative six weeks after the delivery of her fifth child. Her husband explained her actions to me by saying that she was suffering from *sutaka vayu*, a humoral imbalance requiring purification medicine. A friend confided that she was *tali bisi*, anxious, about her state of poverty, that she did not want any more children, was being pressured by the government midwife to get sterilized, and was afraid. Neither this woman nor two female neighbors used the term *sutaka vayu* to describe the woman's condition.[13] It occurred to me that use of the term *sutaka vayu* by the husband might have less to do with diagnosis of his wife's condition than constitute a means of coping with her expression of distress. Reference to a specifically ambiguous illness label like *sutaka vayu* served to structure an uncontrolled emotional display in humoral terms amenable to somatic treatment. The husband's use of the term when speaking to me also served an indexical function well recognized by my research assistant. In an interview with the husband, the term was clearly used as an end point of our conversation. My attempts to probe for specificity were met with silence and I was told by my research assistant that this was not a subject (category) that I should pursue. One could openly speak of *sutaka vayu*, but not of a woman's sadness or anger after delivery.

Diagnostic categories are not static. They are dynamic with a fair amount of latitude for elaboration, invention and reinterpretation. This may be illustrated by the illness category *kempu*. All informants whom I interviewed described *kempu* as red rashes accompanied by burning, swollenness, and sometimes fever. Cases of herpes zoster were identified as a variety of *kempu* as were cases of reddish cellulitis, advanced oedema, staphylococcus infections and articaria. Some informants, however, were far more liberal in their identification of *kempu* than others when allopathic treatment did not appear to be effective. In some cases, their use of the term designated that only a specialist *kempu vaidya* was able to cure their particular skin problem. For example, the term *kajji* is widely used to describe scabies and a variety of itchy, burning skin diseases. In one instance, when a skin ailment originally diagnosed as *kajji* became seriously inflamed and resisted an antibiotic cure, members of my neighbor's household spoke of the condition as *kempu*. My research assistant assured me that the condition was not *kempu* because *kempu* did not produce weeping sores. Reviewing my notes of this household's prototypical description of *kempu* and *kajji* the year before on an illness taxonomy survey, I found that their elicited characterization matched that of my research assistant. Their present use of the term *kempu* indexed the type of practitioner being seen.

I consulted several *kempu* specialists who practice in southern South Kanara to collect taxonomic data on *kempu*. I found both convention and invention in their categorization. All *vaidya* consulted, listed several sub-classes of *kempu* which subsumed almost any type of inflamed swelling (red or otherwise) I had observed or could describe. Categories which they mutually agreed upon were identified by descriptive names such as:

shita kempu (cold redness) red swelling, cold to the touch
sarpa sutu (snake circling) herpes zoster
kalu kempu (foot redness) red swelling of the foot.

Many other classes of *kempu* were individually named and invented by *vaidya*. The invention of illness categories was strategically important for when one *kempu vaidya* could not cure a case, he referred it to another *kempu vaidya* as a type of *kempu* which he could not cure. The same pattern was noted among *sanni vaidya*; *vaidya* who treated high fevers. It was found that in villages where a specialist *kempu vaidya* resided, the range of types of *kempu* known to villagers was more elaborate than in other villages.

Negotiation of an Illness Identity

A taskonomy approach to the study of illness classification, in contrast to a strict taxonomy approach, requires that emergent cognitive models be studied in the context of social interaction and performance. Needed is an approach which accounts for embodied knowledge as well as the production of knowledge and the negotiation of illness identities within action sets.[14]

The identity of an illness becomes important in a context where treatment decisions need to be made, often after sympomatic treatment has failed. An illness identity may be negotiated among significant others and the afflicted or between a practitioner and the afflicted or their representatives. In South Kanara, some practitioners strictly adhere to professional language (Cicourel 1982, 1985) as a means of establishing legitimacy. Others have gained popularity by conceptual translation in response to popular health culture. For example, some ayurvedic *vaidya* whom I observed operated within and across multiple illness traditions. They negotiated illness identities while switching codes between an ayurvedic disease taxonomy, folk illness categories and popular use of biomedical categories. I may provide a case in point.

One ayurvedic *vaidya* whom I observed for several months had undergone a short apprenticeship with a relative trained in ayurveda, but in actuality was self taught. He regularly referred to ayurvedic medical texts written in Sanskrit as well as Kannaḍa, and Malayalam. In order to treat a patient with an appropriate medicine discussed in his ayurvedic texts, the *vaidya* first had to ascertain the name of the patient's illness within the ayurvedic taxonomic system concordant with humoral imbalance. While his choice of medicine was determined by the ayurvedic taxonomic system, he communicated to many of his patients within their folk illness classification system. The practitioner was idiosyncratic and flexible in his use of illness terms. In some cases, he correlated folk and ayurvedic terms, while in other cases, he subsumed a local term as a class or a prodromal stage of an illness named within the ayurvedic system. When confronted, as he often was, by a patient already diagnosed by an allopathic doctor, he would translate a biomedical diagnostic category into an ayurvedic one. The point of such translation was not to come up with an exact correlation, which he denied could be done, but to identify humoral imbalance which underlay biomedically named problems. The practitioner's illness classification system was treatment task responsive.

An issue which may briefly be considered is the extent to which contact with this *vaidya* effected the identification of illness among his clients. We may consider a case example. The *vaidya* used the localized Sanskrit term *cavi* when speaking to patients to designate illnesses caused by poor digestion. His own interpretation of *cavi* etiology was much more complex. Blood became impure due to improper digestion resulting from 1) undereating, 2) eating incompatible foods, 3) overeating or 4) eating in inappropriate places or at inauspicious times. According to ayurveda, reported the vaidya, *cavi* was caused by undigested fats and vitiated *pitta dosha*; *pitta* being the body humor "responsible for fat catabolism." The *vaidya* labeled cases of protein-calorie malnutrition, various menstrual and lactational disorders, infertility, and debility with nausea as *cavi* diseases associated with *ama*, undigested food substances in the blood.

Three points may be noted. First, despite a shared disease taxonomy with other ayurvedic vaidya, this practitioner maintained idiosyncratic ideas about this and other diagnostic categories. Ayurvedic practitioners interviewed in South Kanara used the term *cavi* to indicate distinct sets of symptoms despite the fact that all linked these symptom sets to indigestion and humoral imbalance. The above practitioner's use of *cavi* in cases of infertility was unique among the practitioners I interviewed. It was derived from his reading of a biomedical text which spoke of hormonal deficiencies. He perceived a complementarity between deficient humors and hormones, both resulting in a blockage of flow within the body.

A second point is that when patients consult a *vaidya* with an illness and it is named *cavi*, they often take this to mean that their specific symptoms are *cavi* and not that *cavi* refers to an underlying condition related to improper digestion. Many have no idea that the term *cavi* may be used to indicate other syndromes. Others, however, come to perceive *cavi* as a type of blood disorder from interactions with the *vaidya* which involve courses of blood purification medication.

To document this I kept an inventory of descriptions of *cavi* gathered from informants who had been diagnosed as having *cavi* by *vaidya* from six different locales.]Descriptions of *Cavi* Cited by Different Informants[:

a) Blackish spots on the behind;
b) "children's sprue" characterized by weight loss, steattorhea, foul smelling diarrhoes was undigested fats;
c) laziness in children accompanied by oversalivation, weakness in hands and legs, loss of appetite;
d) spots which appear on the skin at the time of delivery;
e) menstrual pain;
f) decrease in breast milk.

Presented with this inventory of ailments, informants were asked which were *cavi*. Few informants claiming experience with *cavi* recognized more than two of the other conditions listed as *cavi*. The point is that knowledge of an illness category is often personalized. A practitioner's diagnosis comes to fit one's individual experience which becomes prototypical for concerned others.

The *cavi* case illustrates a third point. The nature of an illness is often known in relation to the medicine one receives for it. One embodies meaning with medication. Those informants who broadly linked *cavi* to indigestion or blood impurity did so with reference to their medication. Because their medicine was known for or labeled as a cure for impure blood, *cavi* took on this meaning. Another example may be presented which extends this point and illustrates the notion of a textually transmitted disease. "Liver" has emerged as a popular illness category in South India. It is a condition associated with the humor *pitta* given modern form by cosmopolitan practitioners and a proliferation of medications. These products link "liver" to indigestion, weakness, poor sleep and a range of symptoms even the French would be hard pressed to associate with this favorite bodily complaint. Tonics marketed as good for liver are routinely prescribed by doctors for convalescence.[15] Some patients prescribed these medicines interpreted them as specific to their complaints which they referred to as "liver". Others associated "liver" with indigestion in a specifically ambiguous manner. In both cases, household members come to know when someone suffers "liver" when the medicine for "its" treatment needs to be procured. A form of diagnosis by treatment is in play.

Patients interpret what a practitioner tells them verbally and through treatment modalities in terms of their preexisting ideas about illness categories. In cases of illness where treatment is not deemed effective or complete, an illness identity may be questioned or reinterpreted. Shifts in thinking about illness catgories occur and new categories of illness are introduced during interactions with practitioners.

A case study may be presented illustrating the negotiation of an illness identity among family members and neighbors which comprise a therapy management group (Jantzen 1978). The case may be outlined in six stages:

1. A Shudra child aged two, suffering from malnutrition and symptoms labeled by a Primary Health Center doctor as "tropical sprue," experienced fits on the day of a new moon. The father considered this to be indicative of the illness *bala graha*, caused by a *bala pide* spirit. After taking the child to the health center, the father took him to an exorcist and received treatment by chant, *mantra*, and ash, *busma*. He also purchased locally prepared tablets known as *bala graha matre* from a local provision shop. These tablets are taken as both a preventative as well as curative medicine for *bala graha*.

2. Three days later, the child was visibly weaker, developed foul mucus laden stools and exhibited difficulty in moving his limbs. The father returned to the exorcist, received a *yantra*, a protective device, and was told that the spirit causing the illness was now powerless to attack the child. The exorcist suggested that the child be taken to a *vaidya*.

3 The child's condition did not improve. Fits reoccurred and during these fits, the family noted that the child expelled phlegm from his mouth. A visiting relative diagnosed the condition as *krani* and prepared folk medicine which she administered to the child for one week with little effect. Her diagnosis was questioned by a neighbor who said that the condition was not

krani because in *krani* the skin became thorn like and the eyes developed a film over them. She called the disease *cinne dosha*.

4. The family consulted a *vaidya*. When the father described the child's symptoms, he did not intially mention fits. He rather stressed the expulsion of phlegm from the mouth, diarrhoea, and weakness. The *vaidya* specifically asked about fits and was told that the child had been taken to an exorcist and received a *yantra*. The *vaidya* gave the father medicine for eight days and told him to return with the child after the period had elapsed for additional medicine. The father asked the *vaidya* if the illness was *cinne dosha*. The *vaidya* said that the illness was *cavi*. This name was accepted by the father without comment and repeated to neighbors afterwards.

5. After the father and son left, I discussed with the *vaidya* the terms *bala graha, cinne dosha, krani,* and *cavi*. He described these terms as prodromal stages of a syndrome. *Cavi* was a first stage, characterized by malnutrition, the inability to digest fats, crying fits, and the dissolving of bones in the urine. *Krani* was a possible next stage of *cavi*, characterized by the former symptoms and in addition thorn like skin, a white casting over the eyes and muscular complaints. The next stage was *bala graha*. In this stage, fits would become frequent, be accompanied by vomiting, diarrhoea and temperature change in the body. The body would be cold from the navel downward and hot from the navel upward. *Cinni dosha*, he claimed, was a synonymous term for *bala graha* derived from the fact that ayurveda prescribed *cinne busma*, gold oxide, as a medicine for children's fits. He then stated that *bala graha* could lead to two other conditions, *pakki kadapu* (bird crossing over) or *apasmara*. *Pakki kadapu* is a condition in which a child's limbs are weak and tightly bent in towards the chest. A wheezing sound, like that made by a bird, is heard during breathing, and fits or a low fever may be present. *Apasmara* is an ayurvedic as well as a local term referring to intermittent fits and loss of consciousness among adults and adolescents. These illness categories are described in greater detail in Chapter 5 where I consider the folk classification of states of malnutrition.

6. I interviewed the family of the patient and neighbors two months later, after the child's health had improved. I found that a good deal of ambiguity existed as to the distinctive characteristics of *bala graha, krani,* and *cavi*. The family now thought that *cavi* indicated the symptoms remaining after a *bala graha* attack. I queried the idea that the other children's illnesses might be stages of one another as the *vaidya's* had noted. Family members responded that *bala graha* could lead to *apasmara* in later life, but the suggestion that *krani* could lead to *bala graha* or that *bala graha* could lead to *pakki kadapu* were met with ambivalence. The father noted that *krani* was caused by diet or the stars, *bala graha* by a spirit, and *pakki kadapu* by a bird.

Clearly illustrated in this case study is the ongoing process of negotiating an illness as it influences and is influenced by health care seeking. The identity of a set of illness episodes are reevaluated in relation to symptoms, signs (when fits occurred), treatment modalitites, and the prototype constructs of folk illnesses maintained by different members of the therapy management group. A point worth highlighting in this case is that the suspected etiology of the initial illness episode contributed significantly to its presentation for diagnosis. The father of the child was not sure of the defining characteristics of *krani*, *bala graha*, and *cinne dosha*, other than the fact that they all involved fits. However, when his child developed fits on a new moon, he suspected malevolent spirits and therefore presumed the case to be *bala graha*. His personal diagnosis was contextual and based on assumptions about etiology. Also noteworthy, household members continue to be unclear about the nature of the child's illness. They have altered some of their ideas about illness categories (e.g. *cavi*) but retain prototype ideas about other categories which are quite distinct from those maintained by the *vaidya*.

I have not intended to belittle the specificity of a number of folk illness terms by discussing ambiguity. My discussion of ambiguity serves two purposes. First, it highlights ambiguity as a feature of classification systems in general. Second, it enables me to point out that illness classification is dynamic. This has significance for international health. The existence of substantial ambiguity within folk illness taxonomies provides some latitude for negotiating health education messages. It enables the introduction of new information about illness through the elaboration of existing illness classes as well as the introduction of new classes of illness without confronting established "cultural illness" having metamedical associations (Obesekeyere 1976). This point is addressed again in chapters five and six.

Illness Labeling and Social Relations: The Context of Power

The negotiation of an illness identity within a therapy management group is not a neutral process. As Frake has observed the level of contrast (specificity) in illness discourse is based on life contingencies and as Good has emphasized, illness identities carry with them powerful cultural meanings. Two people having similar sets of symptoms, or manifesting similar forms of behavior may be labeled as having different illnesses or as being effected by different causal agents. As social labeling theorists such as Waxler have pointed out, the social position of the afflicted, relative to the person(s) defining a sickness or experiencing distress must always be considered.

An example may be provided to elaborate this point. It involves a contrast between *huchu*, madness, and uninvited spirit possession. *Huchu* may be a temporary state caused by sorcery or an extreme derangement of humors, or it may be hereditary. Having a family member who is *huchu* is not overtly shameful to a family, but it indexes possible irregular sociomoral relations or a history of madness. Translated into everyday life, this means that marriages are more difficult to arrange in families having a member known to be *huchu*. There are many forms of spirit possession. Spirit possession, of a patron deity or ancestor may occur for a wide range of reasons and involve anybody although it is believed that some people are more prone to spirit possession because of personal or social characteristics. Planned possession may confer status, depending on the status of the deity. Involuntary (unplanned) spirit possession is not shameful. Then again, it is not a feature of one's life that is directly mentioned during marriage negotiations. Any special relationship with a spirit comes with a set of responibilities and expenses related to ritual performance.

The overt characteristics of spirit possession and madness may resemble each other.[16] These characteristics range from silence and seclusion to wild displays of affect, visions and grandiosity. Differentiation between madness and spirit possession at a time when spirit possession is not invited or anticipated is made on the basis of performance. One is labeled possessed by an exorcist or spirit cult leader if they exhibit symbolic behavior responsive to a ritual structure associated with a particular spirit form. If one does not abide by the "performance requirements" of possession for a particular spirit (e.g. reciting the legend of the spirit or responding to ritual cues), than one of two possibilities exist. Either the person is possessed by a different kind of spirit or the person is deemed *huchu*, mad.

Providing legitimization for the afflicted person's behavior and structure for the interpretation of their behavior lies with the family. They may either expend resources in locating a traditional specialist able to negotiate an identity for/with the afflicted person or label the person mad and deal with them accordingly. Important determinants in this process are family pedigree, household composition and social relations between the afflicted and significant others. I investigated several cases where a person was clearly suffering from a psychological disorder.[17] In some cases, a family created a structure for "possession" around the person which family members maintained through rituals. In some of these cases, the structure invented was quite idiosyncratic with priests and exorcists paid a handsome fee for their supportive legitimating role.

In other cases, family members were all to eager to label a member *huchu* and socially distance them as a means of transforming relations of power. In one such instance, intergenerational conflicts between an elder woman and her grown children were involved. The *huchu* label was applied to the elder in an effort to take over the management of the household. The elder engaged the signs of possession (eyes turned upward, trembling) as a silent means of protest indexing the special relationship between the elder and the household patron deity. This was dealt with in a curt fashion by her children. To recognize her behavior as possession by the household patron deity would be to return power to the elder. The label of madness minimized her power.

My point in introducing the possession-madness example is to argue that illness labels index and disguise social relations. The study of the language of illness entails more than a description of conventional illness categories: it involves strategic, performative and constitutive dimensions of labeling and language use.

Contagion and Resistance

Of key importance to those engaged in international health in South Asia is infectious disease. The language of contagion may be considered in relation to local concepts of contagion and contiguity as well as infection and resistance. The importance of metaphor and metonymy in the construction of cognitive models of contagion and resistance will become apparent.

The notion of contagion is expressed both directly and indirectly in Kannada. All illnesses considered to be contagious are referred to as *antu-roga*, sticking illness. During an epidemic, contagion is often spoken of in relation to a bad wind. Villagers either refer to this wind as *sonku*, a term associated with the turbulent movement of spirits,[18] or use the general term for wind, *gali*. Some villagers describe *sonku* as sand thrown by a *bhuta* spirit at a person causing sickness.

Contagion is also expressed subtly by the use of the term *mailige*, a term which denotes various types of impurity. One who is *mailige* should not be touched since contact transfers pollution.[19] Menstruation is spoken of as *mailige* as is the touching of a defiling substance, animal, or person. A contagious pox disease may likewise be referred to as *mailige roga*. Both metaphor and metynomy underly an association between contagion and impurity.

Use of the term *mailige* to refer to contagious illness indexes a range of ideas about the processual nature of the illness and appropriate treatment. The term explicitly conveys the idea of pollution and implicitly connotes shared structural characteristics between the course of the illness and other *mailige* pollutions, such as menses. This may be demonstrated by looking at the treatment of pox disease and measles. These diseases are not treated by local medicine for several days after their onset. Villagers consider pox scabs to be the outcome of internal poisons and heat being pushed out of the body to the surface.[20] The course of a pox disease is analogous to the course of menses which is also a time of pollution and overheat, a time when impure blood is being expelled from the body.

Menses: Overheating: Internal poisons ejected via menses blood
Pox: Overheating: Internal poisons ejected via pustulates

The suppression of either the course of the pox disease or menses is regarded as dangerous[21]. Contagious illnesses are metaphorically like menstruation in several ways.

The pus or scab of a wound or pox disease is considered capable of spreading disease and to be a dangerous substance. This is not merely because it is defiling. Metynomy underlies notions of contagion more than a folk notion of germs (discussed below). One may be exposed to illness not only by touching, but crossing/stepping over (*kadapu*) such substances placing one in a contiguous relationship with the qualitative state of the afflicted. In this sense, ideas about contagion are similar to ideas about contagious magic underlying rituals used in witchcraft and exorcism.

Cultural notions of contagion effect illness behavior. Villagers with pox diseases or measles do not bathe for fear of suppressing the natural course of the body ridding itself of internal poisons. They also do not bathe because if pox scabs are washed off they can spread the disease. Likewise, if a person dies of a pox disease they will be buried and not burned to insure that the disease will not be spread by the wind via smoke and come in contact with others.

The terms *krimi*, miniscule worms, and *kita*, miniscule insects, are also used to communicate the idea of contagion as well as describe an infected wound, or comment on a variety of tickling or crawling sensations in one of the body orifices. Of late, an increasing number of ayurvedic *vaidya* have adapted these Sanskritic terms to subsume the allopatic terms germ and virus which are becoming more popular as a result of school and the media. What is understood by these terms and "germs" varies considerably. Important to consider are *krimi*/ germ differentiation in relation to specific etiology as well as notions of agency and volition.[22]

While some villagers were found to maintain an idea that many different kinds of germs or *krimi* exist, many others perceived "germs" as being capable of causing any number of illnesses much like spirits. With respect to agency, some villagers viewed germs as hungry directionless creatures attracted by impurity, undigested food, bad blood, bad smells and the opportunity availed by weakness and vulnerability. Others perceived germs/ *krimi* as agents of spirits. Exploring multilevel notions of causality (Glick 1968, Nichter 1987) in the context of illness episodes, I found that rural Kanarese folk often perceived spirits to be the efficient cause of a serious illness and germs the instrumental cause. In illness narratives entailing this idea, a form of sociomoral transgression or impure state was often identified as a predisposing cause.

The extent to which minute creatures are associated with various illnesses may be documented by data collected during two etiology surveys, one in 1974 and the other in 1979. In 1974, one hundred illiterate/semi literate villagers were interviewed about the two most common causes of a set of six infectious diseases as identified by local illness terms. The 1979 survey contrasted the ideas of 25 village and 27 town informants of similar educational status.

The survey reveals that less than one third of the samples surveyed at two

TABLE I. *Krimi* as the Cause of Six Contagious Diseases.

	Percentage of informants citing germs, *krimi* or *kita* as causative factors of an illness		
	1974 Village	1979 Village	1979 Town
Chickenpox	17%	16%	11%
Whooping Cough	11%	20%	24%
Measles	9%	4%	7%
Mumps	23%	16%	15%
Tuberculosis	28%	20%	24%
Sanni-high fever (typhoid, pneumonia, etc.)	14%	16%	15%

points during a five year period of time linked germs to the cause of six common infectious diseases. Also noteworthy, the opinions of village and townsfolk were quite similar.

It is important to point out that although the terms germs, *krimi* and *kita* are used by South Kanarese villagers, this does not mean that they have adopted a notion of a specific etiology or that they had given up traditional ideas of illness causality in favor of new concepts. Although it is true that a number of villagers have come to accept the notion that miniscule creatures are involved in causing an illness, several questions remain to be answered. Why is it that at a particular time *krimi* entered a person's body? How do *krimi* penetrate one's body space? Why does one individual contract a severe case of a contagious illness while another is not effected or gets only a mild case? The western layperson answers these questions through vague, if not specifically ambiguous reference to stress, fitness, vitamins, resistance and antibodies. The South Kanara villager answers these same questions with respect to indigenous notions of body constitution and resistance phrased in terms of a balance of body humors (*tridosha*), blood quality, the control of heat in the body and the maintenance of purity as a protective sphere. Reference to these constructs comprises an important part of local discourse about promotive and preventive health.

How do such notions effect behavior during an epidemic? Villagers in the process of making offerings to *bhuta* spirits at a shrine were interviewed during a Kyasanur forest disease epidemic (Nichter 1987). Several correctly stated this disease was caused by ticks and *krimi*. During a group discussion an analogy was offered to me from agriculture to elucidate reasons for ritual activity. If one man's rice field is attacked by insects, but a neighboring field is free of attack this may cause the owner to think that witchcraft has been performed against him and by extension his field. Field, person and crop are co-extensive.[23] A domain of social space connected to the agriculturalist, the field, can be rendered open by witchcraft and made susceptible to an attack by insects. For this reason, fields are protected against both malevolent influences such as evil eye and sorcery as well as insects. Similarly, illness may be precipitated by *krimi*, but be caused by other factors which have reduced one's resistance, opening one to attack. A *bhuta* spirit may be either directly or indirectly responsible for an illness caused by *krimi*. A patron *bhuta's* failure to protect one's social space and leave one vulnerable leads to illness as well as the *bhuta's* direct wrath. An important international health message may be gleaned. Health education which does not pay credence to a "closed domain" concept of resistance as it is culturally constituted, in addition to a "pathogen" concept of illness causality and contagion will no doubt be perceived as simplistic by villagers in South India. The concepts of vulnerability and resistance have metamedical connotations deeply embedded in culture.

The Strategic Reporting of Symptoms

Just as the negotiation of an illness identity is not neutral, the reporting of sets of symptoms to practitioners is not neutral nor strictly objective. Villagers frequenting practitioners during illness were observed to either make brief one to two symptom statements or to articulate a conventionalized set of symptoms including reference to weakness, digestion, shaking of the hands or feet, heat, and sleeplessnsess. An analysis of symptoms cited revealed four patterns of symptom reporting. Reported were: 1) symptoms associated with acute pain; 2) symptoms impeding work capacity and the ability to maintain a daily routine; 3) symptoms closely linked to key health concerns and notions of risk (e.g. menstruation); and 4) symptoms which villagers learned evoked desired responses from practitioners in terms of examination time and powerful medicines. The dynamics of symptom reporting at once reflected cultural concerns and was strategic. An example may be cited to illustrate this point.

For several months while observing practitioner patient interactions, I heard patients cite fever, *jwara*, as a major symptom complaint. I thought little about this as fever was common enough as a symptom. I did observe, however, that a patient's temperature was rarely taken. It wasn't until I moved to an interior village and had neighbors request first aid assistance that I found out that fever was often not fever as I knew it. Fever, *jwara*, often referred to heat in the body. Heat might be manifest to the touch, constitute a latent cause of weakness, or be associated with a wide range of other symptoms. Sometimes fever was reported to be in the stomach, yet I felt a neighbor's head in what appeared a most mysterious ritual. As for sticking a thermometer under someone's arm, well this was deemed a most peculiar form of diagnosis when fever constituted a burning sensation on the palms and soles.

Learning from my experience with neighbors, I observed doctor-patient interactions involving fever more closely. I found that busy doctors who spend 2—3 minutes with a patient rarely questioned fever as a symptom and usually responded with medicine as a form of positive feedback. Those who touched a patient's head and felt no fever often assumed fever was intermittent and sometimes asked a question about duration. Patients with manifest fever commonly received an injection from private doctors and in cases of intermittent fever some analgesic tablets.

Interviews with patients who did not have manifest fever revealed that some cited fever to practitioners because they had learned this symptom was responded to with attention and powerful medicines. Of these, some felt that fever medicine would provide a quick fix for other ailments in the body associated with heat. For other patients, complaints of fever and or heat were more general statements about non well being. They were much like complaints of pain in the U.S. which are difficult to verify by doctors. Heat and pain constitute relative scales of well being. For South Indians, heat is an experiential state. It is not precisely measured against of a norm of 98.6 degrees Fahrenheit. Indeed the idea that everyone has the same temperature amused village informants. Heat was relative to person, among people and was not necessarily continuous throughout the body. One might have a hot head and cold feet or fever with chills. Heat was something one sensed and was only explicitly obvious when one was extremely hot — burning with fever or cold and shivering.

The complaints of heat and fever were polysemous — they referred to many things and indexed a sense of vulnerability. Like pain in the west, complaints of fever often communicated as much about the person as the characteristics of an ailment. Just as a western patient may complain of pain to receive stronger medication and/or increased attention, some Indian patients complained of heat and fever for similar purposes. In both cases, feedback loops are established which lead to the medicalization of psychosocial problems, an issue taken up below. The opposite pattern also emerges. I observed one young doctor who was affronted by "false reports" of fever and broadly interpreted these reports as "psychosomatic". He failed to probe for other symptoms associated with heat and tended to dismiss as psychological vague somatic complaints like "stomach fever". Experienced rural doctors whom I observed followed up upon such complaints often identifying significant pathology.

Medicalization, Psychologicalization and Ambiguity

As noted above, ambiguity in illness conceptualization and symptom reporting may result either in the medicalization of the psychosocial expressed in somatic terms, or the psychologicalization of health problems having medical and nutritional, and ultimately political economic bases. Another example may be provided illustrating this point. Doctors at South Kanarese clinics commonly respond to specific ambiguous complaints such as nerves (*nara dosha*) or dizziness with ambivalence or they interpret these complaints as involving malnutrition or general anxiety.[24] Often the use of these terms is indexical of social relations and feelings of alienation, powerlessness etc (Nichter 1981). Reference to these somatic "states" communicate cultural meaning at a body to body level among a population for whom reference to the somatic constitutes an idiom of distress. These states are the felt experience of the psychosocial within the body. Cultural meaning is embodied, it influences and in turn is influenced by physical states.

Frequenting doctors with simatic complaints is part of a process of problem articulation to significant others setting in motion the social relations of care. The doctor legitimates the claim of disorder through the distribution of medicine. Care may then be articulated by significant others through additional health related actions be they the purchases of tonic (chapter nine), or the frequence of multiple practitioners. On several occasions, I observed doctors giving patients with vague symptoms B_{12} injections and Calmpose (Valium). The justification given for the administration of this mix of medicines is revealing. When questioned doctors often made reference to "widespread malnutrition among the masses" and the "worries of poverty". Political economic problems (hunger, poverty) and social relational problems were identified and treated as medical and psychological problems. If the masses cannot eat rice, let them eat medicine or at least be calm enough to sleep.

SECTION FOUR

The Implicit Meaning of Verbs and Tenses

In sections two and three, I focused on the interactional aspects of the language of illness. Let us now turn to structural features and the manner in which implicit knowledge is subtly expressed through grammatical constructs. A structural semantic analysis of verbs used to describe illness may be presented. A basic tenet of such an analysis is that the meaning of words are a product of the relation among them and not simply their relation to the cultural world each describes.[25]

Verb usage in illness discourse has been little explored. Lienhardt (1961: 147—150) in his writing on Dinka religion, observed that Dinka talk about an illness in a manner significantly different from that of Europeans. A Dinka will say that illness or power seizes a person and not that a person catches an illness. Whereas in the English realization, a person is the subject, the doer, and the illness is the object, in Dinka (as in Kannaḍa and other Dravidian languages) an illness is the agent (subject) working on or in a person. This appears to be both a structural feature of the language and an indication of the speaker's world view. At issue which arises is whether a more extensive analysis of verb usage might reveal insights into the way a population contrasts illness experiences at different levels of specificity. The following analysis, based on conversations between villagers and ayurvedic *vaidya*, explores this possibility.

Verb Choice

Three verbs commonly used in descriptions of sickness were examined. The first verb studied was the Kannaḍa verb *uṇṭu*; a verb which generally expresses existence apart from the consideration of time, place, character, or other conditions of being. Thus, when used with the dative in the sense of possession — a sense in which the word is very commonly found, *uṇṭu* draws attention to the fact of possession rather than to the possessor or to the thing possessed. *Nanage holavuṇṭu* "to me there is a field" lays emphasis on the fact that I am a man of property whereas *nanage holaide* draws attention to the particular kind of property which I possess, namely a field. The timeless-ness of the existence implied by *uṇṭu* renders this word unsuitable for expressing what is merely temporary or recent, but suitable for expressing what is essential or habitual.[26]

The types of illness which are explained by the use of *uṇṭu* include sleeplessness, bloodlessness, weakness, and urinary problems. These are illnesses where the speaker is stressing his integral relationship with the illness, his possession in the sense that he is not seperable from it. When a patient comes to the hopital, the doctor commonly asks, *yen uṇṭu?* "what is there" (what do you possess?). Patients, in their description of symptoms, may reply using verb forms other than *uṇṭu*. Let us consider other verbs which may be used.

The Kannaḍa verb, *baru* has many translations, but in general usage means to come or to know. In the language of illness, the meaning of *baru* is dependent on context. For example, a man may say, *nanage shita bandide* "to me a cold came", to imply that he has a cold but he does not know how he contracted it. The use of *baru* further implies that the cold had a sudden onset.

If a patient wants to convey the impression that a cold developed gradually over a period of days, the verb *agide*, "happened", would be utilized. The shift in verb choice signals information about the onset and course of the cold. In describing the symptoms of a particular skin disease, a person may say *bigu barutade, binki barutade, resi agide* "swelling comes, burning comes, pus happened". Swelling and burning sensation occur suddenly, and thus take the verb "come," pus developed gradually and thus takes the verb "happened."

In another context, a form of the verb "to come" is used with a serious illness which is linked to the wrath of spirit. Examples of diseases which fall into this category are smallpox, cholera, and epilepsy. To say *nanage mailige roge bandide* "smallpox came to me", is to indicate that the disease actually came to the body from a spirit or force outside the body. The use of the verb in this context places emphasis on an external agent.

External factors interact with internal factors of the body to cause an illness and verb usage may reflect this fact. While the verb *baru* may express the external or precipitating factor of an illness, *biddide* "fall" marks its internal development. These two verbs provide a level of contrast by which speakers may mark both the onset and course of their illness. When a speaker says "smallpox fell on the child's body", he implies a sudden appearance of spots. Fall does not mean that spots fell from outside the body to the surface of the body, but rather from inside the body spots fell to the surface.

This does not contradict the notion that smallpox is caused by a spirit attacking one externally, but rather denotes what happens after the initial attack. The spirit causes an imbalance within the body causing bodily heat and poisons to be pushed to its surface causing pustulates to appear. One of the names given to smallpox, *sidubu roga* "shooting up disease", also conveys this notion. Dreams also take the verb "to fall". Dreams are thought to be caused by both external factors such as visitations by ancestor spirits or deities, and internal factors such as indigestion or imbalances in heat or body humors. A swollen sprained ankle is described by the phrase *kolpu biddide* "sprain fell". This does not denote that one has fallen and therefore incurred a sprain. The phrase rather means that swelling has fallen from the inside to the outside.

Perhaps the largest range of illnesses are linked to a form of the verb *agu* "to happen". In general this verb is used to express an ongoing illness which has gradually developed in the body from a point in the past. Many skin diseases are described by the verb *agide* "happened" as are illnesses relating to stomach problems and mental weakness. For example, a form of the verb *agu* is used with rashes on the skin that develop gradually from within the body. To say *avala kaialli kajji agide* "on her hand an itching rash happened", implies that the rash happened gradually and is not extensive. If the verb *biddide* was used as in *maguvina mai mele kajji biddide* "rash fell on the child's body", it would indicate a sudden appearance of spots all over the body. Although the initial cause may be different, as signalled by use of *agu* or baru, the verb *biddide* may be used to provide contrast or explanation. If a villager takes medicine and gets a cure he may say: "Since medicine was given, the *kajji* form inside the body fell outside."

Contrasts in verb choice may further be noted in the following example: *hunnu inali hula agide* "in the wound there were worms". This refers to the entrance in the past and continued development (up to the present) of worms inside the body which are travelling outside to the surface. This is in keeping with a prior discussion of *agide* and the notion of internal worms. *Hula hunnu madide* "the worms made a wound", refers to worms from the outside environment which are "chewing" the feet and thus causing infection. This is

in keeping with the indigenous notion that worms cause athlete's foot. The
condition is literally referred to as "worms eating".

A level of contrast may also be noted in regard to indigenous descriptions
of desirable and undesirable possession states. The verb *hiddide*, in general
usage, is synonymous with *baru* and implies catching or sudden holding.
Among Kannaḍa speakers in South Kanara, one often hears the expression
male hiddiyutade "the rain is catching or holding", to imply that the rain
during monsoons is beginning or about to fall. A form of the verb to hold is
also used to express an unwanted involuntary possession by an ancestor
spirit, wandering *bhuta* spirit or *pide* (a malevolent spirit which troubles
children). *Avanige buta hiddide* "*buta* held him", implies that it did so by
force, not by invitation.[27] Madness, leprosy, and *bala graha* also take the
verb *hiddide* to stress their severity.

In contrast, if a person was describing the desired or anticipated possession by a priest or a patron deity, he would not use a form of the verb
hiddide. In this context, he might say *avarige mai mele devaru bandide* "to
him, on his body, a *deva* came". *Deva* does not possess in a violent sense; it
does not catch or hold: rather, the spirit comes on the body. In the Tuḷu
language, similar contrasts between desired and undesired possession states
are made incorporating differential use of verbs and terms for possession.

TENSE

In the first few months of field study in South Kanara, I elicited information
from villagers by asking about hypothetical symptoms or illnesses with which
I was not yet familiar. When I used this technique, informants answered the
questions utilizing the present tense. However, I noted that during actual situations or illness, speakers often did not use the present tense in describing
illness, but used the past tense. For example, a young man and his father
came to the ayurvedic practitioner's house where I was living. The *vaidya*
looked at the boy and said: "Is it that fits came to him?" *Apasmara bandideyo?*
The boy was having fits at that very moment.

The *vaidya's* use of the past tense in this case seemed unusual and I began
to investigate tense as a further indicator of specific states of illness. In
Dravidian languages the colloquial use of the present tense acts in the
capacity of the English present-continuous and future tense while the past
tense indicates both the English past and the present-perfect tense. Accordingly, the Kannaḍa speaker utilizes tense as a means of specifying how an
illness has come about. For a symptom, such as sudden headache or stomach
ache, the present tense is utilized, indicating that it has just happened without
a series of precipitating or developing symptoms. When the past tense is
utilized, it indicates that the present symptoms are actually part of a known
sequence of events established in the past.[28]

CONCLUSION

Both denotative and connotative, referential and indexical dimensions of the language of illness have been identified and discussed in this chapter. An investigation of the language of illness in South Kanara has revealed that ambiguity as well as specificity are important aspects of classificatory schema, idioms of distress and illness discourse. It has also been pointed out that the way in which illnesses are, and are not, spoken about in South Kanarese culture is related to multiple criteria including ideas of illness causality and responsibility; consideration of the magical power of words; etiquette; and social relations. Emphasis has been placed on the negotiation of illness identities and the power relations involved in illness labeling. The strategic reporting of symptoms has been raised as a form of behavior influenced by patterns of treatment and the interactional dynamics of medicine giving. Ambiguity in symptom reporting, as perceived by practitioners, has been noted to foster both the medicalization of psychosocial problems articulated though a somatic idiom and the psychologicalization of vague somatic complaints associated with weakness, malnutrition etc.

An examination of contagion and resistance has revealed that both metaphor and metynomy underly culturally constituted cognitive models. Contagion is thought about and communicated in a number of different ways including the use of terms indexing impurity and social distance. It has been noted that recognition of "germs" as an etiological factor and source of contagion has not meant that villagers have rejected the doctrine of multiple causality or traditional ideas about etiology. Germs have been incorporated into the existing conceptual universe as another extrinsic cause of illness. As such they are subject to metamedical notions of resistance as a closed domain of personal/social space and purity.

An examination of structural features of the language of illness has revealed that verb choice and tense are means of conveying implicit ideas as to the onset, course and etiology of an illness experience. Verb usage is influenced by both the range of a verb's overt meaning as well as its structural meaning in contrast to other verbs. Here we find verbs employed as markers of various features of an illness experience, not mirrors of thought.

Issues have been raised in this chapter which are relevant to international health practice as well as social science theory. Currently, a social marketing approach to health education is growing in popularity. Lessons learned from early attempts to market health products have led to increased attention being directed toward the identification of local illness categories and terminology. At this point it is prudent to identify both specificity and ambiguity in the use of illness terms and the distribution of term usage as well as meaning. It will be necessary to determine whether the use of local terminology in health messages per se, the redefinition of local health terminology, the introduction of new terminology or approaching illness through prototype symptoms (e.g. the sounds of respiratory distress) is the best means of enhancing health communication.

In terms of anthropological theory, an approach to the study of the language of illness has been advanced which weds a cognitive model approach to the study of knowledge forms to a social interactional approach to knowledge production sensitive to tasks, performances, and power relations. The study of vantages and stakes in describing and naming illness in particular ways has been shown to be essential to an understanding of illness discourse. While I have emphasized the emergent and processual aspects of the language of illness in Sections One, Two and Three, structural aspects are acknowledged in Section Four.

Issues identified in this paper have been sketched in broad strokes. Needed at this juncture are studies which examine illness, health and risk related conversation. Attention needs to be directed toward the transformation of the language of illness at a time when a new vocabulary of illness and health are being introduced through education, the media, and a proliferation of health commodities. Code switching between traditional and popular — modern illness categories will be important to study as will the medicalization of folk illnesses and the creation of neologism categories like "liver". Also needed are sociolinguistic studies of illness discourse strategies which attend to language performance; the distribution as well as consequences of alternative means of articulating distress; and expressions of power and vulnerability entailing reference to health and illness.

NOTES

1. Another example of social relations influencing illness labeling would be differential uses of the terms allergy, sniffles and a cold. When one wishes to be physically close to another person in the west, sniffles may be labeled just an allergy in contrast to a cold.

2. It is beyond the scope of this paper to consider prototype therory in relation to cognitive semantics and the process of categorization. No doubt this theory will give rise to a new generation of studies on illness classification. For a review of recent developments in cognitive model theory see Lakoff (1987).

3. It is beyond the scope of this chapter to consider the connotative dimensions of language as tacit ideology present in discourse (Barthes 1972). Engaging in such analysis would lead to analysis such as that proposed by Foucault where knowledge and power are contingent and domination is embodied through illness classification systems.

4. On the importance of linguistic indeterminancy, creativity and change see Friedrich (1986).

5. For other examples of specific ambiguity in illness discourse see McCombie's (1987) analysis of flue in the U.S., Kendall's (1987) analysis of Naeng among Koreans, and Low's (1987) discussion of "nerves" in Latin America.

6. The category stress has multiple meanings. It is beyond the scope of this presentation to consider competing and coexisting metaphors underlying its conceptualization. From the vantage highlighted in the text, stress is an ambigious category. As a catch-all term, stress is understood from a vantage of similarity. From other vantages stress may be distinctive and specifically characterized. For example, stress may take on a distinctive meaning as a state specified in contrast to anxiety.

5. Carr (1978) uses the term 'final common pathway' to denote culturally sanctioned behavioral pathways through which distress is articulated. They may or may not involve pathology in a biomedical sense.

6. Baker (1987) has recently used this term to describe "bogus" ailments created by Madison Avenue to sell consumer cures e.g. "acid skin," "girdle urb," "tired blood," "middle aged skin."

7. Two limitations of social labeling theory may be noted. Social labeling theorists often emphasize culture without fully appreciating the interplay between culture and processes of pathology. They also fail to consider context specific forms of social interaction among those so labeled. Those labeled deviant or ill in complex societies may act one way in some contexts and another way in other contexts where performance expectations differ or are absent.

8. Generally, the first pregnancy is the source of great embarrassment to young women. Pregnancy is an overt sign of sexuality.

9. The power of a name to call into presence that which is signified has been noted by Tambiah (1968). This same idea underlies the Brahman wife's usage of a sound to call her husband from the field as opposed to his name. Not calling her husband by his name is not simply a matter of being respectful. Calling his name is thought to shorten the husband's life by calling him into presence while engaged in other activities. Metonymy may likewise underly the reluctance of Americans to speak of uncontrollable diseases like cancer or AIDS.

10. On the use of one illness label to mitigate the connotations of another see Kleinman's (1986) study of the social and political relations of neurasthenia in China.

11. Use of the same term by different people to denote either a respiratory or gastrointestinal infection is also found in the west. See McCombie (1987) on the use of the term "flue" in the U.S.

12. The opposite phenomena was also recorded. Some villagers used English disease names as a means of securing powerful medicines from a chemist shop. Their translation of local symptoms into English disease terms may lead to serious consequences. For example, I recorded the term 'blood pressure' used for feelings of dizziness, typhoid for high fever, and diabetes for frequent urination at night (which may or may not be a sign of the disease).

13. To the best of my knowledge, no scholar has specifically researched differences in male and female use and interpretations of illness terms. Research also needs to be done on gender specific illness terms. In a personal communication, Steinhoff has noted that gender specific terms for tetanus exist in Tamil Nad.

14. I use Adrian Mayer's (1966) concept of action set as those members of a social network who interact in relation to a given activity or task. This accords with Jantzen's (1978, 1987) notions of a therapy management group.

15. Cosminsky and Scrimshaw (1980) have provided a complementary discussion of how "vitamin" deficiency has been culturally interpreted in Guatemala.

16. I am not equating possession with mental disorder and concur with Claus (1979), that all too often possession is interpreted as madness by outsiders when in reality (another reality) it constitutes institutionalized cultural performance by participants. The cases I am referring to here clearly involved psychological disorder recognized by native informants involved with facilitating possession rituals.

17. In each of these cases, I received corroboration that the person's household behavior was abnormal and not structured around a culturally coherent set of ritual performances. I concurred with neighbors who confided in me that the person was *huchu* despite the household's support of an identity indexing spirit possession.

18. *Sonku* in Tulu is associated with "spreading" as well as a dramatic "rising or rushing". One who has had a stiff drink is described in Tulu as experiencing *sonku*.

19. The convergence and divergence of South Indian perceptions of cleanliness and purity, dirtiness and impurity have been discussed by Kharve (1962) and Bean (1981).

20. Morley (1980) has likewise noted that in much of Africa there is a strong belief that the rash of measles must be encouraged to come out and not be interfered with by the administration of medications. He also notes that for centuries measles was associated with the impurity of menstrual blood in Europe.

21. Likewise, folk medicines may not be administered by villagers in the initial stages of wound infections (*nanju*) when blood and pus is being expelled from the body. When medicine is taken, villagers are often more concerned about the internal quality of their blood than caring for an infected wound externally. On this subject see chapter seven.

22. I have been unable to find research conducted in the West on the layperson's perception of germs, bacteria, and virus. From some exploratory research in Arizona and Hawaii, I have found that a wide range of ideas and images coexist in popular health culture. Popular images include a perception of bacteria as a passive mold like thing (a thing which lives off the body like mildew lives off of leather causing it harm); virus as packman like creatures "out to get us"; and germs as "preying off people that are weak or stressed out like vultures circling a weak animal". Popular interpretation of biomedical terminology may draw from much older notions of illness etiology.

23. The coextensiveness of one's person, body, house and the soil of one's field has been elaborated by Daniel (1984) among others. Important to recognize is both the intermingling and flowing of essence and substance between these domains, and the contiguity of these domains such that vulnerability in one results in vulnerability in the others.

24. Town and city dwellers more commonly use the term "nerve" or "nerve defect" than *nara dosha*. Reviewing my notes I find the following symptoms associated with these terms: 1) pain and trembling in limbs especially the extremities, 2) post partum weakness, 3) an inability to lift heavy objects, and 4) anxiety and feelings of general unease, 5) short term memory loss, 6) dullness of affect. *Nara dosha* and nerve defect are used by the educated and uneducated alike to refer to a broad range of complaints some of which are medical and other psychological. A neurousurgeon working in Mangalore city told me that two thirds of the patients requesting to see him were self referred and wished to see him about "nerve defect." Most of these patients he referred to a cardiologist or psychiatrist.

25. A comprehensive analysis of verb usage is beyond the scope of this paper and necessitates extensive research into the history of the Kannada language. For the purpose of this essay, I focus attention on the use of verbs to denote contrasting features of the experience of illness. Mimi Nichter first called my attention to contrasting patterns in the way in which verbs were used to describe illness. Data on verb use represents a joint research effort.

26. There is a distinction between the usage of *untu* and *ide* and its corresponding plural forms, but it is quite subtle and cannot be expressed as a rule. For a discussion of the verb *untu* see Spencer 1914.

27. The Tulu language has an even more extensive vocabulary for possession states which contrast both nouns and verbs to designate different types of possession.

28. This is not limited to verb usage in illness discourse. For example, When someone is called to take meals and is about to come, they may say "bande", I came. This usage indicates "I am coming", as a sequence of events has been established.

REFERENCES

Baker, R.
    1987 Textually Transmitted Diseases. *American Demographics*, December, p. 64.
Barthes, R.
    1972 *Mythologies*. New York: Hill and Wand.

Bean, S.
   1981   Toward a Semantics of "Purity" and "Pollution" in India. *American Ethnologist*
          8(3): 575—95.
Bibeau, G.
   1981   The Circular Semantic Network in Ngbandi Disease Nosology. *Social Science and*
          Medicine 15B: 295—307.
Bourdieu, P.
   1977   *Outline of a Theory of Practice*. New York: Cambridge University Press.
Briggs, C.
   1986   *Learning How to Ask*. Cambridge: Cambridge University Press.
Carr, J. E.
   1978   Ethno-Behaviorism and the Culture-Bound Syndromes: The Case of Amok. *Culture*
          Medicine and Psychiatry 2: 269—293.
Carr, J. E. and Vitabliano, P.
   1982   *Depression and the Culture Bound Syndromes: An Ethno-behavioral View*. Paper
          presented at Annual Meeting of the American Anthropological Association.
          Washington, D.C.
Cicourel, A.
   1982   Language and Belief in a Medical Setting. *In* H. Byrnes (ed.) *Contemporary Percep-*
          tions of Language: Interdisciplinary Dimensions. Washington, D.C.: Georgetown
          University Press.
   1985   Text and Discourse. *Ann. Rev. Anthropol. 14*: 159—85.
Claus, P.
   1979   Spirit Possession and Spirit Mediumship from the Perspective of Tuḷu Oral Tradi-
          tions. *Culture Medicine and Psychiatry 3*: 29—52.
Cosminsky, S. and Scrimshaw, M.
   1980   Medical Pluralism on a Guatemalan Plantation. *Social Science Medicine 14b*: 267—
          278.
D'Andrade, R.
   1976   A Propositional Analysis of U.S. American Beliefs about Illness. *In* K. Basso and H.
          Selby (eds). *Meaning in Anthropology*. Albuquerque: University of New Mexico
          Press.
D'Andrade, R., et al.
   1972   Categories of Disease in American-English and Mexican- Spanish. *In* A. Romney,
          R. Shepard and S. Nerlove (eds). *Multidimensional Scaling*. Vol. II Applications.
          New York: Seminar Press.
Daniels, E. V.
   1986   *Fluid Signs*. Berkeley: University of California Press.
Doughterty, J. and Fernandez, J.
   1982   Afterword. *American Ethnologist*, pp. 820—832.
Doughterty, J. and Keller, C.
   1982   Taskonomy: A Practical Approach to Knowledge Structures. *American Ethnologist*,
          pp. 763—774.
Foucault, M.
   1973   *Madness and Civilization: A History of Insanity in an Age of Reason*. R. Howard
          (Trans.). New York: Vintage.
   1975   *Birth of the Clinic: An Archaeology of Medical Perception*. A. M. Sheridan Smith
          (Trans.) New York: Random House.
   1977   *The History of Sexuality. Volume I: An Introduction*. R. Huxley (Trans.). New York:
          Vintage.
Frake, C.
   1961   The Diagnosis of Disease among the Subanun of Mindanao. *American Anthropolo-*
          gist 63: 113—132.

Friedrich, P.
    1986   *The Language Parallax*. Austin: University of Texas Press.
Glick, M.
    1967   Medicine as an Ethnographic Category: The Gimi of the New Guinea Highlands. *Ethnology 6*: 31—56.
Good, B.
    1977   The Heart of What's the Matter: The Semantics of Illness in Iran. *Culture, Medicine and Psychiatry 1*: 25—58.
Holland, D. and Quinn, N. (eds.)
    1987   *Cultural Models in Language and Thought*. New York: Cambridge University Press.
Jantzen, J.
    1978   *The Quest for Therapy in Lower Zaire*. Berkeley: The University of California Press.
    1987   Therapy Management: Concept, Reality, Process. *Medical Anthropology Quarterly, 1*: 1, 68—84.
Kay, M.
    1979   Lexemic Change and Semantic Shift in Disease Names. *Culture Medicine and Psychiatry 3*(1): 73—94.
Kendall, L.
    1987   Cold Wombs in Balmy Honolulu: Ethnogynecology among Korean Immigrants. *Social Science and Medicine 25*(4): 367—376.
Khare, R. S.
    1962   Ritual Purity and Pollution in Relation to Domestic Sanitation. *Eastern Anthropologist 15*: 125—139.
Kleinman, A.
    1986   *Social Origins of Distress and Disease: Depression Neurasthenia and Pain in Modern China*. New Haven: Yale University Press.
Kövecses, Z.
    1986   *Metaphors of Anger, Pride, and Love: A Lexical Approach to the Structure of Concepts*. Philadelphia: John Benjamin.
Lakoff, G.
    1987   *Women, Fire and Dangerous Things*. Chicago: University of Chicago Press.
Last, M.
    1981   The Importance of Knowing about Not Knowing. *Social Science and Medicine 15b*: 387—392.
Lindhardt, G.
    1961   *Divinity and Experience: The Religion of the Dinka*. Oxford: Claredon Press.
Low, S.
    1985   Culturally Interpreted Symptoms or Culture Bound Syndromes: A Cross-Cultural Review of Nerves. *Social Science and Medicine 21*(2): 1987—1996.
MacLaury, R.
    1987   Co-extensive Semantic Ranges: Different names for   Distinct Vantages of One Category. *In* B. Need, E. Sciller, and A. Bosch (eds), *Papers from the 23rd Annual Regional Meeting of the Chicago Linguistic Society* (pp. 268—282).
Malinowski, B.
    1961   *Argonauts of the Western Pacific*. New York: Dalton.
Mayer, A.
    1966   The Significance of Quasi-Groups in the Study of Complex Societies. *In* M. Banton (ed.) *The Social Anthropology of Complex Societies*. London: Tavistock Press.
McCombie, S.
    1987   Folk Flu and Viral Syndrome: An Epidemiological Perspective. *Social Science and Medicine 25*: 987—93.
Morley, D.
    1980   Severe measles. *In* N. F. Stanley and R.A. Joske (eds), *Changing Disease Patterns and Human Behavior* (pp. 28—36). London: Academic Press.

Nichter, M.
1981 Idioms of Distress: Alternatives in the Expression of Psychosocial Distress in South India. *Culture, Medicine and Psychiatry 5*: 379—408.
1987 Of Ticks. Kings, Spirits and the Promise of Vaccines. *Medical Anthropology Quarterly*, December (pp. 406—423).
Obeysekere, G.
1976 The Impact of Ayurvedic Ideas on the Culture and the Individual in Sri Lanka. *In* C. Leslie (ed.) *Asian Medical Systems: A Comparative Study*. Berkeley: University of California Press.
Rosch, E. and Mervis, C.
1975 Family Resemblances: Studies in the Internal Structure of Categories. *Cognitive Psychology 7*: 573—605.
Schutz, A.
1964 *Collected Papers II: Studies in Social Theory*. The Hague: Martinus Nijfhoff.
Silverstein, M.
1976 Shifters, linguistic categories and cultural descriptions. *In* K. Basso and H. A. Selby (eds) *Meaning in Anthropology* (pp. 11—55). Albuquerque: University of New Mexico Press.
Spencer, M.
1914 *A Kanarese Grammar*. Mysore: Wesleyan Mission Press.
Tambiah, S.
1968 The Magical Power of Words. *Man, 3*: 2, 195— 208, June.
Taylor, C.
1976 The Place of Indigenous Medical Practitioners in the Modernization of Health Services. *In* Charles Leslie (ed.) *Asian Medical Systems*. Berkeley: University of California Press.
Torrey, E. F.
1973 *The Mind Game*. New York: Bantam.
Wagner, R.
1981 *The Invention of Culture*. Chicago: University of Chicago Press.
Waxler, N.
1977 Is Mental Illness Cured in Traditional Societies? A Theoretical Analysis. *Culture Medicine and Psychiatry 1*: 233—253.
1981 The Social Labelling Perspective on Illness and Medical Practice. *In* L. Eisenberg and A. Kleinman (eds) *The Relevance of Social Science for Medicine* (pp. 283—306). Boston: Reidel.
Young, A.
1983 The Relevance of Traditional Medical Cultures to Modern Primary Health Care. *Social Science and Medicine 17*: 16, 1205—1211.

5. CULTURAL INTERPRETATIONS OF STATES OF MALNUTRITION AMONG CHILDREN: A SOUTH INDIAN CASE STUDY

In this chapter, I wish to consider how a set of children's illnesses often associated with states of malnutrition are conceptualized by a South Indian population. My focus will be the meaning accorded to these illnesses and the manner in which this meaning influences health care practice and decision making. Highlighted will be rural mothers ideas about the classification, etiology, prevention, and appropriate treatment of seven children's illnesses in South Kanara District, Karnataka State. Following the presentation of this data, I will briefly consider its applied significance and suggest that culturally responsive approaches to health education may be developed around emic illness categories. I will further argue that ayurvedic practitioners are a primary health care resource in rural South India capable of playing an important role in nutrition education. They are consulted about diet for health as well as during illness and convalescence, times of greatest nutrient need and the most dietary restrictions.

CONTEXT

The region of India which provides the context for our discussion is rural South Kanara District, Karnatake State. Rural South Kanara is characterized by scattered, as opposed to nuclear, rural settlements; a checkerboard of crossroads towns; and a progressive, small city accessible by a relatively good transportation system. The South Kanarese health arena consists of folk herbal specialists; traditional ayurvedic specialists (*vaidya*) and herbal compounders; traditional-modern ayurvedic specialists trained in ayurveda as well as some elements of the biosciences; astrologers, diviners, exorcists, and possession mediums; allopathic practitioners and pharmacists; and eclectic combinations of the above (Nichter 1978).

Points of convergence as well as ideological conflicts and contrasting interpretations of illness crosscut coexisting therapy systems. The layperson when aware of inconsistencies is ambivalent toward them. As noted by Leslie (1983), little attempt is made by the layperson to 'resolve the ambiguity and multiplicity of things to a simple form of clear and certain knowledge.' The ordinary man is not surprised when people hold diverse views, but considers that the contradictions and inconsistencies he perceives are like pieces of a puzzle that would ultimately fit together had he time to learn about all the pieces (Beals 1976).

Three points may be highlighted with respect to the popular health culture.

1. At the core of the South Kanarese health culture is the doctrine of multiple causality. Most illnesses are thought capable of being caused or compounded by any one of a multiplicity of caused factors acting alone or in concert.

2. A variety of health resources and possible solutions coexist for the management of symptoms and for problems related to coping with illness. Villagers make varied use of pluralistic health care resources. Health care decision making is influenced by a complex of predisposing, enabling and quality of service related factors (Kroeger 1983) including: notions of etiology, diagnosis, and perceived severity; previous self-help attempts; practitioner accessibility (social as well as geographic); the micro-economics of health care seeking; the reputation of particular practitioners for curing specific illnesses; and cultural notions of and expectations from therapy etc. The focus of this paper is predisposing factors.

3. For some kinds of health problems, significant patterns of health care resort emerge which are illness and age specific. These patterns are more complex than those previously described — of nonincapacitating chronic illnesses being treated by traditional practitioners and incapacitating acute illnesses being treated by allopaths (Gould 1965).

With respect to the latter point, a previous study of South Kanarese health culture carried out between 1974 and 1976 (Nichter 1978) revealed that many villagers who frequent government and private allopathic clinics themselves, administer lengthy herbal cures (folk and ayurvedic) to their infants and young children for some illnesses. A pattern-of-resort survey for 25 common illnesses conducted in a village which had a Government Primary Health Center and two renowned ayurvedic *vaidya* found that ayurveda was a popular treatment for many children's illnesses, including measles, chickenpox, mumps, respiratory complaints and an illness termed *grahani* (*krani*) strongly associated with marasmic kwashiorkor. These data on the use of traditional medicine for children's illness corroborated the impressions of other South India scholars (Andrew 1973; Djurfeld and Lindberg 1975; Mathews 1979). In 1979, a follow-up health behavior study was carried out. One focus of this study was the lay conceptualization of manifest states of malnutrition among children. This paper reports on the findings of the 1979 study.

METHODOLOGY

The study population was drawn from a cross-section of rural locales ranging from interior villages (V) having no medical practitioners of any type to rural towns (T) having a variety of traditional and cosmopolitan practitioners using allopathic as well as eclectic combinations of commercial medicine. House-hold health interviews were conducted to explore mothers' prototype images of the major symptom attributes of children's illness categories identified during previous household and clinic based research. Mothers were queried about their experiences with seven illnesses. Preventive health behavior, home cures, and actual or anticipatory health care seeking behaviors were recorded. Questions about health care seeking behavior explored to which practitioners informants had taken or would take their children if any of the seven illnesses were experienced in the family.

There are methodological problems in assessing anticipatory data elicited in relation to health care seeking behavior (Leslie 1980, 1983). Data generated by health care resort surveys which ask an informant which kind of medical system is best for specified illness categories must be subjected to scrutiny before being taken as an indication of actual behavior or health system preference. Such surveys are limited on at least two accounts. First, they fail to provide perspective into the negotiation process which occurs within households (and broader therapy management groups) where the process of illness identification is dynamic and responsive to notions of etiology, symptoms and health care alternatives. Second, health care seeking behavior elicited in surveys often reflects the popularity of specific practi-tioners and not a preference for health systems *per se*.

Keeping the limitations of anticipatory data in mind, fifty-two lower economic class, multi-caste, rural mothers having young children under 7 years old were chosen for the study. For the purposes of this paper, data from 27 town (T) and 25 interior village (V) households are contrasted where relevant. The household survey was complemented by observational data, including sittings with Government Primary Health Center doctors and five traditional healers. During these sittings, interactions between practi-tioners and families presenting severely malnourished children were observed. When possible, follow-up case study interviews were arranged with patients. Additionally, interviews were carried out in households where children were identified by health practitioners as experiencing frank malnutrition.

ILLNESS CLASSIFICATION

Illnesses are identified both on the basis of referential attributes — symptom sets (see Table I) — and situational factors including event schema (e.g., sociocultural significance accorded to the type and time of onset), the health history of family, the efficacy of attempted therapies, notions of underlying etiology (causal propositions), and the characteristics of therapy.[3] As noted in Chapter 4, considerable overlap exists between the symptom sets of many folk illness categories, and substantial ambiguity is often displayed by villagers when they attempt to classify an illness. This is particularly true with respect to children's illness. Illness taxonomies constructed on the basis of

TABLE I. Children's Illnesses Commonly Associated with States of Malnutrition.

Lay Illness Category	Informants' Descriptions[a]	Doctors' Diagnoses[b]
Agra	Thickness of tongue; White Coating on tongue; Vomiting; Lip sores and cracking; Poor sucking of breastmilk.	Riboflavin deficiency; Glossitis and cherlosis. Also thrush, oral moniliasis, yeast infection.
Chappe Roga	Bloated stomach; Swelling in arms and legs; Lack of appetite; Apathy; Excessive urination.	Kwashiorkor; Marasmic kwashiorkor.
Tamare Roga	Same as for chappe roga, as well as the following: Dry cracked skin; Eruptions and rashes, decreased elasticity of skin; Dry cough; Dry lips and desire for excessive amounts of water (by cultural standards); Clear water issuing from the nose.	Marasmic kwashiorkor with pronounced vitamin A deficiency, deficiency of essential fatty acids, pyodermatitis.
Krani	Bloated stomach; Thin legs; Visible chest ribs; Night blindness; White film over eyes; Poor digestion accompanied by very foul-smelling white/yellow diarrhea.	Marasmic kwashiorkor with pronounced vitamin A deficiency, folic acid deficiency.
Kamale	Edema of body; Yellowing of eyes and body; Fatigue; Pain in arms and legs; Dizziness; Desire to eat mud or raw rice; Body becoming pale; Yellow urine.	PEM accompanied by jaundice, anemia.
Pakki Kadapu	Bloated stomach; Thin arms and legs; Stunted growth; Weakness; Apathy; No crying; Bowing of legs or legs held close to chest; High-pitched wheezing sound; Fits; Spasm of hands and feet.	PEM with pronounced vitamin D deficiency; Calcium malabsorption; Rickets; Sometimes polio.
Bala Graha	Described as fits. Irritability; Delirium; Stupor; Seizures and Convulsions; Coughing fits; Breathlessness; Failure to thrive; Loss of appetite; Increased heat; Kapha coming from mouth after fits.	Wide range of problems. States of malnutrition; Epilepsy; Dehydration; Pneumococcal infections; Tuberculosis and aseptic meningitis; Rickets.

[a] Symptoms cited by at least 25% of 80 informant families.
[b] Differential diagnosis of indigenous illness categories cited by two experienced Primary Health Center doctors and one children's specialist, all practicing in the District and native speakers of Tuḷu and Kannaḍa.

symptom attributes and prodromal relationships between illnesses (see
Figure 1) are ideal types mediated by sociocultural contingencies which
influence the interpretation of actual states of ill health. Illness identification
of persistent symptom states often sets in motion a hermeneutic process
within which interpretation of the present reflects on the past and anticipates
the future.

The complexity of the process of negotiation of an illness identity within
the family varies with the perceived severity of the symptom state,[4] as well as
with the characteristics of the illness. While some illnesses like *agra, kamale,*
or *pakki kadapu* are more readily identifiable by dramatic symptioms — a

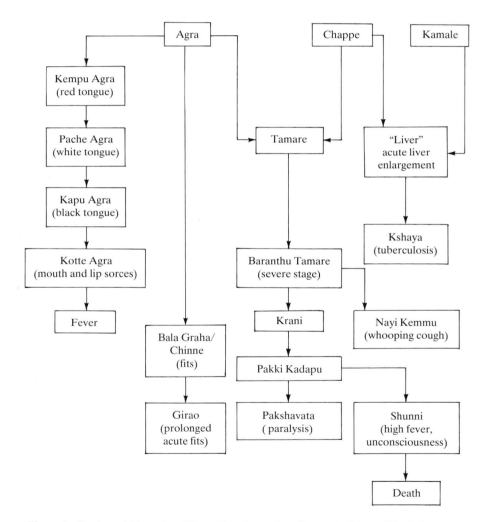

Figure 1. Prodromal Ideas about Illness Transformation. Composite Ideas of Ten Informants.

white pasty tongue, for example — a differential diagnosis between *chappe roga, tamare, krani*, and *bala graha* is more problematic.[5] Lay differential diagnosis (illness reckoning) often focuses on notions of etiology as well as on symptoms. For example, in Chapter 4 I noted that children's illness of sudden onset experienced on or near "no moon day" (a time when spirits are active) is apt to be classified as *bala graha* even if prototypical symptoms of *bala graha* are not manifest.

During the process of negotiating an illness identity a number of home cures may be tried and opinions from neighbors elicited. With each illness identity entertained comes a set of notions about prognosis. Prognosis is an important factor influencing future illness identification. Some illness states are deemed manageable, but incurable. If an illness is considered incurable, manifestations of a wide variety of symptoms throughout one's life (or childhood) may be attributed to this illness. This was found to be the case in respect to the illnesses *tamare* and *krani*. These illnesses once experienced were deemed to remain in the body until adulthood, if not manifest, then latent.[6] Such being the case, therapy was more often sought to manage these illnesses than to cure them. Consequently, villagers considered expensive long-term medication for these illnesses a waste of scarce resources. In one sense this notion reflected accurate observation. High-priced nutritional tonics prescribed by doctors would often remit symptoms temporarily but when the bottle of tonic was finished, the child's symptoms would return before long. In another sense, the notion reflected a self-fulfilling prophecy, for when not treated beyond the symptomatic stage, the illness would return.

ETIOLOGY

A wide variety of causal factors are associated with the 7 children's illnesses. Table II presents survey data on elicited notions of etiology, listing all etiological factors which were cited by at least 10 percent of either town or village informant families. These data provide a useful index of villagers' notions of major causal factors. This index is not definitive, however. It proved to be neither complete nor predictive of actual family reasoning when illness was experienced. Elicited responses related to ideal illness categories, not illness experiences. In the actual cases followed, etiological factors suspected often focused as much on the mother or family unit as on the child. For example, a mother's nonadherence to folk dietetics during pregnancy was commonly remembered and considered an etiological factor when a child experienced illness months later. The qualities of foods a mother consumed while breastfeeding was often deemed to affect the quality of her breastmilk and the health of her child. Notions of etiology were, moreover, extended to the family as a unit — to notions of family vulnerability concordant with such things as unfulfilled promises to deities, the curse of enemies, etc. As the most vulnerable member of the family, a child is viewed as the most likely to be first affected by forces of malevolence directed at the

TABLE II. Notions of Etiology for Childhood Illnesses Associated with States of Malnutrition.

Causal Factors[a]		Illness Categories					
	Agra	Chappe Roga/ Tamare	Krani	Kamale	Pakki Kadapu	Bala Graha/ Chinne
Less Food	Town[b]: 56% Village[c]: 44%	T: 48% V: 20%	T: 48% V: 28%		T: 15% V: 4%	T: 8% V: 12%
Bad Blood (Diet Related)	T: 4% V: 20%		T: 7% V: 20%	T: 26% V: 12%	T: 7% V: 12%	
Overheat or Cold (Diet Related)	overheat T: 70% V: 16%	overheat T: 70% V: 76%	overheat T: 59% V: 48%	overheat T: 14% V: 8%		T: 11% V: 8%
Kapha/Phlegm (Diet Related)	T: — V: 56%	T: — V: 11%				
Pitta (Diet Related)		T: 11% V: 12%	T: 70% V: 72%			
Ancestors, Spirits, Deities[d]					deities/spirits T: 18% V: 80%	deities T: 52% V: 50%
Stars,[d] Planets, Papa/Karma, Heredity	heredity (mother's milk) T: — V: 37%	heredity (mother's milk) T: — V: 50%	para/ karma	stars T: 11% V: —	T: 18% V: 36%	T: 33% V: —
Other		climate T: 22% C: —			climate T:18% V: 14%	
No Answer	T: 11% V: 16%	T: 7% V: —	T: 11% V: 41%	T: 7% V: 16%	T: 22% V: —	T: 11% V: 16%

[a] All causal factors listed were noted by at least 10% of the informants.
[b] Town (T): n = 27.
[c] Village (V): n = 25.
[d] These notions of etiology were compounded with the factor "bird crossing" noted in the text.

family. Because most children's illnesses may be manifested by supernatural as well as natural forces, these illnesses (particularly when sudden) provided an occasion for retrospective thought about obligations and enemies.

Noting the limitation of survey data for etiology, a combination of survey and case study data will be used to highlight some of the major etiological factors associated with the seven indigenous illness categories.

AN INDEX OF ETIOLOGICAL FACTORS

1. *Less food.* Insufficient diet was deemed a probable etiology for *agra, chappe, tamare roga,* and *krani.* It is notable that in the survey far more town informants linked insufficient diet to these illnesses than did villagers. Only in the case of *agra* did a majority of both village and town informants link insufficient diet to a manifest state of malnutrition. Insufficient diet is linked to the etiological factors "overheat," "less blood," and "spoiled blood." One line of reasoning was that when there is less food in the stomach, it becomes overheated — heats the blood — causing it to spoil "the way rice spoils when it is overcooked."

2. *Overheat.* Overheat within the body was associated with *agra, chappe, tamare,* and *krani* by a majority of informants. In all of these illnesses, symptoms of eruption or expulsions are prominent. Overheat can result form a wide variety of factors ranging from climate to diet and from the evil eye to the effect of spirits. Overheat is associated with both the immediate effect and after effect of etiological factors. Reference to overheat, therefore, needed to be followed up by a consideration of those factors contributing to a state of overheat over time. Follow-up on the descriptor "overheat" was warranted to distinguish between the types of reasoning producing knowledge about heat in the body. For example, villagers report overheat in the form of fever to practitioners both when fever is explicitly present and when overheat is implicitly associated with an illness vis-à-vis causal propositions (explanatory models) and interpretations of circumstance influenced by contiguity (co-occurrence), resemblance, or notions of salience (A. Young 1981).

3. *Bad blood.* Bad blood refers to blood which has become "spoiled" or "toxic" as a result of overheat, undigested foods, or impurities (physical as well as moral). Bad blood was cited as a cause of *agra* and *krani* by villagers, and of *kamale* by townsfolk. All causal descriptions of bad blood used in the context of the seven illnesses referred to diet and not moral acts. Reference to morality in the context of bad blood was, however, documented in relation to other illnesses such as leprosy. The concept of bad blood is closely related to diet — an etiological domain discussed below.

4. *Pitta. Pitta* is a humoral substance associated with overheat and yellow excretions from the body.[7] Excess *pitta* is usually related to diet. Unsurprisingly, it was identified as a cause of jaundice, *kamale.* It may be noted, however, that the terms *kamale* and *pitta* are used in the vernacular to refer to a yellowing of the eyes and skin as well as to describe yellow urine. Clear urine is deemed normal for those living on a predominantly rice diet. As will be noted shortly, a child may be given a herbal remedy for *kamale* after taking allopathic medicine which turns the urine yellow.

5. *Kapha. Kapha* is a humoral substance associated with phlegm, used as

a reference in the context of illness. *Kapha* may denote either an accumulation or an aggravation of phlegm and sometimes both. Surprisingly, on the
family survey, *kapha* was ascribed to be a major etiological factor only for
agra, and only by villagers not townsfolk. The reason why this is surprising is
twofold. First, in case studies of children suffering from *agra, bala graha,
chappe*, and *krani, kapha* was commonly cited as an etiological factor.
Perhaps one of the reasons *kapha* was not elicited more often as a survey
response was because phlegm is taken for granted as a problem among
children.

Within popular health culture drawing from ayurveda, each life stage is
thought to be dominated by particular kinds of body humors and associated
health problems. Childhood is dominated by phlegm. In accordance with folk
dietetics, phlegm is increased by sweet foods and reduced by chilies, which
assist in digestion. A child's sweet/bland diet (breastmilk) and the exclusion
of heating chilies make childhood a time prone to mucus-related illnesses.
Swelling and a bloating of the body (*kamale, tamare, krani*) are linked to
kapha, as are a white-coated tongue (*agra*) and mucus-laden diarrhea.
Children are also thought to have more problems with lice, ringworm, and
roundworms than adults, due to an accumulation of phlegm. Likewise,
mucus-related respiratory problems are considered ubiquitous during this
developmental stage. For this reason a child may not be brought to a
practitioner until these health problems become acute. This is not to say
parents are not concerned about keeping *kapha* in check, however. This
brings up a second reason for surprise at the survey data. A number of
preventive home remedies are routinely administered to manage *kapha* (see
Appendix). Moreover, a number of the medicines administered for *agra, bala
graha*, and *krani* have well-known *kapha* expulsion or reducing properties.

6. *Ancestor, spirits, and deities.* The South Kanarese cosmology is composed of a complex of ancestor spirits, patron spirits associated with various
domains of personal and social space, and wandering, hungry, malevolent
spirits, in addition to Pan-Indian deities (Claus 1973, Nichter 1977). Contact
with any of these spirits outside the ritual context, be it through wrath or
affection, is capable of causing a wide range of illnesses. Illnesses associated
with spirits are typically either sudden and acute, or longstanding, even after
the best of treatment has been secured. This means that any illness can be
interpreted as caused or compounded by spirits or deities. Such being the
case, surveys of etiology can at best produce generalizations about which
illnesses are more prone to be immediately linked to spirit intrusion. From
this data one can attempt to look for patterns between particular spirits and
illnesses.

According to survey findings, *bala graha* and *pakki kadapu* are the two of
the seven illnesses most immediately associated with spirits and deities.
However, as mentioned earlier, a child having a set of symptom attributes
more closely matching another illness category may be perceived as having
bala graha if spirit attack is suspected for other reasons (such as the time of

occurrence). From a sample of nine children brought to a Primary Health Center and identified by their families as suffering from *bala graha*, seven had already been taken to an astrologer or exorcist for ritual protection. It is of interest to note that among 71 percent of household survey informants who reported they had children who had experienced *bala graha*, and in six of the nine families observed, a young child in the household had died. The spirit of a child who dies with much desire for life is believed to "touch" living children, causing *bala graha*.[8]

7. *Heredity.* Thirty-seven percent of village survey informants stated that *agra* was hereditary and 48 percent stated that *tamare* was hereditary. The concept of *parampara* — translated as hereditary — has a number of distinct meanings. Follow-up research revealed that in reference to the two illnesses *parampara* indicated that the illness had been passed on from mother to child through breastmilk. No informant linked the illness to the father's bloodline, but two informants (one from a matrilineal and the other from a patrilineal caste) linked *tamare* to the mother's bloodline. In both cases, the mother had herself experienced the illness in childhood. Although several fathers reported experiencing one of these illnesses, this was not explicitly linked to ideas about risk.

8. *Contagion.* A notion voiced by three-informants was that *pakki kadapu* could be contracted by a child stepping over the feces or urine of another child having the illness.

9. *Sin, Karma, Stars and Planets.* As noted elsewhere (Chapter four), most villagers do not speak of their own illnesses as resulting from *papa* (sin) or *karma*. These factors are more commonly an attribution made by others. Elicited survey data is therefore hardly illustrative of feelings about *papa/karma* as an ultimate, as distinct from an instrumental, etiological cause of illness (Glick 1967; Polgar 1972).

Bad stars and planets were deemed instrumental causes of the illnesses *pakki kadapu* and *bala graha*. One cause of *pakki kadapu* (literally, bird crossing), noted on the survey, was a bird crosssing over a child or pregnant women's legs when just awakening from sleep. By the doctrine of correspondence, the child developing the illness comes to look like a bird with wings (legs) tucked in. By analogical extension, one popular astrologer in the region spoke of this illness as caused by a bad star crossing over the child. This explanation had gained regional popularity.

INAPPROPRIATE DIET

By far, folk dietetics proved to be the major cognitive domain of etiological reasoning for five of the seven illnesses. Among all families actually experiencing *agra, chappe, tamare,* and *krani,* inappropriate diet was noted in the illness narrative they related.

While states of malnutrition are linked to inappropriate diet, lay concepts of appropriate diet are markedly different from that of biomedicine. For example, *agra* is linked to indigestible breastmik. One of the most common causes of indigestible breastmilk is an insufficient consumption of chillies and other spicy/heating foods by a mother after delivery. These foods are considered to enhance the mother's digestive capacity (her "cooking fire") and to decrease the *kapha* (mucus) content of her breastmilk, an excess of which can cause *agra*.

In the case of *chappe roga, tamare roga*, and *krani*, a common etiological notion was that the child's digestive system had been disrupted by the introduction of foods too difficult to digest at such an early age. A Westerner would surely concur with the South Indian notion that these illnesses can be caused by hot curry introduced in a child's diet too early. A more common notion, however, was that green leafy vegetables introduced in the diet too early — before a child was a year and a half old — could cause these illnesses. Green vegetables (those deemed to have cooling qualities) are considered too difficult to digest for a young child who is not able to consume chillies as a digestive aid.

Another important notion is that *krani* can be caused by a mother breastfeeding while pregnant. Breastfeeding a child while pregnant is not culturally approved. In reality it is not uncommon among the very poor. This practice is linked to other childhood illnesses such as *kivi soruvudu* — otitis media. Two ideas coexist as to why breastfeeding at this time is bad. In the case of *krani*, the mother's breastmilk is deemed to have become indigestible. In the case of *kivi soruvudu*, it is believed that an unborn child becomes jealous of the nurture being given to its sibling. This jealousy is capable of causing developmental problems in the fetus. *Kivi soruvudu* is considered a developmental defect resulting from this jealousy.

ACTUAL EXPERIENCE OF ILLNESS

Experience of the seven illnesses within the recent past (3 years) was elicited during the household survey. The most commonly experienced illness reported among both village and town informant families was *agra*, followed by *chappe roga* and *tamare*. *Pakki kadapu* (rickets) and *kamale* as acute jaundice (not simply yellow excretions) were the least commonly reported illnesses. Town and village experience of childhood illness was similar with the exception of *agra* which was 60 percent more common in village areas. Due to problems of recall, this data needs to be considered impressionistic.

TREATMENT: PATTERNS OF RESORT

Before considering data on health care seeking behavior for the seven illnesses, it is insightful to provide some background on home care behavior in relation to each. As was well pointed out by Parker et al. (1979), home care is perhaps the most important health care resource in the developing world. This is particularly the case for children in South Kanara. I will briefly focus on preventive-promotive home care first and then move on to consider curative care.

Folk preventive/promotive health behavior has received relatively little attention by medical anthropologists.[9] In fact some anthropolgists have questioned the ability of "traditional people" to conceptualize serious illness as developing slowly without visible manifest symptoms (Foster and Anderson 1978). The aforementioned researchers go on to suggest:

> Since much of preventive medicine is based on the philosophy of taking action before illness appears, through immunization that prevents it, or through early detection that increases the likelihood of successful treatment. traditional peoples are not the best candidates for this branch of medicine.(1978: 232)

In village India, childhood is replete with symptom states. A major health concern of South Kanarese villagers is to prevent existing or anticipated symptoms (such as *kapha*) from becoming worse. A distinction between curative and preventive medicine becomes obscured because prevention denotes both promoting positive health and preventing existing ill health from becoming worse (Nichter 1983).

In respect to villagers having a poor sense of preventive health, I would disagree that action is not taken before illness appears, although in respect to early detection I would concur with the aforementioned researchers. South Kanarese villagers maintain a number of ideas about preventive measures to assure child health, concepts which both converge with and diverge from biomedical conceptualization. Let us take a look at some of these.

In South Kanara, preventive/promotive treatment begins at birth itself, when a child is given a few drops of the juice of *kepala* (Ixorea coccinea) to cleanse its digestive tract, at once preparing the child to receive nourishment and to prevent *agra*. Most preventive/promotive behavior centers around 5 themes: digestive capacity, purification, attuning a child's development to the ecosphere, reducing *kapha*, and controlling worms. There is a saying in ayurveda that hunger is the first disease and the stomach is the source of all disease thereafter (Egnor 1978; Nichter 1977). The digestive process is a central health concern among villagers, especially during childhood. A mother seeks to "kindle" her child's developing digestive capacity by food which does not "smother the digestive fire." The order in which foods are introduced during weaning reflects cultural notions of their digestibility (Nichter 1984b). "Hard to digest" foods are withheld from a child until condiments, most notably chillies, can be consumed as a digestive aid. While condiments are withheld, promotive medicines such as the bark of the *inde* (Caryota urens) tree are given to a child to assist in the development of digestive capacity.

Purification accords with largely hydraulic imagery-cognition of body physiology. Many kinds of illnesses are deemed to be caused by or result in a build up of impurities which impede normal body cycles. Channels (*narambu*) in the body are thought to become obstructed by wastes perceived as "hard" indigestible substances.[10]

Many villagers routinely give their children purification medicines ranging from turmeric and sandalwood paste to commercially available ayurvedic blood purifers. Purification medicines are used to purify the blood, purge the digestive system of wastes, and prepare the body to "take to" herbal curative medicines (Nichter 1980). Up until the last decade, "branding," *suta gaya*, was administered to young children at junctions — joints — in the body as a means of enhancing the flow of blood by breaking down impurities which might become lodged at these points.

Zimmerman (1980) in his description of ayurvedic epistemology notes that a conceptualization of a cosmic flow of ecological relationships within the universe and within man is central to ayurveda. Bodily processes are continuous with the ecosphere. This notion underlies an important form of lay promotive health behavior in South Kanara. During winter season a bitter tonic prepared from the young shoots of auspicious trees is given to young children as a preventive/promotive medicine.[11] This tonic (known as *kanir madhu*) is given to enhance the development of the child's digestive capacity and to purify the blood. Symbolically, by incorporating the essence of development from within nature, the child (according to the doctrine of correspondence) becomes attuned to the flow of development within the ecosphere.

As noted earlier, a health concern which underscores much preventive/ promotive health behavior is the reduction and control of *kapha*. Most families administer some form of herbal medicine to their children to keep *kapha* in check. Common medicines used to expel *kapha* include *baje* (Acrorus calamus) and *tulasi* (Ocimum sanctum). Diet is mediated to control *kapha* accumulation, particularly during times associated with coolness.

A final health concern is intestinal worms, *puri*. According to local health culture, a limited number of "worms of life" are required to assist in the digestive process. These "worms of life" (*jiva da puri*) assist in the "churning of food and the cleaning of the stomach pot." Worms are present from infancy itself having been passed on from mother to child via breastmilk. While a limited number of worms are considered necessary for life, an excess of worms is believed to lead to such health problems among children as stomach problems, fits, and respiratory ailments. As worms are thought to multiply in an environment of sweetness and *kapha*, preventive medicines are given to children to calm the overactivity and overproduction of worms.

The Appendix provides examples of popular preventive medicines for specific children's illnesses. The most common preventive medicines administered to children are for *tamare* and *bala graha*. *Bala graha* pills are the most widely used over-the-counter preventive medicine in the region. They are stocked by ayurvedic practitioners, herbal compounders, and exorcists, and are available in many local provision stores. A number of distinct *bala graha* pill utilization patterns exist. Some families administer this medication on a daily or biweekly basis while others administer it on no moon or full moon days, vulnerable times associated with spirit activity. Still others administer the medication when a child exhibits fear, wakes suddenly at night, or experiences wheezing.

HOME CURATIVE TREATMENT

Survey data (see Table 3) revealed that a majority of village families had knowledge of and anticipated using a home remedy should any of the seven illnesses befall a child. Case follow-up data indicated that 75 percent of

TABLE III. Patterns of Resort for Illnesses Associated with Childhood Malnutrition.

				Illness Categories		
	Agra	Chappe Roga/ Tamare	Krani	Kamale (as jaundice)	Pakki Kadapu	Bala Graha/ Chinne
Illness Experience in Family Within Recent Past (3 months)	T[a]: 30% V[b]: 48%	T: 26% V: 24%	T: 19% V: 24%	T: — V: 8%	T: — V: 4%	T: 15% V: 12%
Case Strategy[c]						
Use or Anticipated Use of Home Remedy[d]	T: 66% V: 92%	T: 44% V: 100%	T: 41% V: 92%	T: 19% V: 68%	T: 22% V: 52%	T: 52% V: 96%
Exorcist	—	—	—	—	T: 33% V: 64%	T: 26% V: 52%
Ayurveda	T: 19% V: 24%	T: 33% V: 40%	T: 26% V: 16%	T: 19% V: 28%	T: 33% V: 48%	T: 26% V: 44%
Cosmopolitan (Allopathic)	T: 33% V: 32%	T: 33% V: 40%	T: 44% V: 20%	T: 67% V: 52%	T: 15% V: —	T: 44% V: 16%
Other	—	—	—	—	T: 20%[e] V: 20%[f]	—

[a] Town (T): n = 27 households.
[b] Village (V): n = 25 households.
[c] Open-ended survey: all care strategies reported were given equal weight.
[d] Obtained from ayurvedic vaidya or exorcist.
[e] Offerings to deities.
[f] Astrologer.

village families bringing a child to a popular cosmopolitan doctor with one of the seven illnesses[12] (n = 40) had first used a home remedy in addition to dietary manipulation. Villagers' knowledge of home curative (noncommercial) medicine was considerably greater than townspeople's knowledge. Only in the case of *agra* did a majority of town informants indicate knowledge of a traditional home remedy.

The most common form of family self-health care, dietary manipulation, was not figured in the survey results reported in Table III. Dietary manipulation was engaged in by all families interviewed where a child was actually experiencing one of the seven illnesses. All survey families explicitly identified dietary change as important for the treatment of the seven illnesses. Generally speaking far more informants had clear ideas about the type of foods which needed to be restricted during these illnesses than about the types of food advantageous to consume. Folk dietetic behavior actually followed was sensitive to the nature of the illness and the qualities of medication taken (Nichter 1986).

Of those children identified as suffering from second- and third-degree malnutrition (measured by mid-arm circumference) this condition was far more often exacerbated by folk dietary behavior than helped. Children exhibiting signs of any of the seven illnesses were typically placed on a bland tasteless diet with most green leafy vegetables and fruits, pulses, oils, and fish restricted. What might start as riboflavin deficiency, thrush, or yeast infection (labeled as *agra*) often developed into a exacerbated marasmic kwashiorkor due to the child's diminished appetite (in response to bland food) and restricted diet.

Two additional dietary restrictions during children's illnesses need to be briefly highlighted. The first involves the child's consumptions of liquids. A child's daily liquid consumption was not uncommonly restricted up to 50 percent during illness episodes where swelling, fever, or diarrhea was present. This was due to a general fear that liquid consumption, particularly when one is immobile, results in a swelling of the body, and an increase in fecal output when one has diarrhea. This fear indirectly contributed to states of dehydration. A second restriction involves the diet of the breastfeeding mother when an infant is ill. This restriction accords with the concept that the quality of breastmilk is affected by the foods a woman consumes. Restriction of the mother's diet may further exacerbate her own nutritional deficiencies.

AYURVEDA (HERBALISTS)

Before reviewing survey and observational data on health care resort (see Table III) to ayurvedic practitioners, three points need be made:

1. The survey results from the first 1978 pattern-of-resort study and those from the second study reported here differ in large part because of the

presence of two esteemed ayurvedic practitioners, *vaidya*, in the first study area and only folk *vaidya* in the second study area.

2. Common folk treatment for six of the seven children's illnesses under study was consistent with common ayurvedic treatment. The regional ayurvedic tradition has been strongly influenced by folk medicine. Popular health culture has been and continues to be influenced by ayurveda. Medicines used in the home treatments for all seven illnesses except *pakki kadapu* were important ingredients in more complex ayurvedic treatments which were "system" as well as symptom oriented. It is therefore advantageous to consider folk and ayurvedic medicine as a composite of herbal therapy, when making generalizations about health care behavior.

3. In a number of cases, ayurvedic treatment is sought after an illness has been treated by an allopathic practitioner. Ayurvedic medicine is sought to purify the body and normalize body cycles after allopathic medicines have been employed to control dramatic symptom states. The survey data presented do not report the use of ayurvedic medicines for this purpose. Case study data collected at stock herbalists, at *vaidya*'s offices, and from follow-up interviews with patients consulting cosmopolitan doctors revealed that use of ayurvedic medicines for this purpose was common.

In terms of anticipatory health care seeking behavior, survey data suggest that over a third of informants would seek herbal ayurvedic treatment early for *chappe roga, tamare, pakki kadapu* and *bala graha*. If self-care and ayurveda are considered together as "traditional herbal treatment" this resource is by far the most popular recourse to treatment for six of the seven, illnesses studied particularly in village areas. Generally speaking, villagers consultation of ayurvedic practitioners for children's illness far exceeds that of townspeople even when the *vaidya* in question practices in town. Observational data revealed that use of modern ayurvedic medicines (commercial medicines) is unsurprisingly greater among townsfolk than village folk as an over-the-counter form of care for children.

COSMOPOLITAN MEDICINE

Cosmopolitan medication was deemed an appropriate health care resource by at least one-third of informants for the treatment of six of the seven illnesses in the town sample and five of the seven illnesses in the village sample. Only in the case of acute jaundice did a majority of informants from both field areas cite cosmopolitan medicine as a resource of choice. This latter pattern of resort was somewhat surprising, for ayurveda is renowned for jaundice medication and villagers not uncommonly seek ayurvedic medication for *pitta* resulting from allopathic medicines which turn their urine yellow or heat the body. Jaundice is associated with *pitta*. A follow-up study of five cases of florid jaundice being treated at a Primary Health Center revealed that consultation of a cosmopolitan practitioner was primarily related to adjunct symptoms, most notably bloody diarrhea, vomiting, and fever. Of the five patients suffering from *kamale*, one child and two adults undertook ayurvedic treatment within a month of their treatment at the Primary Health Center.

Ten allopathic practitioners were interviewed about the prevalence of malnutrition in the district, folk dietetics, and their health education role. All displayed considerable frustration when addressing the topic. Indeed, the most common comment was that while their medications were sought for management of acute symptoms associated with malnutrition, their health and dietary advice was generally disregarded after the symptoms had been managed.

MIXED CARE

Health care seeking for the seven children's illnesses under study was often not limited to one medical system. This is revealed in the *kamale* cases noted above. It also became apparent from clinic interviews. Four children identified by parents as suffering from *tamare* and three as suffering from *krani* were interviewed. Five of these children had received a combination of ayurvedic and home herbal treatment before consulting the Primary Health Center doctor. In a complementary study at the office of a *vaidya*, of five cases identified by family members as *tamare* and three cases as *krani*, four had already consulted a Primary Health Center doctor. Six of these eight children had received home treatment for two weeks or more prior to their visit to the *vaidya*.

EXORCISM, ASTROLOGY, AND OFFERINGS TO DEITIES

According to the survey, exorcists would most often be resorted to in cases of *pakki kadapu* and *bala graha*. Again, it need be remembered that if a symptom set is suspected to be associated with spirits, it is likely to be labeled *bala graha*. Sittings with exorcists and astrologers revealed that all cases of suspected *bala graha* (n = 12) and *pakki kadapu* (n = 2) were divined as the *dosha* (trouble) of stars or spirits. A pattern was observed that the higher the caste and the more educated the afficted family, the more likely that stars and planets would play a more prominent role in divination than spirits. The lower the caste, the more likely it was that spirits would be discussed rather than stars. In all cases observed, the afflicted was given ritual treatment as well as being referred to either *vaidya* or doctors for complementary treatment. Of four exorcists observed, one referred all clients to a particular ayurvedic *vaidya*, whereas the other three differentially referred clients to *vaidya* or doctors. They most often requested a client to seek a practitioner in a particular direction or to think of a practitioner who was then sanctioned by a divination procedure such as a toss of the cowry shells.

Observational data on offerings to two deities renowned as protectors of children revealed that offerings were commonly made for all longstanding illnesses where fever, fits, bloody diarhea, or skin ailments (often associated with the curse of a cobra) were manifest. A separate data set was collected at shrines of village patron spirits during yearly village possession cult rituals (*kola, nema*). During these rituals possessed spirit dancers converse with the family of the afflicted and state reasons for their difficulties. A child's illness of a sudden or persistent nature was commonly linked either to sorcery by an enemy — for which one needed the deities' protection — or to an unfulfilled vow made in the immediate or distant past by an unspecified family member. As the most vulnerable family member, the child was afflicted as a sign of what would befall the entire family if action were not taken. Devotees would most commonly offer a *harike* — a promised offering — and the deity would offer promises that there would be success in treatment currently sought. A typical *harike* might be "if such and such medicine is successful, I promise one cock to 'x', my family patron deity, in addition to any 'y' unfulfilled vow."

SIGNIFICANCE OF THE DATA FOR INTERNATIONAL HEALTH

The data presented suggest that marked states of children's malnutrition are recognized as a complex of illnesses by the South Kanarese lay population. Primary health care for these illnesses among the rural poor is largely a combination of herbal (folk and ayurvedic) remedies and dietary restrictions. Allopathic practitioners were accessible in the study area and popular for the treatment of many other ailments. For states of malnutrition they generally were not consulted for the seven children's illnesses cited until they became acute and accompanied by such symptoms as fever, respiratory ailments or skin complaints which interfere with sleeping patterns. Even then, not all acute symptom states were taken to cosmopolitan practitioners. Fits are a case in point. Research conducted between 1974—76 (Nichter 1978) revealed that fits, be they febrile fits or epilepsy, were commonly taken to exorcists or *vaidya* before doctors.

An assessment of folk dietetic behavior followed during these seven illnesses revealed that food restrictions were more commonly followed than dietary prescriptions among the poor to lower middle class. Food restrictions/reductions associated with the illnesses cited (as well as measles, diarrhea and skin ailments) were found to exacerbate and/or compound existing states of malnutrition, impede catch up growth, and set the stage for interactive infections. For example, dietary restrictions for *krani* and *tamare* exacerbate vitamin A deficiency as well as reduce calorie-protein intake.

Before dismissing folk health behavior as "negative", it is prudent to recognize that folk dietetics constitutes active household participation in promotive/preventive health care. Participation needs to be fostered in an age of quick fixes if dependency and medicalization of health is to be countered. It is therefore worth considering how health education efforts might be tailored to fit popular health culture in such a way as to facilitate better home care. In this regard a few tentative suggestions may be made both with respect to the training of community health workers and the involvement of ayurvedic practitioners in promotive health efforts involving diet.

First, health educators could identify, and health education efforts address, folk illness categories and the major health concerns of the lay population. Emic categories of illness might be a viable springboard from which to initiate meaningful dialogue with mothers about health behavior.[13] Such dialogue might focus on the perceived severity of and susceptibility to clearly recognized illnesses like *tamare*, not culturally distant disease categories like marasmus or protein/calorie malnutrition. This would constitute a "grounded" as opposed to a "paternalistic" approach, to health education. Such an approach would foster a participatory problem-solving process as distinct from a didactic health education monologue. Concordantly, those designing training courses for community health workers might explore the possibility of developing health care decision trees and algorithms oriented toward a differential diagnosis of popular folk illness categories, rather than ignoring local conceptualization.

This suggestion goes beyond the treatment of states of malnutrition. Currently popular in international health are algorithms for the diagnosis and care of diarrheal and respiratory diseases. These algorithms are based on severity and draw attention to degrees of dehydration, rates of breathing etc. While useful as field guides for paramedical staff, these algorithms are less useful to outreach workers engaged in community education. Field staff engaged in health education need to address those sets of symptoms which influence lay health care decision making and health care seeking. Research is needed to identify those combinations of symptoms which influence health care behavior. Algorithms based on emically grouped sets of symptoms are worth experimenting with as an educational tool.[14]

Both the classification of illness and notions of illness etiology are dynamic. Taking this into consideration, innovative health education efforts may be developed based on a convergence model of communication (Kincaid 1979; Rogers and Kincaid 1982) and a negotiation model of health/nutrition education (Katon and Kleinman 1980; Kincaid et al. 1983; Nichter and Nichter 1981; Nichter and Rizvi 1985). The key to a negotiation model of education is paying credence to pervasive lay health concerns, contingent cultural values, and the implications of responsibility attribution. Lay and biomedical health conceptualizations converge on a number of points such as mutual concerns about blood quality and quantity, the quality of breastmilk, a child's digestive power, etc. (Nichter 1986). Approaches to health education which maximize these points of convergence and nutrition programs which build on the mutual accommodation of indigenous and biomedical health concerns work from emic to etic notions of risk and health promotion. It may be possible to present biomedical concerns for calories, protein, and vitamins with or in terms of folk dietetic concepts (e.g. hot/cold, body humors, blood, digestive capability).

Project Poshak provides a case in point. This CARE-sponsored weaning food project found through necessity that nutritional advice and weaning foods could be developed to meet both biomedical and folk health criteria.

The concept of hot and cold food was firmly entrenched in the rural population of Madhya Pradesh and was fairly rigidly followed with regard to foods appropriate for the hot, cold and rainy season and for the maintenance of health as the treatment of illness. These concepts were reinforced by rural practitioners of the ayurvedic and unani medical systems. These beliefs must be known and understood in order to design and carry out a successful program of nutrition intervention, and particularly to overcome the reluctance of mothers to give any form of supplementary food to children under one year of age or to offer solid or semi-solid food to children under age two. Information gathered from the surveys showed that there were various foods and combinations of food that fell within the traditional system and could be recommended for use as weaning foods in appropriate seasons. (Gopaladas et al 1975: 78)

How will traditional practitioners respond to such attempts to contextualize health education? Will ayurvedic *vaidya* be willing to participate in such endeavors? I would contend that they are far less resistant to the incorporation of new health ideas than they are oft times made out to be by self-styled spokesmen. In rural South India, a process of "scientization" is readily apparent among both graduates of integrated colleges of ayurvedic medicine and rural hereditary practitioners often described as conservative. Many *vaidya* are presently making an attempt to interpret, reinterpret, and adapt ayurvedic and folk health ideology to accord with newly assimilated scientific information provided by lay experience with pump sets, electricity, etc. Through analogical reasoning, science is being accommodated if not encompassed by tradition, not rejected. This is a two-way process. In one sense, scientization is a modern-day counterpart to the process of sanskritization. Just as local deities have been elevated to Pan-Indian status, local health ideas are at times elevated to modern "scientific" status. In other cases, the latter take on indigenous meanings and identities. An appreciation of the process of scientization and its relationship to a classical "teaching by analogy" approach may lead health educators to consider how they might employ analogical reasoning in culturally meaningful health communication (Chapter 11). Toward this end the communication skills of ayurvedic practitioners and their knowledge of local referential frameworks could contribute to collaborative health education endeavors.

What about the responsiveness of these practitioners to engage in such collaborative endeavors? On this issue, let me cite data from a survey of 25 *vaidya* (formally and nonformally trained ayurvedic practitioners) conducted in 1976. The survey queried practitioner's attitudes toward modern scientific discoveries. It revealed that a majority (76 percent) of these practitioners were willing, if not enthusiastic, to learn new diagnostic skills and means of treating specific ailments. The six *vaidya* who were disinterested were all above 55 years of age. Notably, when promotive health was discussed, all 25 of these practitioners expressed the view that ayurveda was a far more developed system of promotive health than allopathy. However, when asked about ayurveda's present role in community health, 92 percent of these informants expressed dissatisfaction with ayurveda's public efforts in promoting community health. Most informants stated that the government was uninterested in directly involving ayurveda in mass education efforts although it supported the building of ayurvedic dispensaries and colleges. A question was posed about the need for ayurveda to adapt to changing life conditions in modern India. Most practitioners (84 percent) stated that ayurvedic treatment needed to adapt to changing ecology and life-style in order to make an impact on the public. These data suggest that the term "traditional practitioner" better identifies one who applies traditional knowledge/principles in the service of problem solving, than one who is limited by past and static knowledge.

Given the present emphasis of professional associations and the priority health needs of the country, a paradox is highlighted by the sober views of these "traditional" practitioners.[15] Although ayurveda as the "science of life" is fundamentally oriented toward promotive health — the relationship between an individual and the environment — most of the emphasis of professional ayurvedic medical associations has been on curative therapy. This is indicative of just how medicalized ayurveda has become in its fight to establish credibility in response to the challenge of biomedicine. Indeed one could argue that what is being promoted by ayurvedic associations is a form of ayurapathy (Johannis Laping, personal communication).

In this regard, Leslie notes:

> . . . except for a brief period during the independence movement, they [ayurveda and unani] have failed to project ideas about designing a culturally appropriate system of health services. They have concentrated on problems in curative medicine and on reinterpretations of ancient theories, neglecting the problems of how to use indigenous sources to create a national system of social and preventive care. The ecological character of humoral tradition could have made this their strongest point. (1983: 75)

A health education process responsive to ayurvedic thinking about "acquired appropriateness" (*okaksātmya*) with respect to daily routine (*dinacariya*), seasonal routine (*rtucarya*) and habituation (*avcitya*), might well be more acceptable to the lay population than present health education programs which are largely unresponsive to lay thinking. This would more certainly be the case if ayurvedic thinking could be adapted to the real-life contingencies, economic constraints, and resources of the poor. While I disagree with Opler (1962) that villagers' concepts of illness closely follow ayurvedic doctrine, I concur with Khare (1963) that the ideas — more accurately, the health concerns — of ayurveda stand closer to the elements of popular health culture than those of comopolitan medicine. This makes ayurveda an especially important promotive health care resource, for the lay population is far less impressed with cosmopolitan promotive health than curative medicine. This is readily apparent with respect to nutritional advice. In a two-district survey (n = 282) conducted in 1979 (Nichter 1984) it was found that a large majority of informants deemed cosmopolitan doctors to know much about the treatment of illness, but little about what diet was necessary for the health and well-being of the poor in different seasons. With regard to the seven children's illnesses discussed in this paper, most informants who frequented cosmopolitan practitioners noted that they would follow dietary advice (when affordable) only for the duration of the treatment. Follow-up research on this point revealed that many informants considered their doctor's general dietary advice to be a specific part of medical treatment. Dietary advice was compartmentalized in the context of treatment, not integrated as general life knowledge.

India has implemented a community health worker scheme which is praiseworthy in intention and direction, but vague with respect to specific objectives (Pyle 1981: 144). Community health workers trained thus far have tended to place emphasis on the treatment of minor ailments, activities most desired by the community and easiest to deliver, while allocating little time to health education efforts engendering behavioral change. Nowhere is this more apparent than in the domain of nutrition education. The language of CHW texts is jargon ridden and incomprehensible to the villager (Srivastva 1978). Nutritional advice is culturally insensitive and economically not viable (Bose et al. 1978), a groups-at-risk approach is notably absent, and crucial subjects such as oral rehydration are buried amidst brief discussions of minor ailments (Pyle 1981: 144).

Those nutrition messages which do exist, do not distinguish advice for the healthy from advice for the ill. Mothers with children who are ill or weak, commonly interpret general nutrition messages as being for healthy children, an impression supported by posters depicting chubby, healthy babies. It needs to be recognized that a significant proportion of children under two and between 2 and 5 years, are ill for a significant proportion of the year.[16] Mothers commonly deem ill or weak children to be too vulnerable for the changes in diet advocated by health workers and for preventive health interventions such as immunizations (Nichter 1989).

These children are doubly at risk. They are caught in a malnutrition-infection cycle where the replenishing of nutrient stores and catch-up growth is forestalled by a complex of factors. Often, malnutrition is initiated by illness (e.g. diarrhea, respiratory tract infections, measles). Increased nutrient demands associated with illness (Rohde 1978) are compounded by physiological states which often decrease nutrient absorption. Increased nutrient needs are met by lower nutrient intakes associated with faltering appetite, particularly prominent in diarrheal diseases and measles (Pereira and Begun 1987), as well as patterns of folk dietetics which restrict and reduce nutrient intake.[17] Among the poor the following of food restrictions is more common than food prescriptions. An ill child is placed on a restricted diet during illness as well as during convalescence if the child's digestive capacity, skin erruptions, or mucus production etc. constitute a lay health concern. When the cycle of malnutrition-infection repeats in short order, a child may be labeled constitutionally weak. Where food resources are scarce, the household may come to invest less resources in this child than in others deemed to have a better chance at survival (given such variables as gender, birth order, family composition etc).

This scenario is bleak. A mother's concern for her child often underlies her non compliance with health advice; advice she interprets as possibly appropriate for the healthy, but not the ill. Following new dietary advice or receiving an immunization is deemed risky at a time of existing vulnerability. The point being raised, is that special nutrition and immunization follow up programs need to be developed for those caught in a malnutrition-infection cycle and deemed to be constitutionally weak by mothers.[18] If general nutrition advice is interpreted to relate to healthy children and is not followed during illness, then illness specific nutrition education/intervention needs to be developed to accord with folk dietetics and available seasonal nutrient resources. Attention needs to be paid to the indigenious perceptions of risk understood by mothers if states of malnutrition related to illness are to be reduced by means of diet.

Children caught in a cycle of interactive infections predisposed or complicated by malnutrition suffer from chronic states of ill health not numbers of illness episodes per year (Chen 1986). Mothers understand that these children are vulnerable and need to be treated differently than other children. Rodhe (1978) has aptly noted that :

No therpeutic goal is as important as the rapid recovery of pre-illness weight gain after infection. Since the mother is the only person who can effectively manage convalescent care, she must be given specific tasks with measurable targets in order to reliably oversee the child's rehabilitation. Not generally considered in the realm of preventive medicine, effective homebased convalescent care is the first crucial step in preventing the next round of illness. Rather than a passive recipient of health services, the mother becomes the basic health worker, providing diagnostic and therapeutic primary care for her child. Only the mother can break the malnutrition- infection cycle.

Involving caretakers in primary health care at the level of diet entails meaningful as well as specific tasks. In order to structure tasks which make sense nutritionally as well as culturally, health workers will have to pay credence to emic measures of health and the diagnosis of illness.

NOTES

Acknowledgments. An Indo-U.S. Subcommission Grant on Education and Culture awarded to the author from November 1979 to August 1980 facilitated the research upon which this paper is based. Research was conducted between October 1979 and November 1980 in the Bantval, Vitla, Puttur, and Beltangadi Taluks of South Kanara District, Karnataka State. I would like to acknowledge Dr. K. H. Bhat for his assistance in coordinating the family illness survey noted in this paper and to the local interviewers who participated in this survey from June to August 1980. Special thanks go to Mimi Nichter who assisted in research on the language of illness, and to the many *vaidya* and Primary Health Center field staff who allowed us entry into their clinics and homes. A shorter version of this paper was presented at the Annual Meeting of the National Council for International Health held at Washington D.C. in June 1983.

1. Kakar et al. (1972 raise this point in respect to pneumonia and neonatal tetanus in the Punjab. Nichter (1978) raises the same issue in relation to "fits" and measles in southwest India. These critical incapacitating dysfunctions are commonly taken to traditional practioners.

2. In regard to the routine pattern of resort surveys. Leslie (1980) notes:

   These surveys are misleading because they assume modes of thought that are alien to members of these societies . . . They assume people everywhere use the perspective of cosmopolitan medicine in which specific illnesses have specific causes and therapies . . . The questionnaires assume the universality of individualistic decision-making and of dyadic doctor-patient interactions which are normative for the clinical practice of cosmopolitan medicine in industrial countries, but not for other societies and forms of practice.

   In another paper, Leslie (1983) notes:

   The surveys . . . assume wrongly that laymen have ideological preferences in these matters, and that they consistently follow a disease conception of illness.

3. D'Andrade (1976) has found that in both North America and Mexico, people are more concerned with the preconditions and consequences of an illness than in illness atributes. On the issue of medicine influencing the naming and classification of illness, two examples may be cited. *Chappe* is a term denoting "tasteless." *Chappe roga* is an illness for which ayurvedic *vaidya* recommend a saltless and condimentless diet. A recent illness category, "liver," has symptoms similar to *chappe* and *tamare*. "Liver" denotes an illness for which doctors prescribe such popular B-complex tonics as "Liv 52." The advertisements of companies such as Jammy portray "liver ailments" with pictures of a protruding stomach. This has contributed to the popular conception of the illness. *Bala graha* is called *chinne* on two accounts. In Tulu (the regional language) *chinne* means "sign" as in "sign of spirit attact." In Sanskrit and Kannada (the state language), *chinne* means gold. Gold is an important component of ayurvedic *bala graha* medication.

4. Young (1981) notes in response to Jantzen's (1978) concept of the family as a "therapy managing group" that the family is usually invoked in complex and prolonged cases which involve collective decision making. My own observation is that collective negotiation increases in relation to the expenditure of resources — time as well as money — on care, as well as the general annoyance level of the symptoms in respect to family well-being.

5. This is not to suggest that the differential diagnosis of *kamale* or *pakki kadapu* is straightforward. Yellowing of the eyes may be indicative of either *kamale* or *grahani*. In two cases of rickets where an ayurvedic *vaidya* was consulted, families had doubts as to whether the illness was *krani* or *pakki kadapu*, and *bala graha* or *pakki kadapu*. In one case of rickets brought to a cosmopolitan doctor, the child also had night blindness. This symptom set confounded the family in respect to illness classification, but not cause. The *vak* (curse) of an enemy had been divined by an astrologer. One family I interviewed had a 4-year-old child with bowed legs which the family insisted was a constitutional (*prakṛti*) disorder. During the interview, they noted that the child had experienced *bala graha* for two years.

6. A different notion of illness latency was expressed by six survey informants. They stated that both *agra* and *chinne* were latent in all children, but manifest in only some. These six informants placed particular importance on administering preventive medicines to their children.

7. As I have noted elsewhere (Nichter 1980), *pitta* and *kapha* are terms designating interdependent body humors in ayurveda, but to the layperson they are manifest symptom states.

8. In the Punjab, the illness "*soka*," which Kakar identifies as marasmus, was attributed to supernatural causes by 89 percent of respondents participating in a health survey (n = 60). Eighty-two percent of these respondents expressed a preference for treatment by folk practitioners (Kakar et al. 1972). Kakar notes that the illness was associated with the spirit (literally, shadow) of a child who had died during the breastfeeding stage. A similar idea exists in South Kanara. In South Kanara a few informants stated that *chinne* and *bala graha* were stages of an illness complex. *Chinne* was a sign that the spirit of a dead child (*kule*) was affecting the health of a living child. Their perception was that a *kule* could only control a living child until the age of seven. After this age the child became too strong for the *kule* to control. *Bala graha* could develop out of *chinne* if the spirit was not controlled and the symptoms of *chinne* were not treated.

9. Exceptions are Colson (1971), Paul (1963), and Hughes (1978). Hughes (1978) has emphasized that folk medicine has an important preventive component concordant with a wide range of "social purposes" having broad implications for health. Discussion of the latter are beyond the scope of this paper.

10. As Egnor (1978) has documented, a cooking metaphor for the digestive process is shared by ayurvedic practitioners and villagers alike. Growing rice is likened to being cooked (ripened) in the fields by the sun and rain, again in the kitchen by fire, and then in the body via the processes of digestion. This involves a continuous process of refinement and "softening of substances." Substances spoken of as "hard" by villagers denote substances at once hard to digest and substances blocking the flow of body processes.

11. The winter season, although having the lowest seasonal mortality rate and fewest epidemic diseases, is deemed the worst season for health by many villagers because it is the season of the most extreme temperature fluctuations. The only time period considered worse for health is the month of *Ati* (July—August), during the monsoons, a time when preventive medicines for *tamare* and stomach sores are taken.

12. Lay illness terms were not cited to doctors but were rather elicited by the researcher. Cited were symptoms. Sometimes, symptoms were accurate descriptions of body states, sometimes indicators of distress to impress the practitioner with the seriousness of the case, and sometimes causal presuppositions. For example, *jwara* (literally fever) would be cited when fever was present, or when overheat was suspected as being involved as a causal factor, or because villagers know fever impresses cosmopolitan doctors.

13. On a related note, Nations (1986) has argued that both descriptive and analytic epidemiology may be enhanced by a consideration of folk illnesses. Following Pfifferling (1975), she has recognized the benefits of using a folk illness morbidity profile to enhance morbidity surveillance.

14. Bomgaars (1976) and Nations (1986) have similarly argued that emic perceptions of risk such as "angel eyes" for dehydration, or the folk illness "*runche*" for undernutrition may be used to generate high risk profiles for life threatening health problems. What is important is not only the use of native illness categories but descriptions of symptoms in natural language.

15. More than one *vaidya* pointed out to me that the process of adapting ayurvedic principles to India's diverse and changing socioeconomic contexts was nothing new. Indeed this process was responsible for the generation of regional ayurvedic traditions. According to these *vaidya* discontinuities in ayurvedic practice — not epistemology (Zimmerman 1978) — result from attempts to apply ayurvedic principles and develop regimes appropriate to distinct ecological contexts and life styles.

On a related note, Tarwick (1987) has described ayurvedic physicians as recognizing the "provisionality of knowledge" and struggling to adjust to coexisting theories of health and medical treatment. A responsiveness and affinity toward ecological approaches to health might provide health educators an entry point into dialogue with *vaidya* about promotive health, groups at risk, life style, environmental and occupational health.

16. For example, see illness prevalence data collected by Kamath et al (1969) and Rao et al (1970, 1971) in India; Black et al (1982) in Bangladesh; Martorell et al (1975) in Guatemala; and McAuliffe et al (1985) in Brazil. Rao et al. report a monthly morbidity rate among rural South Indian infants of 77% with a pre-school rate of 71%. The average duration of sickness among both groups is between 5—6 weeks per year.

17. Studies by Martorell et al. (1980); Brown et al. (1985) and Pereira and Begun (1987) have increased our knowledge of nutrient intake during illness. Future studies on illness, diet and catch up growth need to be conducted which ascertain the relative significance of illness on appetite, nutrient absorption and seasonal growth differentials; as well as the impact of folk dietetics on nutrient intake during illness as well as convalescence.

18. Following Chen (1986) these children may more appropriately be seen as suffering from chronic illness (ill health) than being at risk to acute disease.

REFERENCES

Andrews, S.
　　1973　*Feasibility of Involving Indigenous Medicine Practitioners for Family Planning Service Delivery in Kerala, India.* Ph.D. dissertation, Department of International Health, Johns Hopkins University.

Beals, A.
　　1976　Strategies of Resort to Curers in South India. *In* C. Leslie (ed.), *Asian Medical Systems: A Comparative Study.* Berkeley: University of California Press.

Black, R., K. Black, S. Becker et al.
　　1982　Longitudinal studies of infectious diseases and Physical Growth of Children in Rural Bangladesh: Patterns of Morbidity. *American Journal of Epidemiology 115*: 305—314.

Bomgaars, M. R.
　　1976　Undernutrition: Cultural Diagnosis and Treatment of Runche. *JAMA 236*: 22: 2513.

Bose, A., R. P. Goyal, S. R. Grover, K. G. Jolly, D. Madan, V. P. C. Sharma, and C. Singh.
　　1978　*An Assessment of the New Rural Health Scheme and Suggestions for Improvement.* Demographic Research Centre Institute of Economic Growth, University of Delhi, New Delhi, India.

Brown, K., R. Black, A. Robertson et al.
　　1985　Effects of Season and Illness on the Dietary Intake of Weanlings during Longitudinal Studies in Rural Bangladesh. *American Journal of Clincial Nutrition 41*: 343—355.

Chen, L.
　　1986　Primary Health Care in Developing Countries: Overcoming Operational, Technical and Social Barriers. *Lancet*, Nov. 29, 1260—1265.

Claus, P.
　　1973　Possession, Protection and Punishment as Attributes of Deities in a South Indian Village. *Man in India 53*(3): 231—242.

Colson, A. C.
　　1971　The Prevention of Illness in a Malay Village: An Analysis of Concepts and Behavior. *Medical Behavioral Science, No. 1.* Winston-Salem, N. C: Overseas Research Center.

D'Andrade, R.
　　1976　A Propositional Analysis of U.S. American Beliefs about Illness. *In* K. H. Basso and

H. A. Selby, (eds). *Meanings in Anthropology*, Albuquerque: University of New Mexico Press.

Djurfeld, G. and Lindberg, S..
　　1975 *Pills against Poverty*. Indien studenlititteratur. Scandinavian Institute of Asian Studies. Monograph Series No. 23. New York: Cuzon Press.

Egnor, M.
　　1978 *The Sacred Spell and Other Conceptions of Life in Tamil Culture*. Department of Anthropology, Ph.D. dissertation, University of Chicago.

Foster, G. M. and Anderson, B. G.
　　1978 *Medical Anthropology*. New York: John Wiley.

Glick, M.
　　1967 Medicine as an Ethnographic Category: The Gimi of the New Guinea Highlands. *Ethnology 6*: 31—56.

Gopaladas, T., et al.
　　1975 *Project Poshak*, Volume II. New Delhi: CARE India.

Gould, H.
　　1965 Modern Medicine and Folk Cognition in Rural India. *Human Organization 24*: 202—208.

Hughes, C.
　　1978 *Medical Care: Ethnomedicine in Health and the Human Condition*. M. Logan and E. Hunt (eds) pp. 150—158. North Scituate, Mass: Duxbury.

Jantzen, J.
　　1978 The Quest for Therapy in Lower Zaire. Berkeley: University of California Press.

Kamath, K. R., R. Feldman, P. S. Rao et al.
　　1969 Infection and Disease in a Group of South Indian Families. *American Journal of Epidemiology 89*: 375—83.

Kakar, D. N., S. K. Murthy, and R. L. Parker
　　1972 People's Perceptions of Illness and Their Use of Medical Care Services in Punjab.*The Indian Journal of Medical Education 11*(4): 286—290.

Katon, W., and Kleinman, A.
　　1980 Doctor-Patient Negotiation and Other Social Science Strategies in Patient-Care. *In* L. Eisenberg and A. Kleinman (eds), *The Relevance of Social Science for Medicine*. Boston: Reidel Press.

Khare, R. S.
　　1963 Folk Medicine in a North Indian Village. *Human Organization 22*(1): 36—40.

Kincaid, L.
　　1979 *The Convergence Model of Communication*. Honolulu: East-West Center Publications.

Kroeger, A.
　　1983 Anthropological and Sociomedical Health Care Research in Developing Countries. *Social Science and Medicine 17*(3): 147—161.

Leslie, C.
　　1980 Medical Pluralism in World Perspective. *Social Science and Medicine*.
　　1983 *Social Research and Health Care Planning in South Asia*. Project paper for the Social Science Research Council. New Delhi, January.

McAuliffe, J. et al.
　　1985 Prospective Studies of the Illness Burden in a Rural Community of Northeast Brazil. *PAHO Bulletin 19*: 2, 139—146.

Martorell, R., J. P. Habicht, C. Yarbrough et al.
　　1975 Acute Morbidity and Physical Growth in Rural Guatemalan Children. *American Journal of Disabled Child 129*: 1296—1301

Martorell, R., C. Yarbrough, S. Yarbrough et al.
　　1980 The Impact of Ordinary Illness on the Dietary Intakes of Malnourished Children. *American Journal of Clinical Nutrition 33*: 345—50.

Mathews, C.
   1979   *Health and Culture in a South Indian Village*. New Delhi: Sterling Press.
Nations, M.
   1986   Epidemiological Research on Infectious Disease: Quantitative Rigor or Rigor-
          mortis? Insights from Ethnomedicine. *In* C. R. Janes et al. (ed.) *Anthropology and
          Epidemiology* pp. 97—123. Leiden: Reidel Press.
Nichter, M.
   1977   The Joga and Maya of the Tuluva Buta. *Eastern Anthropologist 30*(2): 139—155.
   1978   Patterns of Curative Resort and Their Significance for Health Planning in South
          Asia. *Medical Anthropologist 2*(2): 30—58.
   1979   The Language of Illness in South Kanara. *Anthropos 74*: 181—201.
   1980   The Layperson's Perception of Medicine as Perspective into the Utilization of
          Multiple Therapy Systems in the Indian Context. *Social Science and Medicine 14b*:
          225—233.
   1981   Negotiation of the Illness Experience: The Influence of Ayurvedic Therapy on the
          Psychosocial Dimensions of Illness. *Culture Medicine and Psychiatry 5*: 1—27.
   1983   *Toward a People Near Promotive Health Within Primary Health Care*. Proceedings
          of the First International Symposium on Public Health in Asia and the Pacific Basin.
          University of Hawaii, School of Public Health.
   1984   Project Community Diagnosis: Participatory Research as a First Step toward
          Community Involvement in Primary Health Care. *Social Science and Medicine
          19*(3): 237—252.
   1986   Modes of Food Classification and the Diet-Health Contingency: A South Indian
          Case Study. *In* R. Khare and K. Ishvaran (eds), *Aspects of Food Systems in South
          Asia*. North Carolina: Carolina Academic Press.
   1989   False Expectations and Commanding Metaphors: Immunization Programs in South
          Asia. *In* J. Coreil and D. Mull (eds) *Anthropology and Primary Care*. The Nether-
          lands: Kluwer Academic Publishers.
Nichter, M. and Nichter M.
   1981   *An Anthropological Approach to Nutrition Education*. Newton, Mass: International
          Nutrition Communication Service, Education Development Center.
   1983   *The Use of Analogy in the Communication of Promotive Health*. Proceedings of the
          First International Symposium on Public Health in Asia and the Pacific Basin.
          University of Hawaii, School of Public Health.
Nichter, M., Rizvi N.
   1985   A Negotiation Approach to Nutrition Education. *In* R. Israel (ed.), *Communication
          Answers to Nutrition Problems in Developing Countries*. Newton, Mass: Interna-
          tional Nutrition Communication Service.
Opler, M.
   1962   Cultural Definitions of Illness in Village India. *Human Organization 21*: 32—35.
Parker, R. L., Alexander, A. C. Shah, S. M., and Neuman. A. K.
   1979   Self-Care in Rural Areas of India and Nepal. *Culture, Medicine and Psychiatry 3*(1):
          3—28.
Paul, B.
   1963   Anthropological Perspectives on Medicine and Public Health. *Annals of the
          American Academy of Political and Social Science*: 34—43.
Pereira, S. and Begum, A.
   1987   The Influence of Illness on the Food Intake of Young Children. *International
          Journal of Epidemiology 16*: 3, 445—450.
Pfifferling, J.
   1975   Some Issues in the Consideration of Non-Western and Western Folk Practices as
          Epidemiological Data. *Social Science and Medicine 9*: 655—658.
Polgar, S.
   1972   Health Action in Cross-Cultural Perspective. *In Handbook of Medical Sociology*, H.

E. Freeman, S. Levine, and L. G. Reader (eds.). 2nd edition. Englewood Cliffs, N.J.: Prentice-Hall.

Pyle, D.
   1981   *From Project to Program: The Study of the Scaling Up/Implementation Process of a Community Level, Integrated Health, Nutrition, Population Intervention in Maharastra India.* Unpublished Ph.D. thesis. Massachusetts Insitute of Technology, Department of Political Science.

Rao, P. S., K. G. Koshi, V. Benjamin et al.
   1970   A Longitudinal Study of Morbidity in Rural Areas of South India. *Indian Journal of Medical Research 58*: 7, 927—937.
   1971   Specific Morbidity Rates in a Rural Area of South India. *Indian Journal of Medical Research 59*: 6, 965—973.

Rodhe, J.
   1978   Preparing for the Next Round: Convalescent Care after Acute Infection. *American Journal of Clinical Nutrition 31*: 2258—2268.

Rogers, E. and Kincaid, L.
   1982   Communication in Networks and Convergence. *Inter Media 10*(1): 14—18.

Srivastva, R. N.
   1978   *Evaluating Communicability in Village Settings.* New Delhi: UNICEF.

Trawick, M.
   1987   The Ayurvedic Physician as Scientist. *Social Science and Medicine 24*: 12, 1031—1050.

Turner, V.
   1975   *Revelation and Divination in Ndembu Ritual.* Ithaca, N.Y.: Cornell University Press.

Weiss, M.
   1980   Charaka Samhita on the Doctrine of Karma. *In* W. D. O'Flaherty (ed.), *Karma and Rebirth in Classical Indian Traditions.* Berkeley: University of California Press.

Young, A.
   1981   When Rational Men Fall Sick: An Inquiry into Some Assumptions Made by Medical Anthropologists. *Culture, Medicine and Psychiatry 5*: 317—335.

Young, J.
   1981   Non-Use of Physicians: Methodological Approaches, Policy Implications and the Utility of Decision Models. *Social Science and Medicine 15b*: 499—507.

Zimmerman, F.
   1978   From Classic Texts to Learned Practice: Methodological Remarks on the Study of Indian Medicine. *Social Science and Medicine 12b* (2): 97—103.
   1980   Rtu-Satmya, the Seasonal Cycle and the Principle of Appropriateness. *Social Science and Medicine 14b*: 99—106.

APPENDIX

Examples of popular preventive/promotive folk medicines for children's illnesses

Tamare

1. Medicinal rice gruel containing *adkabare* (Cummis trigonus), *muccilu* (Dillenia pentagyna), and *alamuda* bark (Ricinus communis?) is prepared for three days during the month of Ati (July—August), an inauspicious time associated with overheat and toxicity.

2. Every three months, a child is given a three-day oil bath of *ponne* (Calophyllum inophyllum) oil, especially upon the fontanel.

3. *Alamuda* twigs (milky sap) are ground and applied to the fontanel.

Krani

A decoction is made of *pade mullu* (Polycarpea carymbacia), a thorny plant whose features accord with the thorny skin characteristic of *krani*. By the doctrine of signature, the plant is deemed a preventive/curative medicine for the illness.

Bala Graha/Chinne

1. *Chinne* pills are purchased from ayurvedic *vaidya* (exorcists) and some provision shops for about 15 *paise* (2 cents) per tablet. They are given to children until approximately 12 years of age. Contents vary. Contents of one popular variety include:

— Bile stone of cow
— *Rudrakshi* (Guazina tonutosa)
— Sandalwood (Santalum album)
— *Bhaje* (Acrorus calamus)
— Cloves
— *Bhadra mushti* (Cyperus rotundus)
— Fat of civet cat
— Cumin
— *Tumbe* flowers (Leucas linifolia)
— *Annali* (Terminalia chebula)
— *Shanthi* (Terminalia catappa)
— *Nelli* (Phyllanthus emblica)
— Deer horn
— Gold ash.

2. Decoction of *Ishvara beru* (Aristolocchia indica).
3. *Olle kodi* (Mimecylon amplexicaule) sprouts, *oma* (Trachyspermum ammi), black pepper, and garlic are ground into a paste and given once in 8 days or 2 days before *amavase* (no moon day) till 7 to 9 years of age. This medicine is used to prevent *chinne agra* and the accumulation of *kapha* in children.

Agra

1. Tender sprouts of *renje* (Mimusops elenji), *mader* (Latin name not available), *kotte mullu* (Zizypus iylopyrus), *nekki* (Vitex negundo), *mallige* (jasmine). These sprouts are ground into a paste with water and the juice is given to a baby from infancy to 2 years of age, once weekly.
2. *Kepala* flower (Ixora coccinea), *mader* leaves (Latin name not available), guava sprouts, garlic, and black pepper are ground and the juice is given to a child once weekly beginning in the third month.
3. *Nelli kayi* (Indian gooseberry) is prepared into a decoction and given once weekly from the age of 1 till 4.

Calming of Worms

1. Powdered bark of *pale* (Indigofera pulekilla) tree.
2. Powdered root of *tumbe* (Leucas linifolia).

To control/reduce *kapha*

1. *Ola kodi* (Mimecylon amplexicaule) and black pepper every 15 days after child is seven months old.
2. *Baje* (Acrorus calamus) is mixed with honey and given to the child to lick.
3. *Tulasi* (Ocimum sanctum) leaf juice is squeezed into the mouth of the child.

To Reduce *Pitta*

Decoction is prepared of *goli* (Ficus bengalinsis) and *atti* (Ficus glomerata).

Promotion of digestion

1. Powder of *Inde mara* (Caryota urens) is given from age of 5 months to 1½ years of age.

2. A decoction is prepared of ginger, *oma* (Carum copticum), *ingu* (Ferula asafoetida), cumin, and black pepper.

To Promote General Health

The taste *kaniru*, astringent (like the taste of strong black tea), is deemed to have medicinal value and is linked to health promotion. *Kaniru* tasting decoctions are drunk as a general remedy. *Kodi* decoction, a *kaniru* decoction made from the young buds of auspicious plants (e.g., coconut bud, *ole kode* [Memecylon amplexicaule]), is regularly given to children (6 months—3 years) as a preventive/curative medicine while adults take other *kaniru* substances (e.g., *Goli* bark [Ficus bengalinsis]) when they feel overheat in the body.

Season-Specific Preventive Medicine

Ati Month — Rainy Season

1. *Mara sevu* (Latin name not available), a cooling type of tree fungus, is eaten especially on the no moon day of *Ati* month, an inauspicious month during monsoon season, in order to remove poisons accumulated in the stomach during the year. A leaf steamed rice preparation is consumed for three days.

2. At dawn on the morning of the no moon day of *Ati* month, the bark of the *Pale* tree (Alstonia scholaris) is removed and boiled with black pepper as a medicinal decoction. This decoction is consumed by all family members. *Pale* is a blood purifier, a medicine used to treat recurrent fevers, and a preventive medicine against malaria.

Winter Season

A medicinal decoction is prepared out of the tender shoots of flowering plants:

— *Chimullu* (Caeslalpinia minosoides)
— *Daddala* (Careya arborea)
— *Gamate* (Zenthoxylum rhesta)
— *Kesavu* (Andropogon muricatus)
— *Kene* (Colocasia antiquorom)
— *Kojamb* (Latin name not available)
— *Kukku* (Mangifera indica)
— *Kuntangila* (Latin name not available)
— *Madamala Kare* (Randia species)
— *Nannali* (Heinidesmus indicus)
— *Nekkarika* (Melostoma malabathricum)
— *Nerale* (Eugenia jamblana)
— *Perale* (Psidium guava)

This decoction is regarded to be cooling and good for the stomach sores which are thought to be prevalent in winter season. As noted in the text, by consuming a preparation of budding auspicious plants one is thought to embody the vitality of this time of fertility.

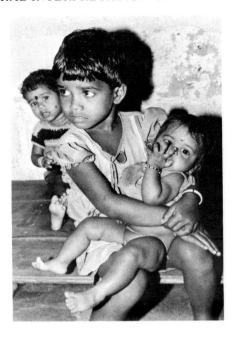

Sibling care: During peak agricultural seasons, older sisters are often given the responsibility of caring for and feeding their younger siblings.

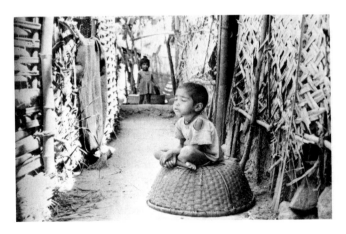

"He is always like that, it is his constitution, *prakrti*." This was the cultural interpretation of this malnourished child's lassitude.

6. FROM ARALU TO ORS: SINHALESE PERCEPTIONS OF DIGESTION, DIARRHEA, AND DEHYDRATION

"We must understand the beliefs conditioning response to diarrhea before an effective strategy can be developed to promote oral rehydration" (Rodhe, 1980).

Despite Sri Lanka's relative success in reducing infant mortality and providing primary health care services to the population at large, diarrheal diseases remain a leading cause of morbidity and mortality in the country. In 1979, diarrheal diseases accounted for 45 deaths per 100,000, 53% of all infectious disease deaths in the country. Diarrheal diseases constituted the third leading cause of death for the population at large. Children under 5 years of age account for 49% of all deaths due to diarrheal diseases (Gaminiratne 1984; Pererra 1985; Pollack 1983).[1]

Environmental, cultural and economic factors interact in determining the prevalence, transmission, and severity of diarrheal diseases. An understanding of diarrhea in Sri Lanka, therefore, requires socio-economic studies of life conditions,[3] epidemiological studies of diarrheal disease transmission, and anthropological studies of popular health practices. In this paper, I will explore the latter. More specifically, I will consider how the phenomenon of infant and children's diarrhea is perceived and acted upon by rural low country Sinhalese. My focus will be the health care behavior of mothers and grandmothers as primary care takers, for as Rodhe has noted:

Only through sympathetic understanding of a mother's attitude towards diarrhea can we develop an appropriate, acceptable and effective strategy that can rely on her active support.[2]

Ethnographic data upon which this paper is based were collected over a 12 month period while I was attached to the Sri Lankan Bureau of Health Education. During field visits, and while residing in rural areas of low country Sri Lanka, I had occasion to observe a number of families in which a child was suffering from diarrhea. These cases were followed up whenever possible. The tacit knowledge of mothers manifest in their habits of hygiene and through patterns of health behavior, was explored during the course of interviews. Mothers were asked to objectify this knowledge while tending to a child experiencing diarrhea. The study was exploratory. Its findings illustrate the range of factors associated with diarrhea among low country Sinhalese. It is hoped that consideration of these data will inspire broader and more rigorous regional studies of diarrhea related behavior, which consider the degree to which health practices, perceptions and expectations are shared and differ among different social strata (defined in relation to social class and educational status).

Two practical concerns underscore my presentation of anthropological data on cultural dimensions of diarrhea. First, attempts are presently being made to popularize oral rehydration in Sri Lanka. These programs are largely *ad hoc* and are supported by a number of international donor agencies. To date, they have not been well coordinated in relation to either their training schedules or educational messages.[4] The immense importance of oral rehydration in the management of acute and subacute episodes of diarrhea, especially among children, is indisputable. For this reason, the social marketing of the oral rehydration therapy (ORT) concept, and the oral rehydration salt (ORS) product, must be done with the utmost care and cultural sensitivity. My impression from the field is that 1) greater emphasis is being placed on popularizing the product ORS than on educating the public about the concept of rehydration, 2) field staff are becoming confused as a result of multiple training programs which employ different health messages, and 3) existing attempts to popularize ORS have not paid sufficient attention to Sinhalese health culture.

Appropriate social marketing of oral rehydration as a concept will need to address popular health culture and home care behavior. I will argue that if the concept of dehydration/rehydration is better understood by the public and if attention is paid to lay health concerns, then ORS may be made more culturally accessible as well as meaningful. The role of anthropology in social marketing must extend beyond the provision of information useful for product marketing (e.g. name, color, taste) to a linking of product to knowledge through appropriate conceptualization.[5] To do otherwise is to participate in the commodification of health and the process of medicalization. By more closely integrating the social marketing of ORS with health education about dehydration, long term popularity for a lifesaving product, which has no immediate demonstration effect in sub acute diarrhea, may be fostered. Moreover, the use of ORS for other health conditions associated with dehydration may be popularized.

My second concern is that diarrhea management programs should not be limited in focus to the treatment of single episodes of disease, but be based upon a careful assessment of both those conditions which contribute to and result from diarrhea. Prudence is necessary. It is important that health planners not become caught up in the success of short term solutions for managing episodes of disease (and dehydration) at the expense of viewing diarrhea as one link in a larger cycle of ill health for people at risk to malnutrition as well as microbes. On this note it is important that as much attention be paid to persistant and chronic diarrhea, diarrheal syndromes associated with malnutrition, as acute episodes of diarrhea. Moreover, there is a need to look beyond diarrhea as an objectified, disease construct to those symptoms which influence popular health behavior both during diarrhea and following diarrhea during convalescence. We must be careful to examine how diarrhea is differentially perceived and acted upon on the basis of stool quality and folk etiology as well as accompanying symptoms.

DIARRHEA AS A SIGN OF TROUBLE AND TRANSITION AS WELL AS A SYMPTOM OF ILLNESS

Let us first consider how diarrhea is perceived by the rural Sinhalese population. Diarrhea is viewed contextually as both a sign of imbalance or transition as well as a symptom or form of illness. This point is especially important to recognize when trying to understand popular health behavior during infant and children's diarrhea. At transitional times such as teething,[6] walking, and weaning, mild or intermittant diarrhea is considered a normal, if not an expected, response to body transition.[7] Should diarrhea occur at these times, it is treated as a trouble, not as an illness. This effects health care seeking. Because episodes of mild diarrhea are expected among under 3s, medical intervention is unlikely to be perceived as an immediate need unless diarrhea is accompanied by complaints such as fever or vomiting. Observations of children with weaning related diarrhea, *bada burulata yanava*, revealed that a majority of mothers administered a home remedy or a commercial patent medicine to these children prior to, or in lieu of, taking them to a practitioner. In none of the families I observed ($n = 12$) was ORS offered to a child for this type of diarrhea. In 4 of these households, however, ORS had been administered to an older child suffering from diarrhea. In each case the reason given for not employing ORS was that this was a medicine for an illness. Loose motion associated with weaning, even of 2 or 3 days duration, was not perceived as an illness. I will return to this point shortly.

Infant diarrhea may be perceived as a sign of imbalance for the breast-feeding mother as well as the infant. There are a number of reasons why a breastfeeding mother may come to question the quality and digestability of her breastmilk. Two reasons may initially be highlighted and expanded upon shortly. As has been noted elsewhere in South Asia,[8] infant diarrhea may be linked to the heaty or cooling quality of the mother's breastmilk. Heatiness may result from several different factors including a mother's immediate diet or her inability to bathe enough to cool her body at a time of environmental heat. On the other hand, she may feel her breastmilk is indigestable and too cool if she has just bathed and has wet hair. Another reason she may come to question the quality of her breastmilk relates to her emotional state. Breast-milk is thought to spoil, become *kirinarakwela*, due to a psychosocial state called *tanikama. Tanikama* is a form of loneliness associated with vulner-ability, fear, and shock.

The point I initially wish to highlight is that diarrhea is a phenomenon associated with multiple meanings. In the next section of this paper, I will identify 4 broad categories of diarrhea as a heuristic device enabling the presentation of data on popular health care treatment and health care seeking for diarrhea. The attributes selected for constructing this typology of diarrhea are stool quality and adjunct symptoms. It is important to recognize that interpretations of specific illness episodes and health care seeking actions are not simplistically triggered by symptoms. The severity and meaning of diarrhea is interpreted in respect to a range of factors including age of the afflicted, season of occurrence, suspected etiology, duration of symptoms, factors influencing persistence or flare up, treatment failure, etc. Natural, social, and moral imperatives related to states of vulnerability enter into the actual construction of illness identities and health care decision making.

Bearing in mind that diarrhea may be perceived as a trouble, not necessarily an illness, and constitute a sign as well as a symptom, we may now consider diarrhea as illness. Following the presentation of an inventory of ideas about diarrhea causality and treatment, I will introduce 3 case studies which illustrate some of the themes highlighted.

DIARRHEA AMONG BREASTFED INFANTS

Among rural Sinhalese women, breastfeeding is ideally continued for 12—18 months.[9] It is not uncommon to see a child breastfed longer than this, particularly if it is the first child. Reasons for early weaning include the ill health of the mother, a subsequent pregnancy, or perceptions that an infant's ill health has been caused by breastfeeding. Among breastfed infants, diarrhea is associated with 1) the swallowing of impurities *in utero* or at birth, 2) a mother's inappropriate dietary behavior during pregnancy or when lactating, 3) climatic changes, or 4) external malevolent forces such as the evil eye.

When a young infant (1—3 months) experiences diarrhea, the swallowing of impurities *in utero* and the mother's diet during pregnancy are commonly suspect. One to two weeks after birth Sinhala (folk herbal) medicines are given to an infant to clean the stomach of impurities acquired *in utero*. A variety of traditional medicines are available for this purpose. Popular medicines (such as *pas panguwa, desadun kalkaya* and *walangasal watera*) are widely available at provision shops and pharmacies as well as from Sinhalese folk practitioners and ayurvedic practitioners. These medicines are given to a child periodically (weekly, monthly) for the first 1—3 years of life.[10] While no common pattern of usage was observed, these medicines tended to be used most frequently in the first 3 months of life. Informants spoke of these medicines as reducing the chance of diarrhea in 2 ways. First, they removed impurities which could impair digestion. Second, they prevented worms from becoming fat and causing digestion problems. We will return to worms as an indigenous health concern shortly.

In actuality, the administration of these and other folk medicines offered to infants and young children may be responsible for causing diarrhea. On 3 separate occasions, rural doctors brought cases to my attention wherein exclusively breastfed children developed acute diarrhea soon after ingesting folk medicines. The point made by these doctors was not the traditional medicines had a direct harmful effect on children, but rather that they increased the risk of infection by bacterial contamination. As one doctor noted:

These medicines are a cultural thing, our people have faith in them. They are a part of being Sinhalese. They are something which even my mother, an educated woman, gave her children. But they are something which must be produced in a hygienic way if they are not to prove harmful.

When a breastfeeding infant under 3 months of age experiences diarrhea, the mother's overconsumption of heaty foods during pregnancy is suspect. An excess of heaty foods during pregnancy can result in the production of indigestible breastmilk. If diarrhea occurs after the third month, a mother's immediate diet is deemed a probable cause. Aside from heaty foods, a mother's consumption of heavy foods or difficult to digest green leafy vegetables may be suspect. For example, in the case of greenish diarrhea, the consumption of green leafy vegetables after noon time, a time of lesser digestive capacity, may be questioned. Alternative explanations are that the condition has been caused by a child gazing too long at green leafy trees or that a mother has breastfed with wet hair too soon after bathing.

Mothers are not only concerned that the properties of foods may be transferred through their breastmilk, but that the properties of medicines may be transferred as well.[11] For this reason a lactating woman may be more reserved in seeking allopathic medications for her own ailments particularly if the medicines are deemed heaty. This constitutes a cultural reason birth control pills are not popular among lactating women. The heaty nature of the pill is reasoned to dry up (reduce) the quantity of breastmilk, as well as cause breastmilk to become heaty. Another factor influencing the quality of breastmilk is pregnancy. Becoming pregnant while lactating is thought to render breastmilk weak and indigestible. Cultural sanctions exist against breastfeeding during pregnancy particularly after the first trimester. Failure to wean a child at this time is linked to the folk illnesses *mandama* and *grahaniya*, both of which are associated with the symptoms of PEM malnutrition.

One behavior pattern engaged in by lactating women who become pregnant may be highlighted for it has serious public health ramifications associated with diarrhea and malnutrition. Some breastfeeding mothers who become pregnant within 1 year of their last birth try to 'bring back' their menses. This is attempted by dietary manipulation, the consumption of herbal decoctions, or popular commercial medicines. In 5 such documented cases, a mother abruptly weaned her infant following her consumption of foodstuffs or medications having extreme properties (either heating or cooling), so as to prevent the transfer of these properties to the infant. In 3 of the 5 cases, the abruptly weaned child developed acute diarrhea when suddenly introduced to powdered milk or rice *kenda* (gruel). When the diarrhea persisted, these mothers either introduced or switched the brand of powdered milk they were using. In addition, they reduced the quantity of powdered milk given to the child. Moreover, in all 3 cases, patent medicines such as gripe water and omam water were administered to calm the child. As the latter causes drowsiness in children, it constitutes an additional factor decreasing fluid intake placing a child at risk to dehydration. Notably, liquid intake was decreased during diarrhea by each of the 3 mothers. However, when these mothers, and a large majority of 22 other mothers were interviewed about feeding behavior for breastfed children with diarrhea, they promptly stated that the child should continue to be breastfed on demand. That is, provided that the mother's milk is not responsible for the diarrhea.

Of the 5 cases where a woman tried to bring back her menses, 2 women were successful and 3 were not. In 2 of 3 cases, where the mother did not regain her menses, and in one of 2 cases where she did, the child entered a cycle of persistent diarrhea associated with malnutrition. Investigations of the case of 1 woman who did regain her menses and who subsequently began to breastfeed in combination with feeding her child rice *kenda* proved instructive. This woman found that when she once again started breastfeeding her 10-month-old baby, her milk output was insufficient. She, therefore, continued to feed the child rice *kenda* in addition to breastmilk. The child became weak and its stomach distended. The woman's interpretation of her child's illness reveals a popular folk-health belief. The consumption of breastmilk along with rice or rice *kenda* is thought to lead to the folk illness *mandama* characterized by PEM like symptoms (bloated stomach, lean legs, lethargy). A child develops *mandama* like symptoms, people believe, because the combination of rice and breastmilk is *aguna*, an indigestable mix, a mix which causes worms to rise. In this particular case, more concern was placed on the consumption of an 'aguna mix of foods' leading to worm activity than on dietary insufficiency, a health concern also recognized by the mother. The woman's response to the child's illness was to discontinue breastfeeding, reduce the child's diet to only *kenda*, and self-treat the child's diarrhea with the popular ayurvedic preparation, '*asamodagam spiriti*', purchased at a local pharmacy.[12]

As already noted, when a breastfed infant develops mild diarrhea, the child generally continues to be breastfed. Infant diarrhea is not considered serious until accompanied by other symptoms such as fever or vomiting. These symptoms then influence behavior toward diarrhea and feeding. Aside from being expected at times of transition, there is another reason why cases of subacute infant diarrhea are treated less seriously than those occurring in older children. There is a Sinhalese belief that breastfed infants are not effected by *visa beeja*, a lay term denoting a generalized notion of 'germ'. According to several informants, vulnerability to *visa beeja* is associated with impurity, heat, and body imbalance. In play is the notion that *visa beeja* (literally poison seed) take root only where there are suitable conditions. This notion may be represented as follows:

seed: *visabeeja*;
soil: impurity;
environment: blockage, impaired flow, imbalance;
climate: heat.

Why should a breastfed infant have problems with *visa beeja*, these informants asked? After all an infant only consumes breastmilk, a pure substance. The same attitude is unconsciously extended to infant feces. Infant feces are not deemed polluting or dangerous, a gross misconception considering the limited capability of the child's immature immune system. This misperception leads women to handle infant feces while in the course of food preparation without adequately engaging in handwashing. This behavior would be inconceivable to a woman if the feces were those of an older child. This behavior pattern may well be responsible for the transmission of enteropathogens *vis-à-vis* the contamination of food.[13]

In addition to a mother's health behavior (diet, medication, bathing, etc.) and emotional state, external sources of malevolence are held responsible for causing sudden diarrhea among infants and children. The effect of stars and planets, evil eye, *asvaha*, and the saliva of an unrelated child who greedily watches another child eat, *kila gula*, were the most common external causes of diarrhea which I encountered during explanatory model type interviews. A fear of evil mouth and evil eye affected the breastfeeding behavior of some women. To prevent *karahara dekket*, a form of evil eye causing indigestion to babies, some mothers took particular care to breastfeed only in private. Attributions of *yakka* spirits causing diarrhea rarely came up during interviews with the caretakers of afflicted infants. In all cases where spirits were suspect, a child was experiencing bloody diarrhea. Regional variation in notions of etiology were apparent. I encountered more cases where the role of spirits was suspect in the southern districts of Galle and Matara than in other low country districts.

In sum, when breastfeed infants experience mild watery diarrhea, a mother continues to breastfeed unless breastmilk is considered to be a causal factor. In this case, breastfeeding is discontinued for a few days during which time the child is given powdered milk or rice water/*kenda*. Unless diarrhea is accompanied by blood, vomiting or fever, Sinhala folk medicines and popular patent medications such as gripe water are tried before either a health worker, doctor, or ayurvedic practitioner is seen. When these symptoms accompany diarrhea, health care behavior alters. Patterns of health care behavior related to stool quality and adjunct symptoms are much the same for infants and young children and will be discussed shortly.

CHILDREN'S DIARRHEA

The terms most commonly used to denote children's diarrhea refer to indigestion (*ajeerna*) and stomach trouble (*bade amaruwa, badaelayanawa*). Other terms such as *bada narakwela* (bad stomach) and *ushna* (heat) were less commonly heard in common speech then in the offices of ayurvedic and cosmopolitan doctors. The term *pachanya roga*, a formal Sinhalese term for diarrhea, is rarely, if ever, used to refer to children's diarrhea. An important point may be made in this regard. Children's diarrhea is generally related to individual abnormalities associated with diet, climate, bathing, etc. When diarrhea is epidemic, some informants believed that children could only catch diarrheal illness from other children, not from adults. Likewise, these informants believed that an adult could not catch diarrhea from a child, nor most other children's illnesses. With respect to the term *pachanaya roga*, many informants noted that this term referred to only severe (*bayanaka ledak*) diarrhea experienced by adults. Use of this term by health workers and the appearance of the term on ORS packets to denote diarrhea in general, confused, if not alarmed, many informants.

Diarrhea among children is believed to be caused by a range of factors inclusive of those noted for infants. The following is a brief inventory of factors identified during interviews with mothers having children with diarrhea.

CAUSES OF DIARRHEA

1. Environment: an excess of heat; sudden changes in weather.
2. Water: impure, dirty water particularly during the dry season (January—April) or at the beginning of the monsoon season.
3. Inadequate bathing: a necessary means of reducing body heat which in excess may cause diarrhea.
4. Food: over-consumption of heaty foods, consumption of heavy foods when one's digestive capacity is weak, consumption of difficult to digest foods such as green leafy vegetables when one's digestive system is weak, consumption of too many kinds of foods at the same time, consumption of dirty or stale food, undigestable breastmilk.
5. Worms: an increased number of worms, an increase in the size of worms, worms travelling.
6. Shock and fear: a cause of loneliness/vulnerability (*tanikama*), humoral imbalance and body heatiness (*ushna*).
7. Evil eye: associated with the envy of others (*asvaha*).
8. Poisonous saliva (*kelagilala*): associated with greedy others.
9. Spirit problems (*yakka*): especially bloody diarrhea.

10. Contagion: Touch, contact with food, feces or blood; crossing over body wastes of the sick; germs (*visabeeja*).
11. Stars and planets (*graha dosha*).
12. Sorcery (*ina behet*): especially bloody diarrhea or vomiting.

Most of the etiological factors listed are found in the existing literature on South Asian health culture. The cultural perception of worms, however, is largely unreported.[14] In Sinhalese health culture, several different types of worms are recognized as influencing human health. One type of worm, *ahara panuwa*, food worms,[15] are considered a natural and necessary symbiote of the gut transmitted to a child *in utero* or through breastmilk. These worms, assist a young child to digest food by turning heavier foods into lighter easier to digest substances, by cleaning the stomach of impurities, and by helping to remove toxins. Some informants went so far as to link folk ideas about food worms with ayurvedic conceptualization of body humors, *tridosha*. They suggested that these worms help to balance the *tridosha*.

Food worms are thought to function in a child's best interest when kept lean and in small numbers. Some informants spoke of the necessity of taking regular meals lest one's food worms suffer. Suffering is evident when one hears a gurgling sound in the belly; the sound of worms asking for foods, *panuwa kegahanawa*. Others spoke of the necessity to drink a small quantity of water with meals in the interest of *ahara panuwa*. While beneficial when controlled, worms are considered harmful when allowed to increase in number, grow fat or mature (*mor anawa*). The latter may result from mucus accumulation, blood impurity, over-consumption of sugar or coconut, the consumption of a mixture of milk and rice, and the over-consumption of food at night. If a child is given more food at night than the body can digest, worms are thought to consume this food while the child sleeps causing them to grow fat.

A common health topic discussed by mothers is the necessity of 'making lean', *heeng venawa*, a child's worms through periodic use of blood purifiers, purgatives, and medicinal consumption of green bitter leaves such as *gotukollu* (Centella asiatica) *lunavila* (Cardiospermum), and *karavila* (bitter-gourd). While controlling the number and size of a child's worms is a felt need, the use of commercial deworming medicines is sometimes a source of concern. Although popular, commercial products are used with care and in some instances in diluted amounts. Mothers do not wish to remove all a child's worms for to do so would lead to serious health problems, or possibly result in death. Consideration of one informant's interpretation of worm medications is revealing:

In a paddy field many plants are there. We use weedicides to keep the growth of unnecessary plants down so they do not take the water and nourishment from the paddy. Some weedicides are harmful to some plants, others to different plants. Worm medicine is like weedicide. It is good to choose a worm medicine which will harm only unnecessary worms, not those necessary for a child's digestion. *Aralu* (*Terminalia chebula*) is the best medicine to lean necessary worms and remove others. We know the affect of this medicine on the worms.

Today, however, people go for shop medicine. It is easy to take, but you must not use too much or you may harm the worms. Even when you use shop medicine it is important to use *aralu* now and again. *Aralu* is a medicine of this place and it is effective for the troubles of this place. Shop medicine is good, but it is also a poison. If you take it and you do not purge afterward, this is very dangerous. With *aralu*, it does not matter.

Mothers feel it is important to control as well as safeguard a child's food worms until the child's digestive capacity develops and the work of worms becomes less essential. When worms become mature or are aggravated, a number of symptoms are thought to result. These range from teeth grinding and sleeping in a prone position to nausea, night cough, vomiting and diarrhea. I will note shortly that a concern about worms significantly influences diarrhea related behavior as well as being seen as a cause of diarrhea.

DEHYDRATION

Before describing health actions related to 4 forms of diarrhea distinguished by stool quality and adjunct symptoms, a few words need be said about dehydration. Infants and young children are at particular risk to dehydration for a number of reasons. Two physiological reasons are that infants/young children 1) have a higher percentage of their body weight accounted for by water; this percentage increasing with malnutrition, and 2) have a greater exposed skin surface area relative to their weight. While it takes an average adult who has stopped consuming fluids 2—3 days to become dehydrated, abnormal losses withstanding, it takes an infant only 24 hours.[16]

Rural Sinhalese mothers recognize severe or long-term diarrhea as commonly accompanied by scanty, dark-colored urine; burning urine; dry skin, mouth and lips; and inactivity. However, these symptoms are as much associated with heatiness of the body as loss of liquid. The fatigue and inactivity, *mathagathiya*, characteristic of dehydrated children is also linked to worm activity. Thirst is linked to worm activity as well. Some informants spoke of thirst accompanying diarrhea as 'worms asking for water'. They warned against quenching a child's thirst when weak for fear that their worms would become too strong and active causing additional problems. When a child was weak it was thought best to keep the worms dormant.

Typical signs of acute dehydration which appeared to carry less cultural significance and which were rarely noted in elicited symptom lists, were sunken, tearless eyes, sunken fontanel and loss of skin elasticity. The formal Sinhalese word for dehydration *vijalanaya* used on UNICEF '*Jeevanee*' ORS packages was not recognized by a large majority of the people to whom I and health educator colleagues interviewed after showing them the packet.[17] A number of images were, however, employed by innovative health staff to convey the concept of dehydration in a meaningful fashion. These images incorporated the ideas of a plant fading or withering (*malanika venava; habala; seppanethiva yanava*), the body drying (*anga velenava*) and one becoming drowsy (*rabbayana innawa; hondumandu venawa*).

FOUR FORMS OF DIARRHEA AND POPULAR IDEAS ABOUT TREATMENT

In general discourse, informants tended to distinguish 4 forms of diarrhea by stool quality and adjunct symptoms. I will employ these distinctions to highlight popular patterns of health care behavior.

1. *Mild diarrhea.* Diarrhea of 1—4 days duration; 3—5 watery stools a day. This form of diarrhea (*ajeerna*) is associated with multiple natural causes and is deemed a common childhood ailment. When children experience mild diarrhea, home remedies are generally given, solid food is withheld and normal liquid consumption is reduced. Common home remedies include: weak coffee (deemed a heaty, drying agent) sometimes mixed with lemon juice (another drying agent), coriander water (a cooling agent), a *kenda* (soup) made of fried rice paddy in water; a decoction of *beli* root and *irewerilya*. One reason liquid is reduced is that mothers feel that if too much liquid is given to a child with an empty stomach this will induce vomiting (see below). The notion that more liquid causes more diarrhea is also common.[18]

2. *Acute watery diarrhea.* Over 6 watery stools a day for over 2 days. This form of diarrhea (*hugank burulata yanawa, waturuawage yanawa*) is associated with multiple natural causes as well as evil eye, evil mouth and planet trouble. The treatment of choice for this type of diarrhea is a medicine which will dry diarrhea quickly. Allopathic medicine is thought particularly useful for this type of diarrhea inasmuch as allopathic medicine is generally believed to be heaty. In addition to allopathic medicines, mothers will sometimes feed a child small quantities of heaty liquids such as weak coffee. For evil mouth and evil eye, as well as planet troubles, an exorcist, *kathadiya*, may be consulted, chanted oil secured, or a curing ritual arranged. Grandmother folk healers and some Buddhist priests also administer chanted oil.

3. *Blood and mucus diarrhea.* This form of diarrhea (*ati sara, le badayanawa, le seedam*) is linked to extreme heatiness in the body. As noted earlier, heat is associated with multiple factors ranging from sorcery and witchcraft to environmental exposure, diet, lack of bathing and the stars. While many informants were observed to frequent clinics for this type of diarrhea, some informants considered heaty allopathic medicines to be dangerous, if not inappropriate treatment for this type of diarrhea. I interviewed 8 families who had opted against the use of allopathic medicines for this kind of diarrhea. Six informants from these families said they had used allopathic medicine in the past for watery diarrhea. The remaining two informants stated that Sinhala medicine was best for all forms of diarrhea.

When children experience blood and mucus diarrhea, powdered milk (considered heaty) and heaty home remedies (such as coffee) are generally not given to the afflicted. Deemed appropriate are cooling Sinhala and ayurvedic herbal medicines as well as king coconut water, rice water, and *beli* root decoctions. If a child is still breastfeeding, this practice is continued. While women spoke of indigestible breastmilk as a cause of watery diarrhea, no informant independently linked blood and mucus diarrhea to breastmilk. When questioned, informants stated this was possible if the woman's body was extremely heaty. Blood and mucus diarrhea is deemed a serious illness, a *naraka lede*, and a cause of alarm. Considerable doubt existed among informants as to whether or not this illness is contagious. Some informants spoke of the necessity of burying stools if a water seal latrine was not used. In 6 of the 10 cases of blood and mucus diarrhea which I encountered in rural clinics, a child had been given Sinhala medicine for at least 2 days before being given allopathic treatment. In 5 of the 10 cases, a parent indicated that the child would be treated with Sinhala medicines to cool the body after the diarrhea had been controlled by allopathic medicines.

4. *Diarrhea with vomiting.* The most serious form of children's diarrhea identified by informants was copious diarrhea accompanied by vomiting (*vamanaya yama, badaeliya, pachanaya*). Informants spoke of vomiting as impairing breathing as well as causing headaches and burning sensations in the head. For many informants, the latter symptoms indicated that vomit rose toward the brain, *mole*. A fear of vomiting effects health behavior appreciably. In 6 separate instances, I encountered a mother who reduced liquid intake to a child either because the child had vomited or because the woman had a fear the child would vomit. The latter behavior was underscored by the idea that if a child with diarrhea is eating less food and has an empty stomach, liquid intake will cause vomiting.

In one memorable case, liquids had been reduced for 2 days after a child vomited. According to the mother, the 2½-year-old dehydrated child had been given approximately half the amount of liquid she normally consumed. Only when ORS was described to the mother by a health educator colleague as good for vomiting, did she permit administration of this liquid to the child.

THREE CASE STUDIES

The following 3 field accounts illustrate a number of the points highlighted thus far. My reason for citing these cases is to convey just how complex cultural interpretations of diarrhea can become over time.

Case One

A baby, aged 8 months, developed watery diarrhea with 'white clots'. After 3 days of diarrhea, the anxious mother took the child to a primary health care center to see the doctor. The doctor instructed the mother to continue breastfeeding the child and gave the mother pills to consume herself. While it was unspecified as to whether the pills were for the mother's or the baby's health, they were interpreted as medicine which would be passed on through the breastmilk. The diarrhea subsided on day 5 (from onset). On day 6, the infant's grandmother noticed small red spots on the baby's skin. The grandmother feared this might be a return of *ratagaya*, a folk illness experienced by the infant shortly after birth and characterized by a red rash. She linked the return of *ratagaya* with the heaty effect of the medicine her daughter had taken to 'dry up' her baby's diarrhea. The infant's post-diarrhea constipation was cited as further evidence of *ratagaya*. A folk medicine, *ratagaya kalka*, was given to the child to cleanse its stomach and blood. A few hours after taking the medicine, the child experienced copious diarrhea. After the diarrhea persisted for 2 days the woman returned to the clinic with her child. This time she received advice to breastfeed, but no medicine was given. A family health worker weighed the child and spoke to the mother about feeding the child other foods, a theme which confused her at this time of concern about diarrhea.

Returning home a neighbor spoke with the woman about the problem and offered a different diagnosis. She recalled how the woman had been startled 2 days before the initial episode of diarrhea. While on the way home from marketing, near a clump of trees, the woman and her neighbor's 8-year-old son had been startled by a crashing noise. The neighbor stated that her son had cried out that right in his sleep. In her opinion, the child's diarrhea was caused by the woman's breastmilk having become lonely, *kiri tanivenava*, due to the woman being shocked and having experienced fear in a lonely place. After this talk with her neighbor, the mother visited a Buddhist priest and acquired some chanted oil for the trouble. She also visited a local Sinhalese herb trader and purchased cooling medicines 'to reduce the acidity of her blood'. This is a phrase which has entered the discourse of the 'educated' to denote blood imbalance.

The woman's husband returned home with a packet of ORS which a friend told him was a '*saline watera*' mixture. The grandmother questioned whether the mixture was heaty or cooling. The father responded that it was a light substance which was easy to digest. Food was withheld from the child and the ORS solution was given to the child for a full day. The child's diarrhea subsided on the following day. When asked about the treatment which worked ('answered') for the child, the family gave equal weight to the herbs which cooled and purified the mother's breastmilk, the charmed oil which protected her from *tanikama*, and the *saline wateru* which gave the child strength.

Case Two

A child, aged 11 months had experienced watery mucus diarrhea for 6 days. The family labeled the illness *badeillya*. On the day before I met the family, the child had passed between 7 and 9 watery stools. The child had been abruptly weaned the week before during a time when the mother was ill with fever. She had taken strong heaty medicines (ampicillin) from a private doctor. The child developed diarrhea, was taken off the breast, and was given powdered milk and rice *kenda* to eat. After 3 days of diarrhea, the amount of milk fed to the child was decreased and the child was given a bread rusk as a pacifier. On the fourth day of illness the child was given only a limited amount of rice water to drink. The family feared giving too much liquid to the child as its stomach was empty. They thought that this might cause vomiting by disturbing the worms in the child's stomach. Thirst, therefore, did not serve as a guide to the amount of liquid given to the child.

By way of treatment, the child had initially (second, third day) been given a small amount of coffee to dry up the diarrhea. On the fourth day, the family considered taking the child to the local health center, but it was both a Tuesday and the first day of the month, inauspicious times to seek treatment. Therefore, they postponed a day and took the child to the health center on the fifth day. The doctor gave them an ORS packet to prepare into a solution for the child. He also gave the mother some unidentified tablets for her fever which she still experienced intermittently. While the mother's fever abated, the child's diarrhea continued. On the sixth day, the child's father consulted an astrologer. The father inquired whether the child had some planetary problem, *graha dosha*, which was preventing the medicine from 'answering' (i.e. taking effect). The astrologer explained that it was a *naraka velava*, a bad time, for the child. A talisman was recommended in addition to medical treatment. The father obtained a talisman and the mother obtained some chanted oil from a woman healer known simply as an *achi*, a grandmother healer.

The father next consulted a friend before seeking new treatment for the child. The friend passed along a few tablets which had proven effective for his 5-year-old child when suffering from diarrhea the previous month. Two tablets, given in quarters, were administered to the child over a 2 day period as suggested by the friend. By day 8, the child ceased to pass stools and was given some gripe water and rice *kenda* as food. On the ninth day the child passed one small, goat-like stool. On the tenth day the child's grandmother became concerned that the child was constipated and spoke of giving the child a 'stomach wash'. Instead of using a traditional purgative, *aralu*, the family opted to use a commercial product (milk of magnesia). This was given to the child on day 12. A blood purifier decoction was taken by both the child and mother for 3 days from days 13—16.

I was able to secure a sample of the tablet given to the child. It turned out to be an adult dose of Bactrim DS (Trimethoprim 160 mg, Sulfamethoxayole 800 mg), a potent antibacterial agent used in the treatment of enteritis caused by susceptible strains of shigella. By interviewing the friend who had originally received the medication, I traced the tablet back to a doctor in a nearby town. Without describing his part in the scenario, I presented the case to him during an interview. The following were his comments:

Patients copy doctors' behavior after we give prescriptions, but they don't view the severity of symptoms the same way. For severe diarrhea I give Bactrim to some of my patients. Now, former patients purchase Bactrim from shops themselves and take it after diarrhea is there for 3 or 4 days. They come to see me after the medicine doesn't work. That is the trend. I see a growing number of cases like that, but usually among older children and adults. Now it seems young children are involved. This is most dangerous.

Two types of danger are associated with medicine misuse: the immediate danger presented by the pharmacologic properties of the medicine and the danger which may result from behavior which increases the chance of iatrogenic response. In this particular case, Bactrim was not only an inappropriate and expensive medication, but it was consumed with an insufficient quantity of liquids. Had the medicine been taken for a longer period of time, this behavior pattern could have resulted in adverse symptoms such as crystalluria. When questioned about fluid consumption during the time the pills were taken, the family noted that gripe water had been given to the child as well as boiled cooled water. The family maintained the idea that increased fluid intake should accompany heaty allopathic medicines. However, they were reluctant to give too much fluids to the child after having restricted food and fluids for some days. They feared that this might cause vomiting. They gave the child gripe water to calm the stomach and quench the child's thirst. Their plan was to clean and cool the child's stomach and blood after the treatment so as to rid the body of any accumulated toxins.

Case Three

A child aged 20 months with frank signs of second degree protein calorie malnutrition had been experiencing diarrhea on and off for the last 2 months. The caretaker, the child's grandmother, blamed the child's poor health on the way in which the child was weaned. She called attention to how her daughter-in-law had fed the child rice gruel while she continued to breastfeed. This was *aguna* and had led to worm trouble manifest as diarrhea. When mild, watery diarrhea turned into acute diarrhea, the child's mother discontinued offering rice gruel to the child and only breastfed. After a few days, the diarrhea abated, but the child was left very weak. The mother found that her breastmilk was insufficient and she questioned its strength and quality. After a few weeks she discontinued breastfeeding all together and only fed the child rice *kenda*. She occasionally supplemented this with powdered milk. The child's diarrhea once again returned. Seeing that the child was lean and weak, a family health worker suggested that the mother attend a nutrition supplementary food clinic. The child was weighed and given *triposha* supplement. Additionally, the mother was given advice about introducing the child to a mixed diet. The grandmother did not approve of the advice. According to the grandmother, the child had developed acute diarrhea because her daughter-in-law had offered the child more than one kind of weaning food at each feeding, fed the child frequently, and offered solid food even when the child suffered mild diarrhea. She stated that the child's digestive system had been too weak to digest such food and that the worms had become strong and mature.

Over the course of my observation of this family's health care behavior, the child's care was placed in the hands of the grandmother when her daughter-in-law went back to work as a seamstress. In place of multiple weaning foods, she gave only one kind of food to the child at each feeding. Foods associated with worm growth, like potatoes, were restricted. *Triposha*, which had been fed to the child, was no longer given, but instead the allocation of supplementary food was given to 2 older children. Now that the mother was working, there was enough money to purchase an occasional box of powdered milk. The mother purchased a box of Nespray for her child. When the baby's feces showed signs of mucus, *sema*, a neighbor advised the grandmother against giving Nespray to the child because of its high *sema*-producing quality. She was advised to switch to Bear Brand powdered milk which was considered to have less *sema* and be more digestible. As a result, the grandmother used the Nespray for tea and spoke of purchasing Bear Brand for the child when money was available to do so.

The grandmother began to feed the child only rice gruel. The child had little appetite and was apathetic and sleepy. On my last visit to the household I noticed that the child was dehydrated. When asked if she had given the child anything to drink, the grandmother reported that she had offered the child small quantities of boiled, cool water and orange barley water, a substance she associated with doctor's advice. Latter, I learned that she had not given the child orange barley water, a local soft drink, but wanted to impress me. Given the poor health status of the child, I considered intervention necessary. Only after being given both tablets and ORS from the local clinic doctor would the mother administer the ORS.

ORAL REHYDRATION

"While the scientific community continues its debate on the ideal composition, packaging and delivery of oral rehydration solution, many mothers continue to withhold fluid from children with diarrhea, and why not? They know that when a child with diarrhea is given extra fluid to drink he passes yet more liquid messy stools. This is true even with the most modern rehydration mixtures. Although oral rehydration does save lives, its widespread use will be determined by complex cultural and social factors which are little influenced by scientific advances" (Rodhe 1980).[2]

In low country Sri Lanka most of the rural population and a great many town dwellers are not familiar with ORS. In less than one-quarter of the cases of children's diarrhea that I encountered ($n = 78$) had the child consumed ORS (often termed 'saline wateru') as a part of treatment. Eighteen families had received ORS from a physician or family health worker. Only 7, however, considered ORS therapy effective. This brings up the issue of how ORS is perceived. None of the 18 families who had tried ORS described rehydration or noted symptoms associated with dehydration when describing the function of ORS. The 3 most prominent impressions of the function of ORS were that it was 1) a medicine for diarrhea, 2) a purification agent for the body, like chlorine for a well and 3) a medicine providing strength when a child was weak. Those who thought that ORS was a medicine for diarrhea were least impressed with its efficacy.[19] In this group ($n = 11$), a majority of families had only used 1 packet of ORS salts. In 3 cases, utilization of the salts had coincided with a decrease in diarrhea and 2 families had chosen to continue therapy by procuring a second packet. In 8 cases, 1 packet had not reduced diarrhea and families had chosen not to procure additional ORS packets. These informants called attention to an increased amount of diarrhea following ORS administration. The latter is related to a gastro-colic reflex which no physician or health worker had informed them about. Interestingly, 1 satisfied informant related the gastro-colic reflex to the medicine's immediate 'wash-out' effect followed by significantly decreased diarrhea.

Of the 5 families who described ORS as providing a child strength or energy, 4 were happy with its effect. However, before this image of ORS — as a source of strength — may be considered for broad usage in social marketing,[20] we must take a closer look at the ramifications of this interpretation. When probed, 3 of the aforementioned informants described ORS as a source of strength suitable when a child should not eat other foods. Their impression was that ORS could sustain health in place of food when one had diarrhea. The taking of ORS minimized the need for other sources of nutrition. Two informants went on to note that the quantity of ORS to be consumed by an ill person depended upon the person's age or size, not the amount of diarrhea excreted by the body.

One of the most common comments about ORS which I heard from both health workers and practitioners alike was that people were never satisfied if only ORS was offered to them for complaints of diarrhea. Dissatisfaction was related to a general pattern of medicine taking behavior. The following comments by two practitioners are informative:

When visiting a doctor, sick people carry a bottle. We must give pills to satisfy the people and mixture to satisfy the bottle. People expect this: this is their habit. Our people have come to expect something to eat, pills, and something to drink, mixtures, when visiting a doctor.

If I give only ORS, patients will go someplace else. I have to give at least some tablets, even if it is Panadol, or people will not be satisfied.

Popular health concerns and expectations must be addressed if an ORS program is to prove effective. At present, instruction for ORS usage, such as those initially released by UNICEF, focus on proper preparation. Proper preparation is essential for effective use of ORS. Just as essential is communicating a clear understanding of what ORS is for and those types of diarrhea for which it is useful. This requires both use of local terminology for folk illnesses associated with diarrhea[21] and conceptual translation of dehydration.

Overly generalized use of culturally loaded words like *pachanaya roga* for diarrhea render messages confusing as do sophisticated terms like *vijalanaya* for dehydration. Dehydration, its causes and deleterious effects, must be described in ways and by images which the population can understand. Moreover, the marketing of ORS need be broadened beyond diarrhea to other times when dehydration occurs. For example, I noted during fieldwork in both Sri Lanka and South India (Appendix) that liquid consumption is reduced during some types of fever. In Sri Lanka, I encountered people with fever who decreased fluid consumption at night even when they increased fluid consumption during the day. Moreover, the types of medications they utilized influenced their liquid consumption behavior. Some informants consumed more fluids when taking allopathic medicines, which they deemed to be heaty or poisonous, and less fluids when taking traditional medicines. The point I wish to emphasize is that fluid consumption is a complex cultural concern having multiple dimensions. Rehydration advice must both be specific and responsive to existing cultural concerns.

Care must also be taken to inform people what ORS is not. The ideas that ORS is a medicine for diarrhea or strength are becoming popular. An alternative or expanded identity might be created around coexisting health concerns as well as increasing knowledge about the ramifications of dehydration. Addressing health concerns such as digestive capacity, vomiting, weakness, shock and humoral imbalance might facilitate the social marketing of information about dehydration as well as ORS as a product.[22]

DIARRHEA MANAGEMENT AND NUTRITION EDUCATION

It is important that diarrhea management and nutrition education programs be complementary, if not closely integrated, for 2 reasons. The first reason is that health care practices for diarrhea and diarrhea related illnesses (e.g. measles) influence feeding behavior both during diarrhea and for some time afterwards. It is necessary for both diarrhea management programs and nutrition education programs to pay increased attention to the folk dietetics of illness and convalescence. Once again, it is important for these programs to address indigenous categories of illness and offer illness specific dietary advice (Nichter and Nichter 1981). The second reason for program coordination is that diarrhea and indigestion are health concerns which influence everyday food consumption behavior among infants and young children. Focusing attention on diarrhea management in one context, but not relating to diarrhea and indigestion as health concerns in other contexts, may serve to reduce a health worker's credibility in the community.

An example illustrating the latter point may be cited. It involves a locally prepared 'nutrition' food called *kola kenda* made of green leaf extract, rice, coconut, and sugar. This traditional food preparation has been popularized by Sarvodaya, a grassroots development movement, and incorporated in their preschool feeding programs. *Kola kenda* has received extensive publicity in the press and is commonly praised by politicians during development workshops. What is important to note here is that family health workers are presently being encouraged to recommend *kola kenda* as a good food for weaning, malnutrition and convalescence.

Kola kenda is a nutrient rich preparation maximizing local resources. The simple machinery, the leaf juice extractor, designed by Sarvodaya to produce *kola kenda* is a shining example of appropriate technology. The catch is that appropriate technology does not constitute appropriate conceptualization. Many Sinhalese feel *kola kenda* is not suitable for consumption when an infant is being weaned or when a child is sick despite its acclaimed nutrient value. While strength giving, it is deemed difficult to digest. Traditionally, *kola kenda* is eaten before 8 a.m., a time when one's digestive power is greatest. Moreover, according to Sinhalese folk dietetics, it should not be consumed on rainy or cool days when digestive power may be weaker. *Kola kenda* has never been considered a good weaning food and its consumption by young children is associated with both diarrhea and worm growth.

My reason for drawing attention to *kola kenda* in the context of a discussion on diarrhea management is to emphasize that acultural nutritional advice, even where 'packaged' culturally, loses credibility for health educators. Recommending *kola kenda* as a weaning food one moment and ORS as a medicine good for diarrhea the next, loses credibility for the family health worker as one knowledgeable about diarrhea prevention as well as management. Cultural sensitivity to diarrhea needs to be built into nutrition programs as well as constitute a special focus of an ORS program. If *kola kenda* is going to be recommended as a weaning food then concern about a child's digestive capacity and diarrhea need be addressed. An informant's comments illustrate this point:

Nona (madam, the health worker) told me to prepare *kola kenda* for my son (age 3) because his blood is less. But what leaves should I use? Even a goat does not eat all the leaves. *Kola kenda* was made at the preschool last week. What leaves were in that *kenda* I do not know. My son had indigestion the following day. I know how to make *kenda*. My father ate *kola kenda*. But leaves are also medicines, *kola kenda* is a medicine. I will not give all medicines to my small child. *Gotukola* leaf is good for health, but other leaves like *thora* and *katurumurunga* are used for indigestion and worms trouble. The advice given by *nona* is not useful. If I give green vegetables or green leaves too early, then my child will get *ajeerna* or possibly *mandama*. *Nona* says nothing about this. When my son had *ajeerna* she gave me *saline wateru* (an ORS packet). It did not stop the diarrhea.

Continuity need be established between ORS programs initiated by different training centers and agencies as well as between diarrhea management programs and nutrition education programs. Both need to address popular health culture if the credibility of field staff is to be fostered.

In this paper I have highlighted cultural perceptions of diarrhea maintained by rural Sinhalese caretakers. Additionally, I have pointed out different patterns of home-care behavior and health-care seeking behavior associated with types of diarrhea differentiated on the basis of stool quality, adjunct symptoms and etiology. Perceptions of dehydration and interpretations of the function of ORS have also been considered. By way of a conclusion, I may identify an area of diarrhea related research in need of anthropological research and note a reservation I maintain about the social marketing of ORS.

Research attention needs to be turned to the home use and commercial marketing of antidiarrheal medication. Oral rehydration salts are not being introduced into a vacuum. The pharmaceutical marketplace abounds with ayurvedic, patent and prescription allopathic drugs, all readily available over-the-counter (OTC). More information is required on popular patterns of OTC drug utilization and the way in which these patterns have been established. Data is needed on those advertising motifs effectively used to foster consumption of popular medications. Research is also required on prescription patterns incorporating antimotility agents, absorbents, and antibiotic combinations (such as Bactrim, chloramphenicol, ampicillin, tetracyclin, furozone, and selexid) and the extent to which popular prescription patterns have influenced lay perceptions of diarrhea management and OTC self help efforts. It is necessary to identify those drugs believed to 'dry up' watery diarrhea, cool the body when bloody-heaty diarrhea occurs, and 'calm' or 'lean' worms. Also, of high priority is an investigation into which drugs and adjunct patent medicines (such as gripe water[23]) are employed for children's diarrhea. Pioneering work by the British group Social Audit on Lomotil usage among Indian children (Medawar and Freeze 1982) provides an excellent example of the kind of research medical anthropologists could expand upon at the micro level.

Attention must also be paid to the social relations and ideology embodied in approaches to medical treatment. Within this paper, I have suggested ways ORS might be socially marketed in a more culturally appropriate manner. My enthusiasm is tempered by a reservation I maintain about the marketing of ORS which involves the commodification of health. In this regard two underlying concerns may be highlighted. First, I am concerned that ORS is increasingly being marketed as a technical fix medicine for diarrhea which it clearly is not. While marketing ORS as medicine may no doubt increase its

short term popularity, I have doubts as to how this may effect its long term
utilization. Likewise, I would caution against marketing ORS in relation to
any popular health concern, such as 'strength', until careful pretesting is
carried out assessing the impact of such an association on product utilization
as well as health behavior.[24] Pretesting must consist of something more
substantial than short surveys or a few focus groups. As I have pointed out in
this paper, an association with strength might enhance ORS acceptance while
contributing to malnutrition should people come to think of ORS as a
replacement for food.[25] This is not to say that popular health concerns
should not be used in social marketing, but that responsible social marketing
requires careful anthropological research at the stages of initial message
design, pretesting and concurrent evaluation. The present international health
fervor to "market social marketing" as a technique and ORS as a product
need be balanced by those who are neither converts nor skeptics.

A second concern is that ORS not be marketed as a technical fix which
overshadows the importance of environmental health and hygiene. The
commodification of health is manifest in a growing tendency by people to
believe that health problems may be solved by medicines. This often leads to
the compartmentalization of disease problems which serves to distance them
from those health and development problems in which they are embedded.
Diseases come to be viewed more in terms of individual treatment strategies,
than in terms of broader community management. This trend needs to be
reversed if only on a small scale. Toward this end, I may suggest one
practical means of initiating a broader based community health perspective
discovered during the course of a participatory research project.[26]

During fieldwork in both South India and Sri Lanka I found that a useful
means of heightening villagers' interest in the community management of
disease is through greater awareness of the frequency and costs of ill health.
This may be facilitated by participatory research and the keeping of a village
(or other appropriate unit of social analysis[27]) health diary. In such a diary,
the number of days children are ill (with diarrhea) and expenses incurred for
these illness episodes are noted. I found that when illness episodes of even 1
or 2 months are tallied, villagers are generally surprised and quick to
recognize that what was once perceived as a series of individual illness
problems is in reality a community health problem. It is through such an
active discovery process, not abstract felt need surveys, that a recognition of
individual felt needs may be transformed into community consciousness. The
latter engenders community motivation for change, increasing interest in both
less expensive treatment options (such as ORS) and knowledge concerning
preventive aspects of a recognized community health problem. Given
direction by facilitators, this interest may be transformed into a problem
solving process at the local level where such issues as seasonal prevalence
and groups at risk may be focused upon.

Engaging the community in such a process through the efforts of existing
health volunteers (attached to Government Family Health Workers), private

voluntary organizations (such as Sarvodaya), change agent programs (such as that sponsored by the Ministry of Plan Implementation) etc. may serve to transform the meaning of ORS from that of a temporary fix, for individuals experiencing diarrhea, to a cost effective community resource comprising part of a larger diarrhea management program. This may be accomplished when the present emphasis on the individual control of diarrhea is shifted. This transformation will require not only the presentation of hard scientific data and the soft sell of a social marketing campaign, but a commitment to decentralized problem solving and a form of health education which begins with popular health culture and an appraisal of costs (e.g. morbidity, cash, time).

Opportunities need to be created facilitating a learning process wherein the community takes increased ownership of health problems. This is not something they have gained from the smallpox campaign, nor from supplementary food aid or family planning programs. Diarrhea, the basest of human ailments, might provide people with the chance to learn the most poignant of lessons about community problem solving. This entails a recognition that most health and development problems cannot be compartmentalized and solved by magic bullets, injections of aid, the panacea of education or simple solutions. At issue is not the worth of ORS, but the manner in which it is employed in the context of development. Technical fixes are resources not solutions.

ACKNOWLEDGEMENTS

The data for this paper was collected while I was a Fulbright Professor in Sri Lanka attached to the Post Graduate Institute of Medicine and the Bureau of Health Education. I would like to thank P. G. Jayatunga, B. A. Ranaweera, R. M. P. Ratnayaka, and S. Veeragoda for their assistance with field interviews and for their comments on earlier drafts of this paper.

NOTES

1. Additionally it may be pointed out that 1) there are approximately 180,000 hospital admissions for diarrhea a year, 2) on an average 6500 deaths occur annually due to diarrheal disease, 3) deaths due to diarrheal disease represent 8% of total deaths in the country, 4) 49% of all deaths due to diarrheal diseases affect children under 5 years, 5) 47% of these deaths occur in infants, 6) 25% of all deaths of children under 5 years of age are due to diarrheal diseases, and 7) on an average, 20—30% of hospital beds in pediatric wards are occupied by diarrheal patients (Ratnayake 1985).
2. In the quote cited, Rodhe (1980) makes reference to the attitudes of mothers. More apt would be an emphasis on the health practices of caretakers be these mothers, grandmothers, siblings, or servants.
3. I focus on health culture in this paper. Presentation of data on cultural factors influencing diarrhea related behavior needs to be complemented by socioeconomic studies of how education and economics (disposable income) influence hygiene, sanitation, and nutrition. See Waxler N. et al. 1985.

4. The Sri Lankan Ministry of Health is aware of this problem. In a recent workshop organized by the National Institute of Health Sciences, ways of better organizing ORS and diarrheal management programs were discussed. At issue here is a fundamental international health problem. Multiple divisions of health ministries in developing countries often function reactively to the funding priorities and program objectives of international development agencies. This makes it difficult to plan training schedules or closely monitor the content of training programs.

5. The term 'appropriate conceptualization' was originally used by Fuglesang (1977). Methods for developing conceptual translation have been discussed in chapter 11.

6. The claim that teething is associated with diarrhea is cross-cultural. It is most likely associated with a child's biting of contaminated objects for counter pressure. On this subject see British Medical Journal (1975) and Illingworth (1975).

7. This is often referred to as milestone diarrhea. It must be kept in mind that this is an etic concept. These phenomena are not necessarily viewed as milestones in other cultures.

8. The idea that heat is transferred through breastmilk is found elsewhere is South Asia. See Chapter 2 and Green 1986.

9. According to an analysis of World Fertility Survey data, 96.2% of babies were breastfed in Sri Lanka in 1975. Eighty-nine percent were still breastfed at 6 months; 70% at 18 months; 50% at 24 months; and 39% at 36 months. (Popkin, Bilsborrow, Yamamoto *et al.* 1979) Using the same figures and all children born in the 3 years preceding the WFS survey, the mean duration of breastfeeding was 21 months. (Kent 1985) A more recent age-stratified analysis of breastfeeding revealed that mothers under 35 years of age breastfeed for 16 months; mothers aged 35—44 for 17.6 months; and mothers aged 45—49 for 19.4 months (See Sri Lanka, World Fertility Survey, 1978).

10. Purgatives continue to be used once or twice a year even after infancy to reduce heat in the body, clean blood, reduce acidity, cool the blood, and control the size and number of worms. Traditionally, *aralu* (*Terminalia chebula*) and *lumwilla* (*Bacopa monniera*) were used for children under age 2 while *aralu* and *senikikoli* were used after age 2. While many families use commerical purgatives for most of the year, they occasionally utilize *aralu* for a more complete wash out.

11. Drugs do pass into human milk and consideration of their benefits to the mother must be carefully weighed against their risks to the infant. For example, ampicillin administered to a lactating woman may cause diarrhea in the infant. Antihistamines, as well as oral contraceptives, may alter milk volume yield (Kirksey and Grayiak 1984). The Sinhalese concern about medicines passing through breastmilk is therefore valid in some instances. It is important that the ramifications of this health concern be studied in greater depth. For example, a study I conducted in 1979 in Ankola Taluk, Karnataka, India revealed that 1) a number of useful medicines were not consumed by mothers during lactation for fear of harming the baby, 2) when medicines were necessary some mothers used this as a reason for weaning, 3) in some instances mothers consumed medicines meant for their infants believing the medicine would be transferred through their breastmilk.

12. Traditional Ayurvedic preparations for diarrhea such as *pippali asava* were not widely used among the informants I interviewed. For *mandama*, a few informants utilized *arivinda asava*. Popular commercial ayurvedic drugs were used by some informants, but Sinhala decoctions were more commonly used.

13. Contamination of food is a common cause of diarrheal disease (Rowland, Barrell and Whitehead 1978, Walker and Walker 1978, Cutting and Hawkins 1982).

14. 'Worms of Life' will be the subject of a forthcoming paper which considers how worms are incorporated in cross-cultural notions of ethnophysiology. The idea that worms are a necessary symbiote of the gut is also common in areas of South India as well as Honduras, Guatemala, Indonesia and Ethiopia. Kendall first called attention to cultural notions regarding worms as an important factor in diarrhea perception (Kendall, Foote, and Martorell 1983).

15. These worms are also called *mavu panuwa*, mother worm and *geevitha panuwa*, life worms.

16. See Levine and Edelman 1979, for a concise review of structural and functional reasons why infants and young children are at greater risk to dehydration and electrolyte loss.

17. A colleague from the Health Education Bureau recommended to UNICEF that a more suitable term for dehydration be used on ORS packets and posters. In response, a word denoting body dryness, *anga veleema*, was placed in brackets next to the formal term, *viyalanaya*, on the packets. My colleague aptly commented that it was the local term which should have taken precedence with the formal term placed in brackets, if not removed altogether. The use of formal terminology is pervasive in other health programs as well. Health education colleagues noted to me that they were given the impression during training that the public should learn 'correct terminology'. For example, in place of the colloquial term used by villagers for children's vaccinations, *lamaita bait vidinava*, the formal term *prathi shakithikanaya* is used in health education materials and programs.

18. Food and fluid restriction contribute to malnutrition and dehydration elsewhere in South Asia. See for example, Kumar *et al.* 1985; and Srinivas and Afonso 1983.

19. On the danger of marketing ORS as a medicine, Green (1986) has noted that informants in Bangladesh expected ORT to cure diarrhea and were unimpressed with the product when it did not. Seen as a medicine, ORT may delay treatment of dysentary.

20. Green (1986) has argued that ORS be marketed by addressing strength and weakness as a health concern.

21. Several other anthropologists and public health practitioners have suggested that indigenous illness categories be addressed in diarrhea management programs. See Lozoff, Kamath, and Feldman 1975; Green 1985, 1986; Escobar *et al.* 1983; Kendall, Foote and Martorell 1983, 1984; Kendall *et al.* Nations M. 1982; De Zoysa *et al.* 1984.
    In a forthcoming article, I argue that attention given to indigenous categories of diarrhea may be used in triage messages and algorithms differentiating dysentery from secretory diarrhea. The former requires antibiotics, the latter does not.

22. In Swaziland the notion that diarrhea treatments should return or maintain balance to the body was used in an ORS social marketing program. Hornik and Sankar *A Preliminary Evaluation of the Swaziland MMHP*, 1985. In Honduras, ORT was presented as the latest achievement of modern science: a remedy for lost appetite and an aid to recovery. ORT was not presented as a remedy for diarrhea. Academy for Educational Development, 1984. See also note 20.

23. The following medicines were kept in the house by at least 50% of 20 lower middle-class nuclear households inhabited by parents under 40 having an infant: 1. gripe water — for digestion, worms, diarrhea, crying; 2. *Siddharta tyla* — for chest complaints, mucus (*sema*); 3. *rakta kalka* — to prevent the folk illness, *rakta gaya*; 4. *l'eau de cologne* — to cool the body, for fever. Use of gripe water was widespread, but the range of complaints for which it was used and the manner in which it was used varied.

24. At issue here is not just that ORS be pretested to determine product acceptability. Investigation need be carried out into how the marketing of ORS (or any other health resource) in a particular manner effects health behavior before and after its introduction. It is here that anthropology may play an important role.

25. My concern is not that short term use of ORS as a medicine for strength will lead to malnutrition, but rather that it may lead people to think that while taking ORS during persistent diarrhea other food sources are not necessary. If strength is employed as a health concern for marketing ORS, care must be taken to explain its use in relation to diet.

26. On the potential of participatory research for mobilizing community participation in primary health care, see Nichter 1984.

27. Here I refer to one of the most common problems in development work, the 'unit of analysis' problem. Planners often presume a unit of analysis when designing programs.

Thus, community health workers are designated for geographic units, not social units defined by everyday interactions. Likewise, household surveys are conducted to understand the microeconomics of *x*, or the decision making relative to *y*, when the immediate family is situated within or responsive to larger social networks. If a change facilitator wants to foster community problem solving, what must first be determined-observed are action sets; that is sets of actors within social networks who respond to particular contigencies of activities. A health diary would best be kept by sets of people/families constituting action sets. Examples might include sets of families using a common water source, engaging in a common work actively, or those living in a settlement which is socially demarcated. Sri Lanka's Change Agent Program (Ministry of Plan Implementation) has initiated development efforts around action sets — small groups of people sharing common economic pursuits who have banded together to form problem solving groups.

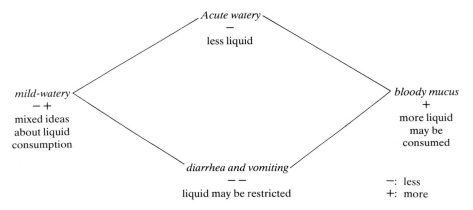

Figure 1. Liquid consumption (other than breastmilk) by diarrhea-symptom type.

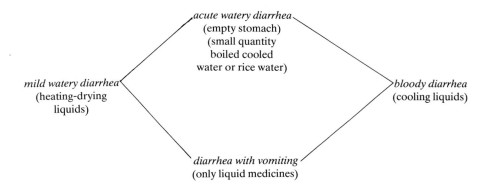

Figure 2. Qualities of liquids consumed.

APPENDIX

In this chapter the point was made that dehydration need be the focus of ORT programs not just dehydration during diarrhea. Data collected in two districts of South India in 1979 suggest why. An open ended health and illness behavior survey was administered to samples of households from town, roadside satellite villages, and interior villages in South Kanara District and a multicaste village population in North Kanara District. Data from two questions involving liquid consumption during diarrhea and fever are presented below.

Question One: How much liquid should be consumed during watery diarrhea (*bhedi*)?

			South Kanara (N = 82) Locale			Education	
	Total N = 82	Town N = 27	Satellite N = 30	Interior Village N = 25	Illiterate N = 25	Literate N = 40	Educated N = 17
Less liquid consumed	89%	89%	93%	88%	100%	88%	78%
Normal or more liquid consumed	11%	11%	7%	12	—	12%	22%

	North Kanara (N = 200)
Less liquids consumed	95%
Normal or more liquid consumption	5%

Question Two: How much liquid should be consumed during fever (*jwara*)?

			South Kanara (N = 82) Locale			Education	
	Total N = 82	Town N = 27	Satellite N = 30	Interior Village N = 25	Illiterate N = 25	Literate N = 40	Educated N = 17
Less liquid consumed	49%	33%	53%	60%	64%	43%	29%
Normal or more liquid consumed	51%	66%	47%	40%	36%	57%	71%

	North Kanara (N = 183)		
	Illiterate N = 26	Literate N = 98	Educated N = 59
Less liquid consumed	100%	78%	83%
Normal or more liquid consumed	—	22%	17%

It is apparent from the data presented that reduced liquid consumption during watery diarrhea is deemed appropriate health behavior in both districts. In South Kanara, this was true within a majority of households, irrespective of locale or educational status, although a higher proportion of the educated deemed normal or increased liquid consumption appropriate. Notably in the case of fever, ideas about appropriate liquid consumption were more mixed in South Kanara. A majority of literate households opted for normal or increased consumption, but a majority of illiterate and interior village households opted for reduced liquid consumption. In North Kanara, a large majority of households opted for less liquid consumption. Literacy did have a positive effect on liquid consumption.

REFERENCES

Academy for Educational Development
    1984   *After Twelve Months: A Status Report on the Projects in Honduras and the Gambia.* USAID, Washington, D.C. January.
British Medical Journal
    1975   Editorial, December 13th.
Cutting, W. and Hawkins, P.
    1982   The role of water in relation to diarrheal disease. *Journal of Tropical Medicine 85*, 31—39.
De Zoysa, I. et al.
    1984   Perceptions of childhood diarrhea and its treatment in rural Zimbabwe. *Social Science and Medicine 19*: 7, 727—734.
Escobar, J. et al.
    1983   Beliefs regarding the etiology and treatment of infantile diarrhea in Lima, Peru. *Social Science and Medicine 17*: 17, 1257—1269.
Fuglesang, A.
    1977   *Doing Things Together: Report on an Experience of Communicating Appropriate Technology.* Uppsala, Sweden: Dag Hammersjold Foundation.
Gaminiratne, K. H. W.
    1984   *Causes of Death in Sri Lanka: An Analysis of Levels and Trends in the 1970's.* Colombo, Sri Lanka.
Green, E.
    1985   Traditional healers, mothers, and childhood diarrheal disease in Swaziland: The interface of anthropology and health education. *Social Science and Medicine 20*: 3, 277—285.
Green, E.
    1986   Diarrhea and the social marketing of oral rehydration salts in Bangladesh. *Social Science and Medicine 23*: 357—366.
Hornik, R., and Sankar, P.
    1985   *A preliminary evaluation of the Swaziland MMHP.* Annenberg School of Communications, University of Pennsylvania, 1985.
Illingworth, R. S.
    1975   *The Normal Child.* Edinburgh: Churchill Livingstone.
Kendall, C., Foote, D. and Martorell, R.
    1983   Anthropology, communication and health: The mass media and health practices programs in Honduras. *Human Organization, 42*: 353—360.

Kendall, C., Foote, D. and Martorell R.
    1984   Ethnomedicine and oral rehydration therapy: A case study of ethnomedical investigation and program planning. *Social Science and Medicine 19*: 253—260.
Kent, M.
    1985   *Breastfeeding in the Developing World: Current Patterns.* Washington, D.C.: Population Reference Bureau.
Kirksey, A. and Grayiak, S.
    1984   Maternal Drug Use: Evaluation of risks to breastfed infants. *World Review of Diet. Vol 43*: 74—79.
Kumar, V. et al.
    1985   Beliefs and therapeutic preferences of mothers in management of acute diarrheal disease in children. *Journal of Tropical Pediatrics 31*: 109—112, 1985.
Levine, M. and Edelman, R.
    1979   Acute diarrheal infections in infants: Epidemiology, treatment and prospects for immunoprophylaxsis. *Hospital Practice, 90*, December.
Lozoff, B., Kamath, K. R., and Feldman, R. A.
    1975   Infection and disease in South Indian families: Beliefs about childhood diarrhea. *Human Organization 34*: 4, 353—45.
Medawar, C. and Freeze, B.
    1982   *Decoding the conduct of a multinational pharmaceutical company and the failure of a western remedy for the third world.* Social Audit, London 1982.
Nations, M.
    1982   *Illness of the child: The cultural context of childhood diarrhea in Northeast Brazil.* Ph.D. dissertation, Dept. of Anthropology, University of Virginia.
Nichter, M. and Nichter, M.
    1981   *An Anthropological Approach to Nutrition Education.* International Nutrition Communication Service, Education Development Center, Newton, Ma.
Nichter, M.
    1984   Project community diagnosis: Participatory research as a first step toward community involvement in primary health care. *Social Science and Medicine 19*: 3, 237—252.
Perrera, P. D. A.
    1985   Health Care Systems of Sri Lanka. *In* S. Halstead, J. Walsh and K. Warren (eds), *Good Health at Low Cost.* Conference Report, Rockefeller Foundation, October.
Pollack, M.
    1983   *Health Problems in Sri Lanka. Part I and Part II: An Analysis of Morbidity and Mortality* Data. USAID, Sri Lanka.
Popkin, B. M., Bilsborrow, R. E., Yamamoto, M. et al.
    1979   *Breastfeeding Practices in Low Income Countries.* Chapel Hill: Carolina Population Center.
Ratnayake, R. M. P.
    1985   *Layperson's Perceptions and Behaviors Associated with Diarrhea and Dehydration. Unpublished report.* Post Graduate Institute of Medicine, University of Colombo, Sri Lanka, May.
Rodhe, J.
    1980   Attitudes and beliefs about diarrhea: To drink or not to drink. *Diarrhea Dialogue 2*: 4—4, August 1980.
Rowland, M., Barrell, R. And Whitehead, R. G.
    1978   Bacterial contamination in traditional Gambian household weaning foods. *Lancet,* 136.
Srinivas, D. K. and Afonso, E.
    1983   Community perception and practices in childhood diarrhea. *Indian Pediatrics 20*: 859—864.

Walker, A. R. and Walker B. F.
    1978   Pure water and infections in Africa. *Correspondence ii*, 639.
Waxler, N., Morrison, B., Sirisena, W., and Pinnaduwage, S.
    1985   Infant mortality in Sri Lankan households: A causal model. *Social Science and Medicine, 20*: 4, 381—392, 1985.
World Fertility Survey (Sri Lanka)
    1978   First Report of 1975 World Fertility Survey, Sri Lanka. Department of Census and Statistics.

SECTION THREE

MEDICATIONS, MEANING,
AND PHARMACEUTICAL PRACTICE

INTRODUCTION

Pharmaceutical related behavior is a subject of increasing international health interest. Anthropologists have conducted extensive research on medical systems. Much less is known cross culturally about medicine taking practice and the meanings accorded to medications. In this section, I examine the user's perspective of medicine; modes of paying for treatment and collecting a fee for curative services, and lay cost reckoning as it influences the practice of medicine. Medicines are assessed in a number of different ways. Highlighted are cultural interpretations of medicine related to their form and power, the processes of habituation and dependency, and the attributes of short term fixes as distinct from restorative medicines promoting health.

Social and economic factors contributing to the commodification of health are also considered. Increasing reliance on commercial medicine products for life's problems is viewed as both a feature of cosmopolitan life and and a practice through which capitalist ideology is subtly embodied. It is argued that models of primary health care need to extend beyond the public to the private sector and address health consumerism.

7. LAY PERCEPTIONS OF MEDICINE:
A SOUTH INDIAN CASE STUDY

INTRODUCTION

In most developing countries, multiple therapy systems, a variety of types of medicine, and a diversity of health behavior patterns coexist despite the efforts of governing bodies and the vested interests of dominant therapy systems to regulate the health behavior of populations. Numerous social scientists have studied the status and relative popularity of coexisting therapy systems. Typically such studies have focused on one of four themes. The first theme contrasts the demonstration effect and "curative" efficacy of bio-medicine on disease with the meaning centered "healing" efficacy of traditional medicine on folk illnesses having broad cultural significance. While descriptions of traditional medical systems place emphasis on meaning, caveats are made about the curative qualities of some medicinal plants. Similarly, the placebo response and the performance efficacy of impressive biomedical techniques are noted. A second type of study shifts attention toward enabling factors influencing health care seeking such as the geographic, economic and social accessibility of various types of practitioners. The third type of study considers interactional and psychosocial factors influencing medical system popularity. Attention is drawn to the influence of opinion leaders, the social status of medical systems and the process of identification. Also considered are the impact of expanding social networks resulting from factors such as women's education and disenchantment with or the romanticization of values associated with therapy systems. The fourth type of study considers the political economy of medical systems. Focused upon are the distribution of medical resources and class structure as it is reproduced in medical systems. Also considered are nationalist and revivalist movements identified with medical systems, world system penetration of local health care markets, changing trends in consumer behavior, and the relations of power associated with the processes of professionalization and specialization.

With all of this attention placed on the relative popularity and politics of medical systems it is easy to overlook two fundamental issues related to health care evaluation and demand. The first is how medications in and of themselves are assessed. The second is how interpretations of medicine influence pharmaceutical related behavior. To address these issues, it is necessary to consider yet look beyond medicine system labels. This is especially important in a day and age when a wide assortment of medicines hailing from pluralistic therapy systems are marketed in similar ways to appeal to consumer demand.

187

There is a need for medical anthropologists to consider the manner in which biotechnical fixes are understood and culturally assessed. While anthropologists have long investigated interpretations of folk illness, they have only recently begun to explore popular interpretations of the qualities of medications, the manner in which they are perceived to function, their impact on health etc. On these issues the international health literature is largely mute. In the west, the bulk of studies on medication use and nonuse have been dominated by an overriding and shortsighted concern with compliance. Compliance studies are replete with statistical analysis of patient characteristics (e.g. age, gender, education, economic status). Commonly neglected, are the social relations of taking medicines and precisely those physical aspects of medications which have attracted the attention of pharmaceutical marketing firms.

In the process of producing popular medicine forms and developing appealing images for their products, marketers of commercial medicines have been engaged in reproducing and transforming popular knowledge about both medications and illness. This knowledge is rarely paid cognizance in international health. A narrow focus on compliance has resulted in a health education literature which advocates better etic education about medicines (e.g. when and how often to take them), but overlooks the emic perception of medications and health concerns associated with them. The cart is all too often placed before the horse.

AIMS OF THE STUDY

In this chapter I will explore popular views of medicine in South Kanara District, Karnataka, India. My vantage point will be that of a rural layperson having access to a rapidly expanding pluralistic health arena. I will focus attention on ways in which the layperson thinks about medicine and how these perceptions effect medicine taking behavior. My emphasis will be on the most common ways medicines are spoken of and thought about. This data has been gleaned from conversations with numerous villagers seeking medical aid and observations in the shops and offices of a cross section of practitioner types and pharmacists. Following the presentation of data on lay evaluations of medications, I will comment on the ramifications of this data for international health.

Before discussing the South Kanara villager's perception of medicine, it is necessary to correct a somewhat misleading stereotype of the Hindu villager and describe the contemporary health care arena within the setting of the bazaar. A questioning of the portrayal of the rural villager as "thinking" within an ayurvedic cognitive framework is warranted because social science literature in the 1960's—70's tended to infer that ayurveda was a formal systematic expression of folk health culture in rural India.[1] A brief description of a town health arena, as seen through the eyes of a villager will be presented as a means of highlighting the eclectic practice of medicine in India and the *masala* of medicines produced and advertised. This description is meant to complement observations made by Leslie (1976). Leslie has described the widespread combined use of indigenous and allopathic medicine by cosmopolitan practitioners. He aptly characterizes the villager seeking medical assistance as more concerned with questions of cost, time and empathy than types of therapy systems.

While I agree with Leslie to a large extent, his remarks on choice of therapy need to be qualified. I will argue that pharmaceutical behavior is significantly influenced both by patterns of illness specific curative resort (e.g. those reported in Chapters 5 and 6), and the layperson's demand for and concern about specific medicine forms. As we shall see, the latter are evaluated in relation to the recipient's relative strength, age, previous experience with medicine, and special considerations (e.g. during pregnancy and early childhood). Perceptions about the immediate and long term action of medicines on health, not only illness, influence health care behavior.

FOLK HEALTH CULTURE, AYURVEDA AND POPULAR HEALTH CULTURE

In many ways a discussion of the relationship between the ayurvedic system of medicine and South Kanarese folk health culture is similar to a discussion about the Brahmanization of the South Kanarese pantheon (Nichter 1977). I may exploit this comparison while noting that ayurvedic and Brahmanic world views are closely aligned philosophically (Zimmerman 1987). The South Kanarese pantheon is composed of numerous indigenous Tuluva deities *bhuta*, as well as pan-Indian gods, just as the popular health sector is composed of numerous folk healers and a few influential ayurvedic pandits (a majority of whom are Brahmans or Keralites steeped in Brahmanic tradition). Just as Brahman priests have, over the years, encompassed Tuluva deities within a distinctly Brahmanic cosmology and organizational structure, so ayurvedic pandits have encompassed folk health notions and practices within a highly elaborate and accommodative ayurvedic conceptual system. The legitimacy of encompassment has been facilitated by the high and to some degree sacred status accorded to ayurveda by Brahman priests.

What is important to note here is that while Brahmanic tenets about hierarchy and order in the cosmos and ayurvedic statements about humors and illness are accepted as authoritative, the actual impact of both Brahmanization and ayurveda on local Tuluva culture has been limited although pronounced. While the principles of ayurveda are publicly acknowledged as eternal truths, the layperson's comprehension of ayurveda is limited to a few names of illnesses and medicines which for the most part have taken on local significance. For the typical villager, the understanding of ayurveda's central most principle of body humors; the *tridhatu/tridosha*, is limited to a notion of *dosha*, troubles, and not body processes. Humoral nomenclature, *vata*, *pitta* and *kapha* have, like the term "liver" (more recently introduced by cosmopolitan physicians) become synonymous with illnesses and symptom complexes.

Three points may be made about ayurveda which I feel have fairly widespread validity in rural India. First, the response to illness by the non-Brahman lay population does not reflect an ayurvedic approach to health care despite the fact that ayurveda and folk medicine share points of commonality, e.g. a concern about hot-cold, a hydraulic model of the body, concern about the blood and digestion, etc. I do not mean to belittle the impact of ayurveda on popular health culture by this statement anymore than I would want to disregard Brahmanic elements of local Tuḷuva ritual. What I wish to emphasize is that discrete ayurvedic practices, and medicines, not a systematic ayurvedic model of health and pathology influence popular health care behavior.

A second point is that the practice of orthodox ayurveda represented in classical texts is not presently, nor has been (in recent history) a popular form of therapy available to the majority of the rural poor. Moreover, systematic ayurvedic treatment is not affordable by most people. The notion that systematic ayurvedic therapy, based upon ayurvedic diagnostic principles, is readily available and inexpensive in village India is unfounded. This myth is propagated by surveys which classify all herbal practitioners as practitioners of ayurvedic medicine confounding herbal medicines with ayurveda. This is misleading. The third and related point is that the system of ayurveda as presented in texts and by authoritative pundits is not understood by most folk herbal practitioners. For that matter, a great many practitioners administering ayurvedic medicine rely more on the commercial medicine catalogues provided to them by ayurvedic medicine companies than ayurvedic texts when determining treatment. Increasingly, these catalogues have been inundated by popular biomedical terminology indicative of the "scientization" of ayurveda. Ayurveda is being dressed up for modern presentation, while at the same time biomedical syndromes are being encompassed within a humoral conceptual framework. A mixing of metaphors and images of health as well as medicines is occurring in India today. Popular health culture is a bricolage, an assemblage of ecletic conceptual and material resources.

QUALIFIED AND UNQUALIFIED MASALA MEDICINE

Let us imagine a villager who travels to a nearby town to obtain health care after exploiting more accessible sources of aid. Numerous medical shops are found in most fair sized towns and the villager strolls past a few. As the villager looks into each shop, he pays little attention to the qualifications boldly written or scribbled under the names of each practitioner. This is hardly surprising given the proliferation of abbreviations which are displayed. Abbreviations for licenses from regional and foreign medical schools as well as integrated medicine courses of allopathy and ayurveda (from different states at different points in time) are intermixed with initials designating homeopathic correspondence courses, the possession of university certificates (in some cases, certificates of attendance not completion!), foreign training or residence, and membership in little known and oft-time bogus professional societies. During my first visit to the small city of Mangalore, I counted nineteen different abbreviations under the names of practitioners, nine of which I was never able to identify.

Rather than look at qualifications, the villager focuses attention on the types of medicines and paraphernalia exhibited in medical shops. By looking at the medicines and paraphernalia in these shops, however, it is difficult to distinguish the type of therapy system which a practitioner is practicing. Many institutionally trained, as well as non-institutionally trained, registered medical practitioners engage in an eclectic form of therapy which draws from all existing therapy systems. Their shops display hypodermic sets and stethoscopes as well as hand labelled bottles of ayurvedic tonics, tins of metallic oxides and a few vials of homeopathic pills. The offices of recent graduates of ayurvedic and homeopathic colleges commonly display stethoscopes as well as a carefully laid out stock of commercial ayurvedic/homeopathic medicines bottled and packaged in much the same ways as allopathic medicine. In most offices, a syringe and a collection of allopathic and ayurvedic injectables (indistinguishable to the villager) are conspicuous. It is also not uncommon to see joint clinics where both allopathic and ayurvedic drugs and services are found under the same roof. As Leslie (1976) has noted, many of these joint clinics are managed by two generation medical families adapting to a competitive medical market.

Passing by the office of an MBBS doctor, our villager may see in addition to a stock of allopathic medicines several different varieties of patent ayurvedic medicines, most of which have English names. If the villager could read English he would find these labels replete with the language of biomedical science. The same medicines are on display at the chemist shop. Approaching the chemist shop he may not see familiar ayurvedic medicinal tonics on the shelf, but if he asks there is a high likelihood that the *arishta* he wants for his postpartum wife will be produced from the backroom. The *arishta* may be a commercial product of a company from Kerala, his own district, Bombay or Calcutta. He will be asked a brand preference.

The villager walks through a bazaar, where the medicines and paraphernalia of coexisting medical systems are displayed to attract the passerby. The practice of medicine, particularly by less expensive practitioners who are attractive to the villager is eclectic, and in the words of one informant. "*masala*" — mixed to the taste and pocket.

Let us imagine that the villager inquires of relatives about the type of treatment given by various practitioners in the town. What types of description would he receive? While listening to numerous descriptions of practitioners, I found that comments were often made either about the general cost of a practitioner's treatment, or a practitioner's healing capacity "power of the hand". The latter was often discussed in relation to the curing of specific illnesses or specific age groups. Comments also center on a practitioner's medical paraphernalia and the kind of medicine he dispensed. It was not uncommon to hear practitioners discussed in relation to the form of medicine they gave for a particular ailment, e.g. single injection, "double" injection (distilled water and a vial of medicine), injection-powered pills (capsules) or tonics for a particular type of ailment. In the mid 1970's it was not uncommon to hear villagers speaking of practitioners in terms of the type of stethoscope, "dekree", which they possessed. German, English and Indian stethoscopes were credited with having varying capacities to locate illness. To some extent, the villager's faith in the reading of the pulse by ayurvedic professionals was transferred to the stethoscope; the achieved ability of medical technology being given similar status to the ascribed ability of the practitioner. Villager's requests of practitioners to touch the body near the location of illness with the stethoscope resemble requests for the laying of hands. Thus, an aspect of *kayi guna*, "the power of the hand" was transferred to the stethoscope.

Other descriptions of practitioners by laypersons portray them as agents of pharmaceutical firms, distributing particular brands of medicine. Some villagers spoke of going to a practitioner in the town as going to the "company". Their attitude is reflected in the fact that when a therapy administered by one practitioner was not considered efficacious, the appropriateness of the medicine for the patient was as often questioned as the skill of the practitioner. A prevalent idea was that the medicine might be appropriate for another person manifesting similar symptoms (if not the same illness category) because of differences in body constitution or life style. In such cases, a patient might request a different kind of medicine from the same practitioner or go to a different practitioner for a different "brand" of medicine. Observations of 150 illness episodes (diarrhea, respiratory tract infections, fever) revealed that the average length of time a villager taking medication was willing to wait for symptoms to diminish or disappear before seeking an alternative treatment was four days, the equivalent of 1.5 visits to the practitioner. A survey of 50 rural households proximate to a town revealed that in 75%, an established relationship with a particular family practitioner did not exist.

As the villager circulates within the health arena he is, as Leslie has suggested, more concerned with time, cost and empathy on the part of the practitioner than the type of medical shop/office (if not therapy system) consulted. This trial and error approach to the seeking of health services creates a client dominant medical market (Friedson 1970) characterized by low compliance and high pressure for practitioners to produce demonstration effects through medicines administered. In such a context, health care provision is significantly influenced by client demand. An important aspect of client demand, are illness and age specific ideas about and preferences for forms of medicine having particular characteristics. Interest in the form, and increasingly in the brand, of medicine often supercedes interest in a medical system per se.

Let us next consider ways in which medications are perceived. We may focus attention on the themes of habitation and power, dietary advice offered in conjunction with medicine use, and overt characteristics of medicine (form, color, and taste).

HABITUATION (ABHIYASA, AUCITYA)

That plant is a good medicine for fever; it was used by my father. I do not use it ... I have taken many injections ... herbal medicine does not "take to" my body (excerpt from fieldnotes).

The concept of *abhiyasa*, habituation, is a counterpart to the concept of body constitution, *prakṛti*. One is born with a particular *prakṛti* subject to the characteristics of age and humoral predominance, but one gains *abhiyasa*. In the words of one villager:

"Some people are born with the capacity to gain weight easily, others eat but gain little, this is due to their *prakṛti*. Health, their age or the seasons may influence their digestive power, but they always have this capacity, it it their *prakṛti*. *Abhiyasa* is the way a rice eater adjusts to be able to digest wheat after some period of time. As a parboiled rice eater if I eat wheat it is heating to my body and I become constipated, even raw (polished) rice causes these problems. But to one with *abhiyasa* these foods are neutral and they do not suffer."

An analogy was drawn by another informant between the concepts of constitution and habituation and one's fate and *karma* — the fruit of one's work:

nontransformable:	*transformable*:
hanne baraha (unqualified fate, what one is):	*karma*, reaping what one sows, inherited obligations and responsibilities (what one has).
prakṛti (one's constitution):	*abhiyasa* (what one gains through experience), habituation.

An appreciation of *abhiyasa* is important for an understanding of health and medicine taking behavior. It is common to hear a villager describing why a medicine has not been useful for him because he has no *abhiyasa* for that kind of medicine. This comment is made of both cosmopolitan and traditional herbal medicine. During a health behavior survey in 1974, I asked 100 adults stratified by caste and class whether they thought herbal medicine (folk as well as ayurvedic) was as effective as it had been 20 years prior. Over 90% of informants answered that herbal medicine was less effective. The reasons given for this phenomena included changes in diet, the decreased potency of raw drugs and increased tea drinking. The most frequently mentioned reason was the increased use of "English" medicine. According to the concept of *abhiyasa*, for the body to "take to" a new food or type of medicine it must first adjust to its properties. For this reason, mothers feed a young child minute quantities of food prior to weaning so that the child will become accustomed to the food. In the case of medicine, a young child regularly receives herbal preventive medicine for a number of culturally defined illnesses. Cosmopolitan medicine is generally not administered unless a crisis occurs. Likewise, a breastfeeding mother avoids the extensive use of cosmopolitan medicine, lest it be transferred to the child through breastmilk. Cosmopolitan medicines are thought to be too powerful for a child's body to be able to accommodate. Moreover, they interfere with a child's capacity to "take to" the herbal medicines used in the home for preventive and common curative functions. Children are gradually introduced to cosmopolitan medicine through crisis involving illnesses which the villager believes to be managed faster by "English" medicine. Thus, the young lose their habituation to herbal medicine and gain habituation to cosmopolitan medicine. But at what cost?

When one is habituated to cosmopolitan medicine, herbal medicine is thought to be less effective. Many villagers think that english medicine offers a quick cure but eventually harms the overall intergrity of one's health. This concept is expressed by the statement that "english" medicine is heating and its continued use leads to bloodlessness and weakness. One educated informant drew the following analogy between chemical urea fertilizer and "English" medicine:

"English" medicine and urea are both powerful, heating, and harmful after some years of use . . . But, they are popular. Urea makes crops green overnight and increases yield until one day you find that the earth is hot, acidic, and useless. Injections are like that too. You take them and feel better quickly but later your body turns weak . . . Yes, the agricultural extension officer tells us to balance urea with potash and other chemicals and that this will prevent the soil from becoming hot. The doctor tells us to eat good food, drink milk, and take tonic and we will not have side effects from the injections he gives us. But this is not how we live . . . We don't drink milk or take tonic daily, nor do we use fertilizer the way they tell us . . . This is not our habit — such things are costly and we have other needs.

The comment that the use of "english" medicine eventually leads to weakness indexes other concerns. In developing an *abhiyasa* to "english" medicine, the villager enters into a dependency relationship. In the words of one ayurvedic vaidya:

Allopathic medicines are like eyeglasses. Once you put them on, your eyes do not improve, they become dim with continual use and you come to depend on them more and more.

Eyeglasses are not bad, they are useful for those who grow old. They are a good crutch, but if one does not need a crutch this may be a bad thing. One leans on the crutch and does not strengthen the leg, one wears the glasses and does not strengthen the eyes, one takes medicines and does not strengthen the body, one becomes dependent on the medicine bottle. The company becomes strong, the body remains weak.

A sense of understanding health in terms of a routine set of bodily signs and processes is forfeited as a result of medicine taking, a change in life style or diet. This results in a feeling that one has lost control over one's long term health, a sense of alienation which impacts on health behavior (Chapter 9). In some instances, attempts are made to regain this sense of health through becoming rehabituated to herbal medicine and traditional diet. Patients who have an ailment which cosmopolitan medicine has failed to cure may use substances such as blood purifiers, purgatives and diuretics, to realign themselves to herbal treatment. Other people seek realignment with ayurvedic medicine as a means of identifying with or embodying Brahmanic values (Nichter 1981). This latter group includes revivalistic Hindu leaders who have championed ayurveda for political as well as personal purposes.

POWER

Comments about a medicine's power are common when therapy is discussed. Villagers consider medicine in relation to both its inherent power and the ability of the patient to accommodate to this power. Powerful medicine is desired by those whose body can stand the "shock" which it entails. The shock factor is considered carefully when a person is deemed to have constitutional weakness, when a chronic illness renders one weak but demands long term treatment, and during times of vulnerability such as pregnancy and postpartum. Shock is also an important health concern for infants and children who have experienced multiple illnesses. This is particularly true in seasons interpreted as having a negative impact on health, blood purity and digestive capacity (e.g. monsoon season).

As a category, "english" medicines are spoken of as powerful yet dangerous. Let us consider what the concept "powerful" means to the villager. Conceptually, power is regarded as unstable, vacillating, and requiring control; a factor evident in ritual healing as well as in the worship of deities (Nichter 1977). While english medicine is praised for its fast action, it is commonly spoken about as having "uncontrolled" side effects. Ayurvedic medicine, on the other hand, is referred to as a controlled medicine engendering balance. Ayurveda is typically spoken of as "causing no side effects", a statement having symbolic significance.

Gleaning my notes on these two general catetories of medicines, a set of oppositions emerged which was complementary to a set of oppositions noted between classes of deities by Brahman priests (and others). Contrasted were more stable Brahmanic gods receiving vegetarian offerings and more rash, blood demanding deities of local *bhuta* possession cults. Presented below is protypical knowledge emergent from the discourse of one of my key *vaidya* informants. These oppositions were cross validated in interviews with other informants.

Local *bhuta* deities	:	Brahmanic deities
Uncontrolled power/desire	:	Controlled power/balance
Immediate action, often rash action	:	Ultimate justice overtime
Requires blood sacrifices	:	Vegetarian offerings
English/cosmopolitan medicine	:	Ayurveda
Heating	:	Balanced, *sama*
Reduces blood	:	Produces blood

"English" medicine is commonly referred to as heating and ayurvedic medicine as *sama*,[2] neutral, although individual medicines within each system are recognized as having heating and cooling properties. The term "heating" is multivocal, its meaning varying by context. Saying that "english" medicines are heating is in one sense a statement about the speed at which they act. It also indexes association with uncontrolled activity and heightened danger. *Sama*, as the term is applied to ayurvedic medicine expresses balanced action and the concept of control. Stating that "english" medicine is heating also infers something about its perceived effect on the blood. The notion exists that heating the blood causes it to evaporate. In Tulu, the expression used to explain this process is *netter ajune*; *ajune* is the verb used to describe water evaporating from a boiling rice pot. Since digestive capacity is related to the quantity of blood and to general strength, the statement that "english" medicine is heating conveys a sense that one is at risk to general symptoms of malaise as well as symptoms such as burning skin rashes and burning urine associated with heat.

Some villagers frequent ayurvedic vaidya or folk herbalists weeks or even months after taking cosmopolitan therapy for medicines to cool the body and replenish blood loss. Here, herbal medicine is taken to complement "english" medicine by restoring the integrity of body processes which has been disrupted by powerful medicine. The notion that powerful medicine disrupts body processes and causes weakness is one reason why "english" medicine is not favored for the very young or old. It is not because villagers "have not experienced the wonders of cosmopolitan medicine" that they may choose to use such medicine sparingly for sickly children or the elderly. It is precisely cosmopolitan medicine's display of power that leads some adults to commonly use such medicines themselves while maintaining a more cautious set of medicine taking behaviors for individuals they deem at risk.

Medicines administered for one purpose are sometimes used for other purposes on the basis of assumptions about how they effect the body.[3] For example, menses is thought to be a state of overheat in the body — "like a rice pot boiling over." When a woman suffers from amenorrhoea a cosmopolitan practitioner or chemist shop often prescribes a hormone booster such as E. P. Forte to induce her period. The popular interpretation of the drug's action is that it causes the blood to heat up and the *vayu* (wind principle) to push the blood out of the body. Accordingly, a popular notion is that if two tablets are powerful enough to induce menses, than a double or triple dose will heat the body enough to induce an abortion. A flourishing trade exists in towns with women purchasing four to eight tablets when they think they are pregnant and want to abort. College girls take these tablets as a morning after pill. Cloroquine tablets also believed to be heating are used the same way. Another dramatic instance of the action of a medicine being interpreted beyond its biomedical intent involves antishistamines. In both India and Sri Lanka some women consume antihistamines as a powerful drying agent for body secretions manifest as leucorrhea. In Korea, Kendall (1987) describes a similar usage of antibiotics.

Villagers view medication based on perceptions of power gradation in relation to dose and medicine form. Tablets are perceived as weaker doses of medication than injections and a notion exists that a single injection is a weaker dose of medication than a double injection — a term referring to a test dose and an injection, or to an injection where the villager observes a vial of distilled water being mixed with a vial of medicine powder. Accordingly, some people try to enhance the power of recommended doses of medication against the instruction of practitioners. If one tablet does not yield satisfactory results, two or three tablets are taken simultaneously and if a single injection is given for an ailment for which a friend has received a double injection, another practitioner may be frequented for another injection without mention being made of prior treatment. I never saw or heard of this strategy being applied to herbal therapy. One reason, perhaps, is because it is not merely the power of the drug which is considered in indigenous therapy, but notions such as balance, purification and digestive effect.

With respect to cosmopolitan medicines' "display of power", it may be noted that common acts associated with the administration of cosmopolitan medicine are also interpreted as increasing the power of the medicine. For example, the heating of a needle before an injection is interpreted by some villagers not as a sterilization procedure, but as a method which increases the power of the medicine and the speed at which it travels through the body (*vis-à-vis* heat).

Going to a practitioner is a learning experience for the villager. The villager listens, watches, and interprets what transpires at the clinic in terms of preexisting knowledge. Conventional knowledge is reproduced in such settings. New impressions are also formed. The perceived action of a medicine causes the villager to extend or interpret notions of physiology and bodily processes. For example, according to South Kanarese notions of physiology, many channels, *narambu*, run throughout the body. When talking to villagers about *narambu*, I found that some explanations about the structure of *narambu* networks were based on experiences with medicine.

Some informants noted to me that *narambu* were all connected. When I asked how thy knew this I was told that an injection was given in the left arm despite where an illness was in the body. Therefore, the medicine must travel through all the *narambu* to get to the location where it was required. Unlike herbal medicine, an injection did not go to the stomach first. It is important to recognize that experiences with medicine draw from and expand explanatory models of physiology and health. Medicines are more than fixes, just as foods are more than nutrients. They are thought about as well as consumed.

DIET AND MEDICINE

"Disease is a hunger, food a medicine for that hunger."

In a culture having an elaborate multidimensional food classification system and set of folk dietetic norms (Nichter 1986), diet is viewed as an essential part of the treatment of illness. One of the few questions a villager asks a practitioner during a consultation is what types of food should and should not be consumed. The question refers both to the patient's illness and the type of medication administered by the practitioner. The villager already maintains a number of folk ideas about diet during illness which include both restricted and prescribed foods. The patient expects that a practitioner will offer specific advice about diet after considering the illness, the patient's body constitution and the qualities of the medicine administered.

Foods are thought to enhance and facilitate the action of medicines as well as to provide a means of balancing the extreme qualities of medicines. For example, most impoverished villagers in South Kanara drink milk only during times of illness and when taking medicines. Traditionally, ayurveda placed great importance on milk, buttermilk and ghee both in the preparation of medicines and as a vehicle, *malpudi*, to assist a medicine "take to" the body. Milk is thought to enhance the action of medicine. This notion has been incorporated in folk therapies to a lesser extent. With respect to cosmopolitan medicine, however, milk drinking plays a different role. Milk is thought to reduce and control the heating side effects of cosmopolitan medicine, particularly when administered in injection form. This impression is fostered by the nutritionally orientated advice offered by cosmopolitan practitioners for patients to drink milk. Villagers have interpreted this advice to mean that cosmopolitan medicine is so very heating that it requires milk as a counterbalancing agent.

Milk is not only thought to be a necessary commodity to be consumed after an injection or capsule,[4] but a substance which may be used by villagers attempting to limit the action of medicine. For example, piperazine citrate, a deworming medicine is considered to be very heating for the body. According to indigenous notions of physiology, an optimum number of worms existing in a symbiotic relationship with the body are necessary for the digestive process. When villagers are told that piperazine will remove all worms, they become concerned. In an effort to retain at least a few worms, villagers drink milk to constrain the medicine's action. Milk is consumed a few hours after taking piperazine as a means of limiting the heating action of the drug.

The importance given to milk by villagers effects compliance behavior. I have spoken to many villagers who were reluctant to take cosmopolitan medicine for long periods of time if a supply of milk was not available to them. Other villagers reduced the quantity of medicine which they took because milk was unavailable. This was particularly the case where a large number of tablets were prescribed each day (e.g. 6 sulfamadizide tablets) followed by a practitioner's advice to drink plenty of water (to flush the kidneys). More sensitive practitioners, recognizing the importance villagers place on balancing heating medicines by the use of cooling substances, advise the drinking of tender cocount water or lemon juice as substitutes when milk is unavailable.

The ambivalence paid to diet by many cosmopolitan practitioners has resulted in patients disassociating diet from the curative process engaged by "english" medicine. Some have come to view cosmopolitan medicine as requiring no specific diet. For example, village women who deliver at primary health centers are offered a diet which runs counter to traditional dietary restrictions followed during postpartum. A good example of this involves blackgram, classified as toxic, *nanju* and traditionally avoided during illness (Nichter 1986). In the hospital, protein rich blackgram preparations, such as *idli*, are commonly served. Patients will often eat such foods when they are in the hospital, but abstain from them once they have returned home to convalesce. Patients interviewed stated that while taking hospital medicine, diet did not matter because the medicine controlled the body. It was observed, however, that if infection manifested post hospital discharge, it was common to hear family members blame inappropriate foods consumed at the hospital as the cause. Follow up interviews revealed that the effects of *nanju* food were thought to be suppressed but not eliminated by cosmopolitan medicine.

The cosmopolitan practitioner's lack of sensitivity to diet has important public health ramifications. The cosmopolitan practitioner is viewed by villagers as knowing about technical cures, medicines which reduce symptoms, but not much about health. Such practitioners are not thought to understand the population's everyday and special seasonal dietary needs. While this impression has not decreased their popularity as a treatment resource for illness, it has effected the villager's evaluation of these practitioners as sources of appropriate advice about preventive and promotive health. This is unfortunate for most villagers do think it is the practitioner's duty to know about and offer advice about diet for health (Nichter 1984).

PHYSICAL CHARACTERISTICS OF MEDICINE

The form in which a medicine is administered is highly significant to the villager. It is not uncommon to hear a village patient request a liquid mixture, pills or an injection during a consultation. In addition to interest in medicine form, patients articulated interest in or questioned the color or taste of medicines prescribed. Let us consider why it is that medicines having different forms and physical characteristics are requested or deemed appropriate at different times.

Injections, as I have already noted, are considered powerful and heating. Like stethoscopes, some villagers have classified injections on the basis of their power (Indian, English, German) the most powerful injection being those manifesting the greatest "burn sensation" (German injections). Injections are preferred by those who want quick symptomatic relief. For those patients who fear that they may be too weak to withstand the shock of an injection, injection-powered pills (capsules) are sometimes requested. Alternatively, mixtures are desired for infants and those experiencing chronic debility and weakness. This is due to ease in administration as well as the fact that they are considered to be less powerful and "shocking" to the body.

Illness specific "medicine form" preferences exist and are cross cut by age specific preferences. In instances where there is a felt need for dramatic curative action, preferences are suspended. Such cases are not necessarily acute or life threatening. For example, injections which are not generally popular for toddlers are deemed especially effective for the cure of pus (*raci*) in wounds and swelling. "The heating action of injections dry up rashes and wounds". I interviewed several rural lower middle class mothers who were in the process of taking children with weeping scabies (*kajji*) to doctors. Most wished to secure injections. Five cases were followed over a three month period of time. In all five cases, injections of antibiotics were received for these children without topical treatment (benzol benzoate is standard treatment) or instructions for mothers to boil clothes, cleanse the skin routinely, or have the child sleep alone. In three cases, the children frequented doctors six or more times for injections during this time period, while in one of the other two households the child was taken for follow up treatment to a chemist. He sold the mother tonic for blood purification and an appropriate topical treatment providing instruction for its use. In the other household, the child's condition improved, but a subsequent urinary track inflammation was attributed to the treatment.

Mother's interpretations of '*kajji*' illness associated this ailment with heat in the body or impurities in the blood. Irregardless of their perceptions of etiology and despite their concern about the power of injections, mothers sought the acknowledged ability of injections to dry weeping rashes rapidly. Their impression was that pus originated from within and had little to do with hygiene from without. A topical prescription was not a felt need, but dietary restrictions were followed against foods thought to increase *raci* (*nanju* foods). In some cases, cooling foods were consumed to reduce heat in the body after injections were taken. In two cases, herbal medicine were taken following a drying of the rash to clean the blood.

Irregardless of age, injections are popular for diarrhea with vomiting, and high as well as persistent fevers. These are ailments requiring immediate and dramatic relief. In general, however, injections are not popular for infants and pre-school age children deemed to have weak and developing constitutions. For all but acute ailments, mixtures are preferred for these age groups. For complaints associated with poor digestion, liquids are a clear preference. Tablets are popular for respiratory complaints among adults, but observations of the elderly revealed that when a number of pills are prescribed at once, concern is expressed about medications interfering with digestion and resulting in debility. The same is true of adults asked to take tablets for long periods of time for illnesses like T.B. associated with debility.

Weakness experienced by a patient during an illness in which pills have been administered is sometimes attributed to the interference of the pill with the patient's digestive process and not the illness. If tablets cause thirst or a practitioner tells the patient to drink plenty of water with the tablet, the medication is suspected as not only being difficult to digest, but being heating. Liquids are preferred for bloodlessness (anaemia) and weakness because they are believed to readily join the blood. Medicine in liquid form is especially desirable by pregnant women who not only feel that injections are too powerful and heating (capable of inducing abortion), but fear that pills might sit in their stomachs. According to indigenous notions of physiology, (described in chapter two), the fetus grows in the "stomach pot" and shares the stomach space with food. Some women perceive pills as not only being difficult to digest but causing ill effects for the fetus.

Among lactating women there is a concern that the medicine taken by the mother is transferred to the baby through breastmilk. This was observed to be related to two behavior patterns having public health significance. First, when taking "strong" medication some women cease breastfeeding temporarily if not permanently. In two cases where this was observed, a concern about medicine led to sudden weaning and subsequent histories of infant diarrhea. On a breastfeeding survey, to be discussed elsewhere, more than a quarter of 80 rural women surveyed associated illness and medicine taking with the cessation of breastfeeding.[5] The second pattern, observed more commonly in neighboring North Kanara District, involved women consuming medicines intended for their baby as a means of transferring the medicine's qualities to their child. By in large, doctors interviewed about this behavior pattern were unaware of it. I first observed mothers consuming their infant's medicine while conducting a first-aid clinic in the village in which I lived.

Table I presents survey data on preferred forms of medications for specific types of illnesses. It may be noted that different forms of medication

TABLE I. Preferred Form of Treatment, South Kanara District.

Illness	Adults						Children			
	Injections (I)		Pills and capsules (P) H = herbal		Liquid mixture (M)		0–3 years		3–7 years	
	V	T	V	T	V	T	V	T	V	T
I Fevers										
Sita jara A cold with fever	*	+		*	*	+	+(M)	+(M)	*(I) *(M)	*(M)
Chali jara High fever with chills	+	+			*	*	*(I) *(M)	+(M)	+(I) *(P)(M)	*(I)(P) *(M)
Sanni Prolonged high fever	+	+			*	*	*(I) *(M)	*(M)	+(I) +(M)	*(I) *(M)
II Respiratory										
Kemmu Wet cough			+	+	*	*	*(P)(M)	+(M)	*(I) *(P)	*(I) *(P)
Ubbasa Wheezing			*	*	*	*	*(P)(M)	+(M)	*(I)(M) *(P)	*(I)(M) *(P)
TB	+	+							+(I)	*(I)(P)(M)
III Digestive/urinary										
Loss of appetite					+	+	+(M)	+(M)	*(M)	+(M)
Ajirna Poor digestion			(H)	(H)	+	+	+(M)	+(M)	+(M)	+(M)
Nitrana Bloodlessness			*	*	+	+	+(M)	+(M)	*(M)	+(M)

Table I (Continued)

| | Adults | | | | | | Children | | | |
| | Injections (I) | | Pills and capsules (P) H = herbal | | Liquid mixture (M) | | 0–3 years | | 3–7 years | |
Illness	V	T	V	T	V	T	V	T	V	T
Puri Worms					++	++	+(M)	+(M)	+(M)	+(M)
Pipadike bundapune Constipation			*	*	+	+	*(M)	+(M)	+(M)	+(M)
Julab Water diarrhea			*	*	+	+	+(M)	*(M)	+(M)	*(M)
Urchune kakkune Diarrhea & vomiting	+	*	*	+			*(I)(M)	*(I) +(M)	+(I)	*(P)(I)
Uri padike Burning urine	–	–	*	*	+	+	*(M)	+(M)	*(M)	+(M)
IV Skin										
Kajji Weeping rash	+	+					+(I)(P)	*(I)(P)	+(I)(P)	*(I)(P)
Nanji Infected wound	+	+	*	*			*(I) +(P)	*(I) *(P)	*(I) +(P)	*(I)(P)
Udarpu Swelling	*	*		*			*(I)(P)	*(I)(P)	*(I)(P)	+(I)

+ = Very strong felt (> 70% sample); * = Strongly felt (40%–70% sample); (I) = Injections; (P) = Pills and capsules; (M) = Liquid mixture; (H) = Herbal; (V) = Village: N = 30; (T) = Town: N = 20.

are preferred for adults and among children, aged below and over three years. For example, injections were preferred for *chali jwara* (fever with chills) for adults, but mixtures were preferred for young children with differences of opinion existing between village and town populations as to appropriate treatment for children over three years of age. Differences in preference were also found to exist between towns and villages. Interestingly among the poor and lower middle class, injections were as popular, if not slightly more popular in villages than towns. Differences in medicine preference between the illiterate and semi literate were not statistically significant and therefore are not reported.

COLOR AND TASTE

Medicine is scrutinized in terms of its color in as much as colors are thought to signify a medicine's inherent properties.[6] For example, a black medicine is thought to be powerful as well as being good at reducing *pitta*, an ayurvedic term used in local parlance to denote nausea, dizzziness, or yellow bodily excretions (eg. urine, mucus). Black pills are considered appropriate for vomiting, fever and fits, but not for digestive disorders, weakness or bloodlessness. This is one reason black ferrous sulfate tablets are not popular among pregnant women and those experiencing weakness due to anaemia. Both the form and color of this iron supplement are not culturally appropriate.

White medicines, particularly liquids, are generally attributed to have a neutral if not a cooling quality. They are deemed to be more easily digested by the body than medicines of other colors and are trusted more when consumed for the first time. White pills are often interpreted as cooling and appropriate for fever, burning sensation, body pain, headache, and a loss of vitality, complaints all linked to overheat.

Red medicines, particularly pills, are attributed to be heating and good for wet cough and cold. However, liquid red colored medicines are thought to be blood producing despite the fact that cooling foods and medicines are generally attributed to be blood producing. In this case of mixed signals, color concordance, i.e. red substance and blood, supercede an association of the color red and heat.

Yellow medicines are generally thought to be heating and aggravate *pitta* when consumed internally. As a topical medicine, however, yellow ointments are viewed as purification agents. An association is made between yellow and turmeric, a traditional blood and skin purifier used both in the home and for ritual purposes. Burnal, an ointment purchased over the counter, is used for a wide range of skin infections and cuts. Its popularity is in large part derived from its yellow color which villagers associate with turmeric. Here, we have an instructive case where the attributes of a traditional medicine are applied to a commercial medicine having similar physical characteristics.

Taste, like the form and color of medicine is also regarded as a sign of a medicine's inherent qualitative characteristics. The tastes, astringent and bitter, are generally regarded as cooling for the body and are thought to have a positive promotive/medicinal value. Herbs having a bitter/astringent taste (like black tea) are labelled *kanir* and are commonly used as folk medicines. For example, a number of *kanir* astringent herbs and shoots of budding trees are used as preventive medicines (*kodi oshadi*) for young children as well as being used as general medicine for stomach aches, fever, and blood impurities (Chapter 5). Salty medicines, on the other hand, are viewed suspiciously

TABLE II. Associations Between the Color, Taste, and Effect of Medicines.

Color or taste	Associations/ property (guna)	Good for	Negative effect
Yellow	*pitta* *ushna*	as a topical medicine for *nanji* (septic wounds, skin diseases)	turns feces and urine yellow, phlegm turns yellow, *pitta*, heating
Black	powerful, reduces *pitta*, may be very cooling or heating	vomiting, fever, fits	dangerous, causes digestive disorders, black feces
White	safe, *sama* i.e. not heating or cooling.	cleans the blood; bloodlessness, semen loss, septic wounds, fever; Breastmilk	none
Red	powerful, heating, blood producing	cold, wet cough, blood producing	fever, diarrhea *dhatu* loss (especially tablets)
Bitter	cool, health promoting	cough, stomach pain preventive medicine	none
Sweet	cooling	fever, children's illnesses	not useful for skin illnesses, worms
Salty	heating, dangerous for bones		vomiting, joint pain

by villagers and thought harmful for the bones (causing brittleness) if taken for any length of time. Pungent medicines are considered appropriate for cough (as they melt mucus) and as digestive aides, but they are considered inappropriate for skin diseases, urinary tract disorders, or rheumatic complaints.

TEXTURE, LIGHTNESS AND HEAVINESS

Texture and perceptions of the inherent lightness and heaviness of substances also effect the way in which they are evaluated as curative resources. While oily substances are not generally consumed as foods during skin ailments or illnesses entailing skin eruptions, externally applied medicinal oils are popular for skin ailments, wounds and for head related ailments. The latter range from headache and sleeplessness to anxiety, sexual overstimulation and the improvement of mental capacity. Taken internally, oils are considered to increase the production of pus as well as to be difficult to digest. Used externally, they are believed to transfer the qualities of medicines contained in them directly to the regions where they are applied.

The taking of oil baths is a popular promotive health activity in South Kanara at once associated with cleanliness and ritual purity as well as the stimulation of flow within the body.[7] It is for this reason that oils are placed on the skin as a means of purification and to promote healing. A differentiation is made between light oils (e.g. sesame seed oil) and heavy oils (e.g. coconut oil) with light oils preferred as a vehicle for medicines to be internalized through the skin and heavier oils popular for purification. In preference to soap, oils are often a first line of purification.[8] A wound will be covered with oil in which medicines have been ground or fried. Moreover, after using insecticides agricultural laborers will demand that employers supply oil for an oil bath to remove itching and burning sensations. Infection will rarely be attributed to the external care of a wound or open sore. Attention is directed to the quality of the blood within, digestive capacity and diet. Medicinal oils are also popular for the head with cooling oils (e.g. *Bhrami tyla, Tripaladi tyla* used to lessen overheat in the head at large causing hair loss, and in the brain resulting in anxiety, confusion and sexual stimulation as well as poor sleep.

Medicines as well as foods are attributed to be inherently heavy or light. Light is a term which denotes relative digestibility and low shock impact on bodily processes. Those who are young, pregnant, weak or convalescing are thought to require restorative medicines and supplements which are light and easy to digest. The healthy who wish to enhance their present state of health or improve their weight are attracted to medicines which are associated with heavy and strength producing substances.[9] An important distinction is made between substances which are appropriate for the ill as resources promoting convalescence when one's digestive capacity is weak, and medicines and foods promoting positive health when one's digestive capacity is strong. An analogy provided by one informant was that one's digestion is like an internal fire. A weak fire must be protected and fed small twigs (light foods) until it catches while a burning fire may be fed branches (heavy foods) causing it to blaze. This distinction impacts on medicine taking behavior. Tonics and supplements are taken during illness and convalescence as much to protect digestive capacity as to provide nutrient resources. Products like glucose powder have become immensely popular in India as health supplements marketed as "light" sources of energy which are easy to digest as opposed to sugar or gur which are heavy. In medicine advertisements attention is often drawn to the digestibility of the product, a central concern in popular health culture.

POLYPHARMACY AND THE INTERPRETATION OF MEDICINES IN RELATION TO BODILY PROCESSES

Combinations of medicines with different physical characteristics prescribed simultaneously are sometimes interpreted as part of the practitioner's strategy to counterbalance the adverse effect of one medicine by another. For example, red tablets issued with white tablets may be interpreted as cooling tablets issued to counterbalance heating tablets. Likewise, pills prescribed with red color mixture may be interpreted as heating medicine to dry up one bodily secretion with a liquid medicine to promote blood production. I have observed such reasoning in play at chemist shops when impoverished clients come in with a medicine chit from a primary health center doctor. Presented with a list of medicines which the client can not afford, a selection is made influenced by cost as well as a folk evaluation of the overt qualities of the medicines prescribed. In some cases, the client will ask the purpose of various medicines. In other cases, it will be the form or color of the medications which influences which combination of types or the amounts of medicines which will be purchased. I have also observed a client presented with prescribed medicines who feels that these do not constitute a good mix. A client prescribed only pills, capsules or an injection may ask the chemist for a suitable tonic or mixture to complement or counterbalance the medicines prescribed. In such cases, the labeling of products plays an important role. Medicines marketed in terms of digestion, blood, the liver, regularity etc. are popular and come in a variety of forms (Chapter 9).

Polypharmacy, while popular, is not always viewed as beneficial. When a combination of tablets are taken, but not deemed efficacious, the quality, *guna*, of the medicines are sometimes spoken of as being in opposition. In such cases, the colors or tastes of medicine may be scrutinized by villagers in respect to the types of associations thus far described. Ayurvedic and folk practitioners generally take greater care than doctors to explain the medicines they administer in terms of common health concerns. This increases the

"performance efficacy" of the medication prescribed as a fit is established
between cultural expectations and the therapy administered. This is perhaps
one reason why villagers are often willing to take a longer course of
medicines from these practitioner than from doctors of cosmopolitan medicine.[10] This is particularly the case when symptoms have abated and patients
feel convalescence requires a balancing of the humors and regularization of
body processes. A illustration of this pattern and its clinical consequences
has been provided in an ethnographic study of Kyasanur forest disease
(Nichter 1987). In this study, a relapse of the illness three weeks after
symptoms abated was attributed to patients, particularly the elderly,
discontinuing medication. The elderly perceived that taking a number of
tablets for weeks after fever abated interfered with their digestive process.
Anorexia, a significant feature of the disease, supported this impression.

For acute illnesses, medicines are evaluated on the basis of their demonstration effect on dramatic symptom states which take precedence over long
term health exigencies. In the case of chronic illness and old age the
demonstration effect of medicine fixes is often less dramatic and the side
effects of medicines are often more notable. Experiential, age related health
concerns reemerge as important. It is here, in particular, that medicine
combinations are evaluated in relation to culturally defined states of normality; body signs and biological processes accorded ethnophysiological and
metamedical significance. Medicines are evaluated on the basis of how they
impact on health defining bodily processes (e.g. digestion, defecation, sleep)
and work activities. Where medical treatment impacts negatively upon bodily
processes deemed of social importance, it is discontinued. This is certainly
not unique to India. It is a pattern I have commonly encountered in my
anthropological research in North American clinical settings. Constipation
among the elderly, reduced libido among the mentally ill, and the side effect
of sleepiness among taxi cab drivers and construction workers cause these
people to discontinue their medications. The point I am raising is that
medicine is interpreted in relation to social and work related activities as well
as deep seated health concerns. The dysfunctional effects of medicines on
routine life are evaluated against those of illnesses. The effect of medicines
on "healthy" meaningful parts of one's life, not just dysfunctional body parts
or processes, are considered.

Biological processes are culturally evaluated on the basis of health
concerns which index images of ethnophysiology and the dynamics of social
interaction. In situations where health concerns are high, negatively valued
changes in biological processes, be these digestion or menstruation trigger an
interpretive process which calls attention to the properties of medicines.
Medicines are scrutinized on the basis of their overt characteristics and
implicit qualities as well as power of the hand and power of the brand.

CONCLUSION

In this paper, I have focused on the user's perceptions of medicine and tried to illustrate how such perceptions underlay consumer demand, medicine taking practices and adherence to medicine regimes prescribed. A greater appreciation of how medications are viewed by the lay population provides valuable clues as to why illness specific and age specific patterns of medicine taking behavior exist. Such data is clearly different from that generated by studies which focus on patterns of curative resort in terms of therapy systems per se. Such studies are not without merit, but are limited in contexts where eclectic treatment is common and commercial forms of traditional medicines and patent medicines are undistinguishable from allopathic medicine in the cosmopolitan market place.

Data on popular perceptions of medicine also provide clues as to why specific forms of medicine are produced for regional pharmaceutical markets, an issue taken up in chapter nine. The study of the user's evaluation of medication has rather obvious applied significance at a time when social marketing has become a buzz word. It is worth examining what it is about specific types of medication, or a combination of medications, which make them popular or unpopular for the treatment of a particular illness or a range of illnesses. This is no simple task. It requires investigation into issues ranging from indigenous notions of etiology and ethnophysiology to symbolic analysis of color, the cultural evaluation of manifest power and images of health. It also requires study of what supplements and/or foods are thought necessary to consume while taking medication for short or extended periods of time. This includes both substances to enhance the effect of the medicine, reduce its immediate side effects, or restore bodily processes once medications have managed symptoms.

Are such studies warranted? When they provide insights into why pregnant women do not find black ferrous sulfate tablets an appropriate form of therapy for bloodlessness (anaemia) during pregnancy, I believe they are. If types of medicine (supplements etc.) being distributed to high risk segments of the population are not being maximized, it behooves those engaged in health service research to consider why. Is it the characteristics of the medicines administered which are deemed inappropriate, or is the system of therapy itself deemed inappropriate? In lieu of black ferrous sulfate tablets, it is worth investigating whether an appropriately colored liquid tonic might be more acceptable and cost effective if bottles were supplied from home.[11] Popular ayurvedic promotive medicines (*aristhas*) are available which are rich in iron. It might be worthwhile studying patterns in the consumption of these *aristhas* and the possibility of producing a local promotive health tonic for groups at risk to anaemia. Studies on medicine taking behaviors are also warranted if they help identify dangerous medicine taking practices, such as the taking of E.P. Forte as an abortive, associated with popular reinterpretation of the manner in which modern drugs function.

Public health officials might also benefit from studies on medicine taking behavior by gaining a better appreciation of "timing" with respect to the introduction of preventive health medicine fixes. For example, in South Kanara, it is deemed culturally inappropriate (especially for children) to take helminthcide during monsoons.The heating properties ascribed to piperazine citrate are thought particularly dangerous at this time of general poor health, humoral imbalance and overall vulnerability (Nichter 1986). Elsewhere (Nichter 1989), I have described how the timing of vaccination programs have an impact on acceptability. Timing need be considered in relation to season and climate (rainy or sunny days) as well as times of the day ascribed qualities conducive for, or antagonistic to, the perceived action of medicine fixes.

Anthropologists engaged in health service research can be an immense help in contextualizing health intervention programs as well as evaluating health service delivery problems involving medicine taking behavior. With the opportunity for such research increasing, anthropologists need beware the potential for becoming party to simplistic approaches to primary health care based strictly on compliance as distinct from informed adherence. Like many of my colleagues, I am concerned about the social control and dependency ramifications of biotechnocentric fix approaches to health and disease. While the intent of such programs is often humanistic, the organizational structure may be coercive, and as I will point out in Chapter 9, the implicit ideology fostered by medicine fix based programs may undermine community participation. If anthropologists are to engage in health intervention efforts they must hold themselves accountable. By this I mean they must at once maintain a critical as well as a service based posture which causes them to look beyond the solving of immediate operational health service problems to the context of ill health and the social relations of development.

Clearly, a study of medicine taking behavior need be complemented by studies of medicine giving and medicine producing behavior. Studies are needed on the pharmaceutical industry, medicine distribution pathways, marketing strategies, advertising themes, and the degree to which product production reflects opportunities for profit as distinct from patterns of morbidity and mortality (Chapter 9). In need of study is the manner in which prescription patterns in a client dominant health care arena are influenced by factors having little to do with biomedical efficacy or "cost effectiveness." Factors in need of consideration include patient satisfaction and the dynamic of collecting a fee for medical services, a subject taken up in Chapter 8.

NOTES

1. Assumptions about folk health culture being closely related to ayurveda were common

in the pre-1970 anthropological literature. See for example Opler (1963) and Gould (1965).

2. *Sama* is a shortened version of the Sanskrit term *samadhatu*. In the regional language. Tulu, informants prefaced the use of this term by *wow edde* (that's good) or *dal tundara ijji* (without causing trouble).

3. For other studies on the cultural reinterpretation of medications and the cultural logic influencing the use of modern pharmaceutical see Bledsoe and Goubard (1985), Logan (1973), Mitchell (1983) and Cosminsky and Scrimshaw (1980).

4. It may be noted that the ingestion of milk soon after a tetracycline injection or capsule greatly reduces the positive activity of the drug. In as much as tetracycline is commonly used in India, a study was undertaken to investigate the extent of milk drinking (as a cultural phenomena) soon after tetracycline medication. Twenty patients prescribed tetracycline were followed up and it was found that 16 (80%) had consumed milk soon after the medication at some point during the course of treatment in an effort to cool the body.

5. See O'Gara and Kendall (1985) for a similar discussion of illness, medicine taking and breastfeeding.

6. The colors of foods are likewise thought to signify inherent qualities. The dynamics of color symbolism discussed in anthropological analysis of ritual underlie popular perceptions of foods and medicines. See for example, Beck (1972) and Nichter (1986) on color symbolism in India. Marshall and Polgar (1976) have discussed the importance of colors in the marketing of culturally appropriate fertility medications in the third world. Studies in the West have also documented the impact of medicine forms and colors on the perception of efficacy. For example, Brody (1977) conducted research on medicine form and the placebo response and found that a) placebo injections are perceived to work better than capsules or pills and b) that placebo capsules are deemed to be more powerful than pills. Helman (1985) cites studies by Shapiro which found that anxiety states are managed better by greeen tablets and depressive states by yellow tablets. Evans (1984) found that pink stimulants work better than blue ones and that multicolored capsules and small red/orange or pink pills work better than white pills or pills of other color combinations.

7. Oil massage is famous in nearby Kerala State. It may be pointed out that the purpose of massage is less bodily manipulation than the penetration of the medicinal properties of the oil into the body.

8. Popular use of oils in the care of wounds is unintentionally supported by doctors' recommendations to keep a wound dry. What a doctor often means is 'keep the wound clean' in a context where agricultural labor may demand working in mud. Villagers, however, take this advice to mean keep the wound dry so that water will not be absorbed through the wound resulting in the formation of pus. A related belief is that pus manifests more in rainy season because the body absorbs rain water.

9. Leela Visaria (personal communication) has noted that in Gujarat the term heavy is used for more powerful medicines. When the medicine of one doctor achieves no visible demonstration effect, a patient will ask for more *bhara*, heavy, medicines.

10. I am not suggesting that compliance to *vaidya* is necessarily better than compliance to doctors per se. One would need to study differences in compliance/adherence by illness as well as practitioner type and reputation to account for 'power of the hand' attribution.

11. Nutritional anaemia due to deficiencies in iron and folic acid are major public health problems in India particularly among pregnant women. It has been estimated that 10—30% of the general population and 30% of pregnant women are iron deficient (haemoglobin levels below 10g.). Prophylactic studies have indicated that if pregnant women ingest 30 mg. of ferrous sulfate per day during the last trimester of pregnancy that not only is their haemoglobin level stabilized, but that birth weight of infants rise. Needless to say, more appropriate social marketing of ferrous compounds and folic acid would be an important public health endeavor. See Gopalan, Raghavan, and Vijayan (1974).

REFERENCES

Beck, B.
    1969   Colour and Heat in South Indian Ritual. *MAN*, n.s. *4*(4): 553—572.
Bledsoe, C. and Goubard, M.
    1985   The Reinterpretation of Western Pharmaceuticals among the Mende of Sierra
           Leone. *Social Science and Medicine 21*(3): 275—282.
Brody, H.
    1977   *Persons and Placebos: Philosophical Implications of the Placebo Effect*. Ph.D.
           Dissertation, Department of Philosophy, Michigan State University.
Cosminsky, S. and Scrimshaw, M.
    1980   Medical Pluralism on a Guatemalan Plantation. *Social Science and Medicine 14b*:
           267—278.
Evans, F.
    1984   Unraveling Placebo Effects. *Advances 1*: 3, 11—20.
Friedson, E.
    1970   *Profession of Medicine: A Study of the Sociology of Applied Knowledge*. New York:
           Dodd & Mead.
Gopalan, C. and Vijayan, R. K.
    1971   *Nutritional Atlas of India*. National Institute of Nutrition. Hyderabad.
Gould, H.
    1965   Modern Medicine and Folk Cognition in Rural India. *Human Organization 24*:
           201—208.
Helman, C.
    1985   *Culture, Health and Illness*. Bristol: John Wright and Sons.
Kendall, L.
    1987   Cold Wombs in Balmy Honolulu: Ethnogynecology among Korean Immigrants.
           Social Science and Medicine 25(4): 367—376.
Leslie, C.
    1975   Pluralism and Integration in the Indian and Chinese Medical Systems. *In* A
           Kleinman et al. (eds) *Medicine in Chinese Cultures: Comparative Studies of Health
           Care in Chinese and other Societies*, U.S. Government Press, DHEW Pub. No.
           (NIH) 75-663.
Logan, M.
    1973   Humoral Medicine in Guatemala and Peasant Acceptance of Modern Medicine.
           Human Organization 32: 385—395.
Mitchel, F.
    1983   Popular Medical Concepts in Jamaica and their Impact on Drug Use. *Western
           Journal of Medicine 139*(6): 841—847.
Nichter, M.
    1977   The Joga and Maya of the Tuluva Buta. *Eastern Anthropologist 30*.
    1981   Negotiations of the Illness Experience: Ayurvedic Therapy and the Psychosocial
           Dimensions of Illness. *Culture Medicine, and Psychiatry 5*: 1—27.
    1986   Modes of Food Classification and the Diet-Health Contingency: A South Indian
           Case Study. *In* R. S. Khare and M. S. A. Rao (eds) *Food, Society and Culture*.
           Durham, N.C.: Carolina Academic Press.
    1989   Vaccinations in South Asia: False Expectations and Commanding Metaphors. *In* J.
           Coreil and D. Mull (eds) *Anthropology and Primary Health Care*. The Netherlands:
           Kluwer Academic Publishers.
O'Gara, C. and Kendall, C.
    1985   Fluids and Powders: Options for Infant Feeding. *Medical Anthropology*, Spring
           107—122.

Obeysekere, G.
   1975 Illness, Culture, and Meaning: Some comments on the nature of traditional
         medicine. *In* A. Kleinman, et al. (eds) *Medicine in Chinese Cultures: Comparative
         Studies of Health Care in Chinese and Other Societies,* U.S. Government Press.
   1976 The Impact of Ayurvedic Ideas on the Culture and Individual in Sri Lanka. *In* C.
         Leslie (ed.) *Asian Medical Systems: A Comparative Study,* University of California
         Press.
Opler, M, E.
   1963 The Cultural Definition of Illness in Village India. *Human Organization 21*: 32—35.
Polgar, S. and Marshall, J.
   1976 The Search for Culturally Acceptable Fertility Regulating Methods. *In* J. Marshall
         and S. Polgar (eds) *Culture, Natality and Family Planning,* Carolina Population
         Center Monograph No. 21. Chapel Hill.
Zimmerman, F.
   1987 *The Jungle and the Aroma of Meats.* Berkeley: University of California Press.

8. PAYING FOR WHAT AILS YOU: SOCIOCULTURAL ISSUES INFLUENCING THE WAYS AND MEANS OF THERAPY PAYMENT IN SOUTH INDIA

Illness costs in many different ways: in time, cash, emotions, social relations and choices. Economic considerations are commonly cited as important determinants of when and how people choose to use the services of different types of practitioners in pluralistic health care arenas. Perhaps because economic considerations are such obvious factors influencing health care decision-making, they are often over-looked as a subject for rigorous qualitative research. There is a poverty of research on both how much the poor spend on various illnesses experienced by different family members (by age and gender) and what the costs of illness in time, disposable income and loans mean in terms of family life and health. Even less research has been conducted on patterns of payment for health care services and the social factors influencing these patterns. It is the social relations of paying for therapy and asking for fees which will be the focus of this chapter.

Existing studies on payment for therapy are quantitative, and focus on medical costs in relation to patient characteristics. The details of payment are limited to amounts of time, money, and medicines. This is unfortunate because a contextual understanding of the dynamics of payment sheds light on health care seeking and medicine giving behavior, patient-practitioner interaction, and referral. I will demonstrate this in the course of the chapter while describing modes of payment to traditional, traditional-modern, and cosmopolitan therapists practicing in the pluralistic health arena of rural South Kanara. Focused upon will be direct and adjunct payment by pre-scribed and non-prescribed offerings as well as fees for service payment. Contrasted will be the meaning accorded to payments for therapy by practi-tioners more and less closely associated with the sociomoral dynamics of exchange relationships based on the theme of 'partaking.' The ways in which fees for consultation are collected will also be considered in relation to lay cost reckoning for therapeutic services rendered and medicines received. Public health ramifications of existing modes of paying for therapy will briefly be explored generating issues for additional research. Kunstadter (1978) has rightly cautioned against overemphasizing ideal 'rational man' or 'economic man' type explanations when attempting to understand health care behavior. Bearing this in mind, we may approach the subject of paying for therapy without a fixed economic gaze limited to market exchange.

214

PATTERNS OF PAYMENT

Non-prescribed Offerings

When first visiting a rural astrologer, diviner, or spirit medium, a client will typically initiate the consultation by presenting an offering in cash. For most specialists the size of an offering will vary in accord with the status of the client and specialist, and the severity of the case. The manner in which an offering is made as well as the amount given indicates to the traditional practitioner something about the case. The example of Subramanya, a local astrologer and exorcist will illustrate this point. Sitting on the porch of his mud and tiled house, crouched before a pile of cowry shells used for divination and a chalk grid depicting the day's stellar coordinates, Subramanya tends to the problems of a steady stream of clients. These clients come from a 50 mile radius to seek divination for a variety of problems relating to health, finances, and family welfare. Before each consultation a client places money — usually 2—5 rupees — before the stellar grid. Subramanya observes the non-verbal communication of the client including the manner in which the offering is placed before him and the amount. These observations assist him in ascertaining the probable status of the patient, the urgency of the case and the client's attitude toward the consultation. For example, an offering of 10 rupees (about 2 days wages for a coolie in 1978) thrown down in great haste by a low income client often suggested to Subramanya that 1) the case was urgent, 2) the consultation came at a time when other modes of therapy had failed, 3) debate existed in the family as to the cause of the problem-frustration was high, or 4) the client wanted protection as much as diagnosis. A haphazardly placed smaller sum, on the other hand, might indicate that 1) the client was curious, but not anxious about the cause and nature of the problem, 2) the consultation was more a matter of routine diagnosis/divination than a special event, 3) the client was very poor and was looking for a temporary reprieve from a long standing problem or 4) faith in the practitioner's power was not great.

Once presented, an offering to a specialist such as Subramanya is not generally increased as the consultation proceeds. However, if ritual protection is required in addition to divination, the amount of the offering may prove important. A client usually receives blessings and temporary ritual protection from Subramanya during a time of vulnerability, but the duration of this protection is time bound varying from days to weeks or months.

Two points may be highlighted. First, the size of the initial offering is not thought to affect the quality of diagnosis or divination. The specialist is believed to speak the truth and to entertain questions regardless of the amount offered. Second, although non-prescribed, the size of the offering influences treatment options. The size and manner of presenting an initial offering figures in an exorcist's decision to issue a protective device (*rakshana*). This may be of use as a general preventive or palliative measure against malevolent forces or a decision to ask the client to resolve the problem permanently by way of a ritual. As described by Subramanya, payment capacity and inclination significantly determine whether "a protective fence (*bund*) is placed around an individual's 'life field' requiring continual mending or whether that which is trying to destroy the field is itself destroyed, pacified, or controlled". The traditional specialist collects small periodic offerings for providing short term protection and large offerings (if not direct fees) for ritual services required to dispel malevolent forces permanently.

Prescribed Offerings

In some healing contexts, offerings are prescribed for specific ritual services or as an adjunct to the fees a client pays a traditional practitioner. Prescribed offerings are required for many healing rituals. These constitute both indirect and direct forms of payment. One type of indirect payment involves the procurement of ritual materials by a specialist on behalf of a client. After completion of the ritual, the specialist retains some of these items for personal use or use in the rituals of other clients. Direct payments may be in kind, most commonly grain and coconuts, or in cash.

For some illnesses, offerings of 'service' must be made as an adjunct to the fees a client pays an ayurvedic practitioner. An understanding of the meaning of these offerings requires a consideration of the concept of *karma* and the notion of 'partaking' in exchange relationships.

As Mauss has observed (citing India as an example), an exchange of goods or services may constitute not merely a mechanical, but a moral transaction.

The recipient depends upon the temper of the donor, in fact each depends upon the other. . . . Nothing is casual here. Contracts, alliances, transmissions of goods, bonds created by these transfers — each stage in the process is regulated morally and economically. The nature and intention of the contracting parties and the nature of the thing given are indivisible. (Mauss 1954: 58)

In Brahmanic custom an offering involves the receiver in 'partaking' of the giver. For example, Parry (1980) has observed that when Brahman funeral priests accept gift offerings (*dan*) they absorb the sins (*pāpa*) of their patrons. Ideally, the perfect Brahman who performs *jāpa* (the recitation of sacred verses), can 'digest'/'burn' these *pāpa* without jeopardizing himself. In essence, the priest takes on *pāpa* through *dan* and by *jāpa* burns the *pāpa* of the deceased. If, however, the Brahman priest who receives *dan* is unworthy because he has not performed *jāpa* or because he uses the *dan* unwisely, the sins of the receiver are compounded by the sins of the giver and both may suffer.

The theme of 'partaking' underscores other relationships between ritual specialists and clients. I may briefly examine this theme as it effects the practice of a tradional ayurvedic *vaidya*[1] whom I have described in depth elsewhere (Nichter 1981). According to ayurveda, an individual's ills are ultimately related to *karma*, the results of one's past and present actions. The question arises: If suffering from an ailment is a result of one's *karma*, then how can the *vaidya* justify the alleviation of such suffering? The *vaidya* whom I questioned asserted that *karma* differs from fate (*hanne baraha*-the writing on one's forehead) in that *karma* may be transformed through good deeds such as the performance of service (*seva*). *Seva* engenders merit (*punya*) which counterbalances sin (*pāpa*). As a *vaidya*, it was his duty to treat a patient's illness and to promote health. In order for his treatment to be effective, it was necessary for patients to perform good deeds to mitigate negative *karma*.

For major cultural illnesses (*maharoga*), as defined by ayurvedic texts, this *vaidya* prescribes *seva* as an essential part of a treatment program. If a prescribed *seva* such as the feeding of Brahmans or the poor was not carried out by a patient, then the *vaidya* considered himself liable to receive the patient's *karma*. Numerous stories were related by the *vaidya* about patients with *maharoga* who failed to carry out prescribed *seva* and thus put the *vaidya* in jeopardy. Most stories described how the *vaidya* contracted the same illness as the patient. A favorite story described the *vaidya* experiencing partial paralysis, discovering which of his patients was to blame, contacting the patient to perform the *seva* and being cured of the ailment.

The treatment of *maharoga* requires prescribed offerings, *karma vipaka*, which are fixed by tradition.[2] Such offerings may be considered an adjunct to payment for a *vaidya's* services. For the *vaidya*, these offerings and good deeds mitigate the patient's *pāpa* and thus the *karma* which the *vaidya* partakes of as part of the therapeutic relationship. The therapeutic alliance is influenced by mutual obligation concordant with the theme of gift giving. Moreover, healing is performed in the name of *Dhanvantari*, the patron deity of ayurveda and not directly in the *vaidya's* name. The point to be noted here is that the ultimate responsibility for cure is placed in the hands of the gods. Curing remains a socio-moral activity.

But what of the many minor ailments the *vaidya* treats which are not *maharoga*, ailments for which the *vaidya* does not request a client to perform *seva* or give *karma vipaka* as part of the course of therapy? My *vaidya* informant noted that the *karma* of such patients was also transferred to *vaidya*, but that many *vaidya* failed to recognize this. He cited the case of his deceased elder brother who had practiced ayurvedic medicine without payment as a *seva* and means of gaining merit, *punya*. His brother had not given medicine, but had only offered diagnoses to patients. His logic had been that diagnosis was a *seva* while the giving of medication and the collecting of fees involved a *karmic* relationship with the patient. All patients,

once diagnosed, were referred with a chit describing the type of medication
needed for cure to an ayurvedic compounder. My *vaidya* informant noted
that his brother had deluded himself. His brother's patients did involve him
in their *karma* regardless of whether medication was given. A failure to
realize this and take necessary ritual precautions had shortened his life.

To mitigate the *karma* transferred to *vaidya* from routine clients, a ritual
known as a *Dhanvantari pūja* may be conducted.[3] This ritual also gains for
the *vaidya* the blessings of the deity *Dhanvantari* which is thought to increase
the *vaidya's* power of the hand, *kai guna*. According to my informant, the
ritual also serves to symbolically recycle the payment a *vaidya* receives for
services rendered.

Prior to the ritual, the *vaidya* recites *jāpa* and observes strict purity rules
for a stipulated number of days — the number of units of *jāpa* recited is
thought to correspond to the amount of blessings received. The ritual
contains three important events. First, a *nāva graha homa*, ritual offerings to
the nine planets *vis-à-vis* a sacred fire, is conducted to mollify any bad effects
associated with these sources of celestial power which are to some extent
contingent on one's *karma*. Second, a ritual bath is conducted in which the
vaidya is washed of *pāpa* by a priest. Third, the *vaidya* invites a host of
Brahmans who practice *jāpa* to partake of a meal in the name of the *vaidya*.
By partaking of the ritual meal, the *pāpa* which the *vaidya* has accrued from
patients is 'shared' through the exchange of food. My *vaidya* informant,
incidentally the only *vaidya* whom I met who faithfully carried out the ritual
on a yearly basis, described the ritual as an occasion during which he
invested part of the payment he received from clients in *seva* — the feeding
of Brahmans. We see here a cycle of exchange where *karma pāpa* is passed
on from patient to *vaidya* to priest.

A different sort of relationship exists between patients and practitioners
who do and do not share mutual responsibilities to each other in the curing
process. In the present case, not only is the patient somewhat responsible for
the outcome of his treatment by mitigating *karma* through an offering of
service, but the patient has a moral responsibility to the *vaidya*. One *vaidya*
described this dual responsibility to me by way of an analogy. He stated that
just as landlords and tenants traditionally had mutual obligations to each
other and to the gods if a good crop was to be received, so the *vaidya* and
patient had a mutual responsibility to mitigate *karma* if a cure was to be
realized. In contrast, going to a practitioner whom you simply paid for
medicine was described as like paying for 'contract labor'. The image
conveyed by the analogy is not strictly that of an isomorphic comparison
between *vaidya*: patient and landlord: tenant. The image rather evokes a
complementarity of feeling concordant with mutual responsibility. The moral
investment of a *vaidya* to a patient is complementary in quality to that of one
who shares a moral responsibility to a piece of land and to the deity of that
land.

A point to be highlighted is that some degree of moral bonding exists between patient and traditional specialists. Payment conveys meanings which extend beyond economics defined from within a narrow formalist tradition. Indeed as Marriott (1976) has pointed out, Hindu transactions involve a flowing together of essences between 'persons' who in the Hindu sense are not 'bounded individual units' but rather permeable human lives constantly involved in an 'elaborate transactional and transformational culture'. In contexts where Brahmanic values are prominent, such as in interactions with ayurvedic practitioners and astrologers, sensitivity to the moral implications of 'partaking' and the dynamics of exchange relations are of a different magnitude, if not order, than in more secular contexts such as the setting of the Government Primary Health Center.

FEES FOR SERVICES

Vaidya

Let us now consider fees for services as a mode of payment. We may take up the case of ayurveda first. While the services of some traditional specialists are solely compensated for by offerings of one type or another, others are paid directly in the form of fees. Consultation to *vaidya* are usually not paid for separately, but are included in the cost of medications.[4] What is *explicitly* sold is medication. Inclusion of fees within medication charges is influenced by two variables: 1) lay reckoning as to a reasonable cost range for the forms of medication provided; and 2) the number of days of medicine offered to the patient. The lay population entertains a set of ideas as to how much certain forms of medicine should cost. If a *vaidya's* charges exceed these anticipated costs, chances are that the patient with limited means will not return to the *vaidya*. Anticipated costs for medicinal oils (*taila*), fermented wines (*arishta*) and herbal decoctions (*kashaya*) are each reckoned differently. For example, in December 1979 the general price ranges for three commonly purchased ayurvedic preparations, considered in respect to medicine form, were by unit of reference:[5]

ayurvedic pills (per pill) — 15—40 np   Rs. 1 = 12¢
one day of herbal decoctions — Rs. 1—1.50
100 ml medicinal wines — Rs. 3—4.50
100 ml medicinal oil — Rs. 6—7.50

Vaidya must include their consultation cost within the reasonable limits established by lay cost reckoning if they are to retain a poor patient.[6] This influences the number of days medicine a *vaidya* gives to a patient per consultation as well as the types of medicines they directly administer and prescribe. If costs go beyond the limits of expectation the *vaidya* has two options. The *vaidya* can win the patient's trust by explaining that the medicine is composed of rare or expensive herbs. Or, the *vaidya* may administer only those medicines which fall within reasonable limits established by lay reckoning; medicines which allow the *vaidya* to collect a fee. Other medications which fall outside the limits of lay reckoning are prescribed. For older established *vaidya* having a family tradition and 'power of the hand' associated with self-made medicines, it is easier to convince clients of the worth of more expensive medicines. The higher the status of the *vaidya* and the greater the purchasing capacity of the client, the less of an issue expense becomes. Less established *vaidya*, particularly younger *vaidya*, must win the confidence of poorer patients by sticking within the limits of reasonable cost established by lay reckoning. This is particularly the case if the *vaidya* relies on commercially prepared medicines as opposed to medicines which are self made. This influences the types of medical regimes administered, prescribed and purchased in bulk by such *vaidya*. For example, *amritha aristha*, a medicinal wine indicated in cases of debility and fever, is purchased by traditional-modern *vaidya* from commercial ayurvedic companies for approx. Rs. 16 per 40 oz. (40 paise per oz.). A daily dose may easily be sold to patients for Rs. 1.50 per oz, providing a Rs. 1 hidden consultation fee within the reasonable limits set by lay cost reckoning. Such medicines are purchased in bulk by *vaidya* and rarely prescribed for purchase by the patient from an ayurvedic chemist's shop. Often the brand of medication administered by the *vaidya* is disguised or the label removed. This either leads the rural patient into believing that it is self made or serves to limit their familiarity with a medication they may purchase from ayurvedic chemist shops in towns themselves. Costly medicines, such as those containing minerals (e.g. gold, mercuric oxide) or musk (*kasturi*) are prescribed and not directly administered to the patient as it would be difficult to tag a consultation fee onto a medicine that is already costly. When such expensive medicines are required, the patient is asked to purchase them elsewhere and the *vaidya* initially collects his fees through charges for a set of purification medicines required as a preliminary to the treatment.

Cosmopolitan Doctors

As in the case of *vaidya*, consultation fees are not charged by most rural cosmopolitan doctors but rather added on to medication costs.[7] A distinction may be drawn between the villager's perception of the traditional and cosmopolitan practitioner. Whereas the traditional practitioner is thought to diagnose and tell the truth regardless of the amount of payment, doctors are not uncommonly thought to diagnose in accord with the paying capacity of the patient.[8] A doctor's efforts at diagnosis are judged both in terms of time expended with a patient and the doctor's use of artifacts which take on symbolic importance for the patient, such as the stethoscope, blood pressure apparatus, etc. One patient drew a parallel between doctors and lawyers on this point. He related a popular South Kanarese story of the client who upon asking the fees of a lawyer was directed to a shelf of books of varying sizes. A case argued from larger books, the client was told, would cost more than a case argued from books of smaller size. The story was used to compare a doctor who simply touched one with a stethoscope to a doctor who placed the stethoscope carefully and performed other diagnosis (*tapas*) or who consulted books on one's behalf. A general feeling was that more careful diagnosis was performed on patients who could purchase more expensive medicines.

As in the case of ayurveda, appropriate fees for rural cosmopolitan doctors are crudely reckoned by laypersons on the basis of the medicine form and the number of days a medicine is administered. In 1980, a medicine cost survey (N = 50/low-lower middle class informants) found that a one day's supply of pills was most commonly reckoned at between Rs. 1—1.50, capsules at Rs. 1.50—2.50 and injections at the rate of Rs. 2—5. Differences in the actual charges for medicine were in large part understood by the layperson as being a reflection of the quality and strength of the medication. For example, 'single' injections were thought to cost less than 'double' injections. Double injections are drawn from two vials (suspension in one and distilled water in the other) and deemed more expensive because they are more powerful.

One of the ramifications of lay cost reckoning in an increasingly competitive cosmopolitan medical market, is a pattern characterized by practitioners administering popular forms of medicine: that is, forms of medication which meet patient's felt needs and expectations, fall within the layperson's anticipated price range and facilitate the collection of hidden consultation fees. This pattern is somewhat similar to that of the less established *vaidya*. For example, a cosmopolitan practitioner will dole out 3 days tablets to a patient if the actual cost of the medication does not exceed Rs. 2—3 in as much as the most the practitioner can charge the poor patient within the expected fee range is Rs. 5 (yielding Rs. 2 in hidden consultation fees). If charges exceed Rs. 5—10, practitioners realize that most rural clients will not return. When required, medications which exceed lay estimations of reasonable cost are prescribed rather than provided as a means of disassociating the practitioner from high costs. For example, a Rs. 10 injection of an expensive antibiotic will be prescribed while the practitioner personally supplies aspirin or vitamin tablets for 3 days yielding a profit as a consultation fee. These commonly administered simple drugs (e.g. aspirin, vitamin tablets, flatulence tablets) can be purchased over the counter and are therefore disguised. Labels and names are removed from medication increasing secrecy and dependency on the practitioner.

When medication is prescribed the patient is generally asked to return to see the practitioner with the medicine 1—3 days later. In the case of injections, a practitioner may use the service of 'injection administration' as a means of collecting a fee for consultation. The usual cost for this service when administered by a private practitioner is Rs. 1—2. Collection of this fee as a means of charging for consultation inhibits practitioners from referring patients to the homes or subclinics of Primary Health Center (PHC) staff for follow up injections, even when there is little chance the patient can return to the practitioner for daily injections because of the distance or poor transportation. When villagers do approach PHC personnel living in closer proximity for injections, they offer them payment even when not directly asked for compensation. Aware of this pattern, many local GPs have argued against letting 'less qualified' health personnel give injections, lest their own status be undermined and a source of fee collection be lost to others.

In some cases, lay cost reckoning sets in motion payment behavior even before payment is specified by a practitioner. In clinical transactions in the offices of small town practitioners or PHC doctors having private practices on the side, a charge is often not requested immediately at the close of a consultation. Rather, an uncomfortable silence follows treatment during which time the patient has the opportunity to offer payment. The patient offers a fee on the basis of the cost reckoning guidelines noted above. After the fee has been offered, the practitioner may either accept the fee and act as if money matters of this magnitude are beneath the practitioner's status or the practitioner may inform the patient that the cost of the medicines given exceed the fee offered. The latter causes the patient to either offer more money or promise to give more at the next visit. On many occasions, I observed that the amount offered by a patient exceeded the fee the practitioner had demanded as payment from other patients having similar problems but who waited to be told the charges.

A contrasting pattern of paying fees involves patients who offer money to practitioners at the beginning of consultation. In some cases, this is a presentation of all a patient's funds. In other cases a patient may make a cash offering to a cosmopolitan practitioner as a sign of respect or to establish a bond in much the same way as making an offering to a traditional practitioner when seeking advice. This behavior is commonplace at the Government Primary Health Center. Discussion with patients as to why they offered money to doctors whose services are supposed to be free[9] revealed that the money is given either as kindness (*kuchi*) so the doctor will take interest in the case, or as a bribe (*lyncha*) to enchance the chances of getting medicines instead of a prescription which requires additional expenses of time and money to fill.[10] Giving a PHC doctor a bribe to secure medicine appears no more unusual than offering a ticket attendant a few extra rupees for a seat on a crowded train. Another dimension to this transaction may exist, however. It is suggested that just as offerings serve to establish a moral bond between patient and traditional practitioner, so to bribes and payment of kindness to Primary Health Center doctors constitute weak attempts to establish moral bonds.[11] As one informant noted, customary bribes and customary offerings merge in India.

It is interesting to note that some villagers who frequent a PHC doctor give small offerings not so much for good medicines but for diagnosis. It is much the same as making an offering of a rupee to an astrologer. Some of these patients used the government doctor as a consultant to find out the severity of their sickness. Once the nature of the illness was diagnosed and they were given a prescription, these patients would consult a private practitioner (possibly the PHC doctor at home) for medication and follow-up.

Other doctors directly tell patients what their charges are at the beginning of a consultation. Some negotiate terms with patients who can not afford 'best treatment' but want treatment within a given cost frame. In some cases, practitioners extend credit, particularly during slack work seasons. A majority of practitioners interviewed deemed credit extension a necessary evil with two major drawbacks. While a client initially praises a practitioner for extending credit, it is common for the client to forget the amount of medication received and the number of visits to the practitioner responsible for the debt. The debt then appears large because it is not seen in respect to lay cost reckoning. The practitioner appears like the merchant who advances rice during times of scarcity for high interest rates. The other drawback is that as debt increases so do the chances of practitioner-hopping as patients would rather have many small debts than one large one. The practitioners sampled for interview estimated their losses to be as high as one third their original charges. To cover such fee losses some practitioners develop a Robin Hood-like attitude. Patients with larger funds are charged more to offset losses incurred by treating the poor. Charging more has its own set of dynamics. Being charged more, when greater respect is shown to a patient, can constitute a sign of status. It is not uncommon for wealthier patients to exploit a discussion of medical charges as a means of portraying status.

LAY COST RECKONING, FEE FOR SERVICE PAYMENT AND THE ROLE OF THE CHEMIST

It has been noted that both ayurvedic and cosmopolitan practitioners tend to administer medications which fall within lay cost reckoning parameters, and prescribe medications which fall outside these parameters. Taking a systems analysis vantage point, let us briefly explore ramifications of this pattern by considering the position of the chemist. This will entail a brief mention of the impact of the pharmaceutical representative on chemist-practitioner relationships in the rural health arena.

Rural practitioners tend to purchase in bulk medicines such as vitamins, tonics, digestants, and flatulence tablets because they are popular and cost effective from both a therapeutic and fee collection vantage point. Bulk purchase of these medicines cuts their cost appreciably and administration of such medications to clients affords a reasonable vehicle for collecting consultation fees. Pharmaceutical representatives (reps) of major pharmaceutical companies directly visit popular practitioners in rural India as long as they hold some form of license or degree.[12] Reps aggressively seek direct purchase orders from practitioners as well as promises to prescribe their products. In return, reps offer practitioners information about drugs, free samples and significant discounts on medicines purchased directly from distributors. Important to note is that the same discount is offered to chemists and licensed practitioners. This affects the chemists' drug trade carried on with different kinds of practitioners.

Chemists derive their business from prescriptions written by private and PHC doctors, over the counter sales to the informed public, and sales to non-degree holding registered medical practitioners who are not directly served by pharmaceutical agents. As noted, many prescriptions received from private doctors are for medications which are deemed expensive by lay reckoning. Chemists must face rural patients who come in with a prescription chit and selectivity purchase medications. Chemists have become adept at negotiating with clients who typically ask the prices of the medications prescribed and then proceed to purchase what seems reasonable on the basis of lay cost reckoning. Often the prescribed medication is a product from a major pharmaceutical firm which has 'won over' the practitioner. In cases where the medication is far more expensive than generic drugs of less reputable companies, the chemist may attempt to convince the patient to take 3 days supply of a generic drug as opposed to 1 days supply of a name brand medication prescribed. A point to be emphasized is that it is often the chemist who educates the patients as to the purpose of multiple medicines, the importance of following a course of medication and the dangers of misusing a medication by tampering with dosage. It is the chemist who must reason with the patient within a set of economic constraints. While rarely reported in the literature, the health education role of the chemist may prove as important, if not more important, than that of the practitioner.[13]

Another point may be raised. Chemists stock well-known drugs as well as take a chance with the products of less renowned companies who offer lower costing medicine, no frills packaging, bigger profit margins but less quality control. Aside from being administered to poor patients as substitutes for prescribed brand-name drugs, these drugs are also in demand by registered, non-degree holding practitioners. The latter are not directly served by pharmaceutical representatives, do not receive professional discounts, and must adhere closely to lay cost reckoning.

PUBLIC HEALTH RAMIFICATIONS OF PAYING FOR THERAPY

A number of public health issues arise from a scrutiny of modes of paying for therapy and competition in the pluralistic health arena. I may highlight four issues worthy of further research. First, because the practitioner's compensation depends on fees hidden in medicine charges the practitioner must stock popular medicines and, to some extent, acquiesce to client demands. Practitioners stock and directly administer medicines which are 'fee facilitating' be they essential or nonessential as long as they provide some relief, meet patients' felt needs and are judged potent by cultural criteria. The misuse of calcium gluconate illustrates this point. Calcium gluconate injections are administered by a number of practitioners intravenously not to correct calcium deficiencies, but to produce a "heat effect" which is deemed a sign of power by folk health criteria.[14] India's present pattern of drug production and sales does not accord with an epidemiological profile of India's disease patterns (Chapter 9). It may be speculated that a factor influencing this pattern is practitioner's direct medicine purchases which in turn are influenced by the constraints posed by hidden consultation charges in a medical market influenced by lay cost reckoning. This speculation requires further research.

A second issue raised by an examination of fee for service presentation and lay cost reckoning involves the reluctance of cosmopolitan practitioners to refer patients to PHC staff living in closer proximity to patients for follow-up services such as injection administration. Easier access to assistance could enhance therapeutic adherence by minimizing logistic problems involved in receiving medications. Private cosmopolitan practitioners do not support activities of PHC staff which serve to reduce a service from whence they receive fees (Nichter 1986). To acknowledge PHC staff's capability in an important area of status, such as control over injections, would reduce practitioners' own status. Moreover, in the eyes of many practitioners, to acknowledge the skills of PHC staff would be to invite competition from staff who might then be approached by villagers for other medications and services. Practitioner informants cited multiple instances of former PHC staff who had become registered medical practitioners as cases in point. One probable outcome of this fear of competition is that practitioners contribute to the negative image of PHC staff as incompetent either by word of mouth or non-referral.

The practitioner's collection of fees from the sale of medicine raises a third and related issue. As noted, practitioners can not afford to refer patients to PHC staff for follow-up services associated with status because of economic considerations; considerations often disguised by moral overtures against the poor receiving second-rate treatment. By a similar rationale many local practitioners are against the idea of villagers setting up local medical cooperatives, an idea explored during a community diagnosis project (Nichter 1984).

As a means of exploring the social soundness of the medicine cooperative concept (legality and management were other issues), fifteen rural cosmopolitan practitioners were interviewed about their feelings towards this idea.

While all the practitioners recognized that scarce resources were being expended by patients on transportation in order to secure common drugs, eleven stated that they would not be in favor of the concept of a local medical cooperative. All but three cited quackery as an initial reason against the establishment of a cooperative. Eight of the eleven, however, noted that financial loss associated with the existing pattern of fee collection was a central problem. Only four of the fifteen practitioners, all popular practitioners with secure clientele, supported the concept. Public health advocates of increased community participation in primary care will need to consider the economics of the rural practitioner if they are not to alienate them or threaten their economic survival. This constitutes a priority research area.

One further issue, somewhat tangential but certainly relevant to our discussion of paying for therapy as a public health issue, may be highlighted as an important area for future research. Lay cost reckoning is largely determined by medicine form. In the competitive medical marketplace, it will be worth monitoring the way in which medicine production and marketing accords with consumer demand as influenced by popular health culture. For example, to what extent are medicines produced by allopathic and ayurvedic medical companies made to fit popular ideas of appropriate medicine form as well as cost? To what extent will marketing campaigns be tailored to accord with lay health concerns and popular explanatory models of how medicines works? A study of the advertising of medicines in India as a cultural phenomenon is needed.

DISCUSSION

An examination of how villagers pay for pluralistic therapy services and how practitioners collect fees introduces a number of issues which add depth to our present understanding of health care seeking behavior, practitioner-patient relationships, health expenditures, referral and perhaps, medicine production on a macro-level. We have seen that in the traditional health sector the size of an offering to an exorcist, diviner or astrologer and the mode of its presentation are interpreted as signs revealing the nature of a patient's problem and the relative importance of the consultation. The interpretation of such signs as a form of meta-communication influences diagnosis and therapy management options.

For the traditional ayurvedic practitioner, payment also involves a notion of moral bonding implicit in the dynamics of exchange relationships. Accepting the services rendered by a traditional *vaidya* involves the patient in moral aspects of healing associated with the meanings of illness in the Hindu world. In order for a patient to be effectively treated by a *vaidya* for a major illness, the patient has to pay off a debt of karma to society by way of a service offering in addition to paying the specialist. Such penance serves to reintegrate the patient into the socio-moral order. Within the Hindu great tradition the role and identity of the healer is defined in relation to the meanings of illness. The concept of partaking involves the healer not only with the patient but with society itself. This is exemplified by the rituals performed for the *vaidya*. Priests of the socio-religious order participate in a 'healing of the healer' by dissipating the sins taken on as karma by the *vaidya* from patients.

The ideal moral bonding of healer-patient and society may be contrasted to the typically non-moral interaction between cosmopolitan practitioner and patient in a market economy.[15] Here, patient-practitioner relationships have been seen to be strongly influenced by lay cost reckoning in a competitive health arena which is becoming increasingly client-dependent. Friedson (1970) describes client-dependent practitioners as follows:

1) Like a businessman, a 'neighborhood shopkeeper' whose stock of diagnostic and treatment practices/resources reflects their position between two worlds, the lay health system and that of the professional. The practitioner must on occasion give in to his patients' prejudices if they are to return to him and to refer other patients to him. Such practitioners are likely to honor lay demands for such popular remedies as vitamin B-12 injections, copious use of antibiotics, and prescription of tranquilizers, sedatives and stimulants.

2) Dependent upon laymen for the referrals that provide him his business. Insofar as lay referrals are 'inevitably based on lay understandings of illness and its treatment', the practitioner's survival depends upon the compatibility of diagnosis and treatment with that of the layperson. Here the patient is an 'active participant' in a process of diagnosis and treatment management.

We may consider Friedson's depiction of client-dependent practitioners in the South Kanarese context. With an increase in transportation facilities and a rising number of cosmopolitan and traditional modern practitioners who dispense forms of medicine which appear similar to the layperson, the rural practitioner must win the trade of the lay population by establishing a reputation for having good medicines, and reasonable costs as discerned by lay cost reckoning. Inasmuch as a rural practitioner's compensation depends on fees hidden in medicine charges,[16] the practitioner stocks popular medicines and to some extent acquiesces to client's demands for particular medicine forms. Practitioners stock medicines which are 'fee facilitating,' be they essential or nonessential as long as they provide some relief or meet patients' felt needs. A practitioner's choice of medications is influenced by the practitioner's assumptions as to what a patient's felt needs are and the constraints lay cost reckoning imposes. Adapting treatment to lay cost reckoning constraints engages a market mentality.

Parsons (1976) has noted that describing health care merely in terms of a market model is limited on two counts. First, it undervalues the element of 'confidence' that goes with the professional role of the practitioner which is clearly different from that of shopkeeper supplying commercial products.The second limitation of the market model is that it assumes that practitioners are catering to the 'consciously formulated and rationally understood wants of sick people' — the rational man argument.

In the South Kanarese context, Friedson's depiction of lay referral and of the relationship between patient and practitioner needs to be modified. Lay referrals are only partially based on lay understanding of illness and treatment. Medical practitioners who are popular are often those who understand local illness vocabulary and acknowledge folk health concerns. Other factors however, enter into lay referral ranging from power of the purse and the power of advertising to "power of the hand".

In a context where health is increasingly being marketed as obtainable through medicine products (Chapter 9), the prevailing market mentality is undercut by the tenets of a precapitalist ideology upon which perceptions of healing are based. While curative efficacy is predicated on universalistic claims, (procedures, products) healing is based on particularistic perceptions and relationships entailing an exchange of a different order (Young 1983). Medical anthropologists typically contrast healing and curing in relation to efficacy as seen from the different vantage points of biomedicine and indigenous populations invested in meaning systems. As several anthropologist have pointed out (e.g. Dobkin de Rios 1981, Finkler 1980, Press 1971, Synder 1981) healing does not necessarily entail that a patient understands the actions of a practitioner or for that matter that they share world views.

For routine complaints, a chemist or convenient practitioner is often consulted for the medicine commodities he or she possesses. The medicine cures, it is the active agent. When attempts at symptomatic treatment fails a different kind of health seeking behavior is often initiated. A practitioner is sought for whom one at once feels confidence and faith. Confidence entails the diagnoses of person as well as condition, while faith entails affiliation and a feeling of interpersonal resonance. While confidence and affiliation is often spoken of in the West in terms of competence, in rural India confidence and faith merge in descriptions of a practitioner's "power of the hand." Ascription of power of the hand places primary importance on the practitioner as active agent. "From this practitioner's hand even water will cure."

Healing may be based on a negotiation of knowledge, meaningful signs, and an illness identity which is transformed. It may also be based on what is felt more than what is seen. It may involve sociomoral relations established through the quality of social interactions; the asking of questions which touch and not just probe; and the listening to complaints which speak of life and not merely refer to symptoms. The healer, irregardless of garb or repertoire of medications, is recognized in South Kanara as distinct from the possessor of medicines. Resort to a healer is distinct from resort to a practitioner whose relationship to patients is defined in terms of commodity fixes. As in the case of a pilgrimage, that which evokes faith is often distant. A healer to one person is the mere possessor of medicine fixes to another.

I raise the issue of curing and healing in the conclusion of this chapter to emphasize that the study of medicine taking related behavior is complex and need be complemented by studies of the social relations of treatment (Nichter and Nordstrom 1989). Bearing this in mind, I next wish to critically examine the theme of "health is wealth" in a market economy where medicine is a vehicle for the embodiment of ideology as well as the promise of safe passage through a deteriorating environment (see Chapter 9).

NOTES

1. The relationship between *ayurveda* and the doctrine of *karma* is multifaceted and has been presented differently by the major formulators of *ayurveda* (Caraka, Vágbhata, and Susruta). For a review see Weiss (1980).
2. For a review of exising Sanskrit literature on *karma vipaka* see Thrasher A. Some Sanskrit works on karma and their results. Unpublished paper delivered at the Second Karma Conference, Pasadena, CA, 1978. It is interesting to note that *karma vipaka* texts present abnormality and illness much less as punishments and more as opportunities for prudent men to mitigate past sins by appropriate countermeasures. Penances prescribed involve a reintegration of the afflicted with society and offerings associated with public utility.
3. Few *vaidya* practice yearly *Dhanvantari puja*. Other *puja* are sometimes substituted for *Dhanvantari puja* when a *vaidya* feels he suffers from karma accrued from patients. For example, *Sathyanarayana puja*, a general all purpose *puja* which has grown in popularity over the last 50 years is sometimes performed for this purpose.
4. Some *ayurvedic vaidya* and astrologers charge fixed consultant fees, but this is rare in rural areas.
5. Patent medicines included were the following: pills — Dhanvantari matre, Bala graha (chine) matre, vayu matre. Wines — Dashamoolaristha, Draksharistha, Amritaristha, Ashoka aristha. Oils — Dhanvantari taila, Triphaladi taila, Narayana taila, Brahmi taila.
6. While it is not generally recognized, patient dropout and non-adherence among patients visiting ayurvedic practitioners is common. The costs of receiving systematic ayurvedic treatment are often higher than what a patient is willing to invest or the rigor of treatment is too demanding.
7. In more urban areas of South Kanara and in neighboring Kerala State, doctors consultancy rates range from Rs. 5 to Rs. 15. Middle to upper class patients frequent practitioners with high consultation fees as a measure of status as well as to get better therapy. A local joke among rural GPs is that they are the specialists because higher class patients consult specialists first; specialists see all problems from their own vantage point and when simple differential diagnosis is overlooked, GPs are able to treat successfully when specialists have failed. The trend of visiting specialists prior to local GPs appears to have increased significantly over the last 8 years.
8. This is, in fact, not the case. Diagnosis by traditional practitioners, such as astrologers and exorcists, is often influenced by a patient's paying capacity.
9. I do not wish to infer that all government primary health center (PHC) doctors accept money from public patients or maintain private practices. However, the patterns of behavior noted are by no means uncommon.
10. In one region of South Kanara investigated, filling a prescription necessitated a day off from work and a bus ride costing half a days wages. PHC medical supplies are limited. PHC doctors must either be highly selective in allocating free drugs or ration medicine daily in accord with a supply management plan.
11. See Van der Veen's discussion of the moral bonding aspects of payment for medicine in relation to the issue of 'free medicine' and patient mistrust (1979).

12. In one region of India studied, 48% of the practitioners visited by the medical representa-
    tives of a major pharmaceutical firm had licenses from ayurvedic or integrated medical
    colleges. Thirty six percent of practitioners visited who were ranked as the "most
    popular" fell in this category. Nichter M. Toward a culturally responsive rural health care
    delivery system in India. In *The Social and Cultural Context of Medicine in India* (Edited
    by Gupta, R.). South Carolina Press, 1981.
13. For a complementary set of studies from Latin America which describe the role of the
    chemist in educating the lay population and/or practitioners in the use of medications,
    see Cosminsky and Scrimshaw (1980) on Guatemala, Logan (1983) on Mexico, and
    Ferguson (1981) on El Salvador.
14. Personal observation of the use of calcium gluconate and discussion of this practice with
    Dr Carl Taylor who has made similar observations in North India.
15. For further description of allopathic doctors' non-moral business like manner of practic-
    ing medicine in India, see Madan T. Doctors in a North Indian city: recruitment, role
    perception and role performance. In *Beyond the Village: Sociological Explorations*
    (Edited by Saberwal S.). Indian Institute of Advanced Study, Simla, 1972.
16. Kapsil's recent article (1988) serves to validate my observations on the means by which
    doctors collect a consultation fee through medicine sales in South India. The author
    points out that this practice was common in 19th Century England.

REFERENCES

Cosminsky, S.
    1980 Medical pluralism on a Guatemalan plantation. *Social Science and Medicine 14b*:
         267—278.
Dobkin de Rios, M.
    1981 Social-economic characteristics of an Amazon urban healer's clientele. *Social
         Science and Medicine 15b*, 51—63.
Ferguson, A.
    1981 Commercial pharmaceutical medicine and medicalization: A case study from El
         Salvador. *Culture, Medicine and Psychiatry 5*: 105–134.
Finkler, K.
    1980 Non-medical treatments and their outcomes. *Culture, Medicine and Psychiatry 4*:
         301—40.
Friedson, E.
    1970 *Profession of Medicine: A Study of the Sociology of Applied Knowledge.* New York:
         Dodd & Mead.
Kapsil, I.
    1988 Doctors dispensing medications: Contemporary India and 19th Century England.
         Social Science and Medicine 26(7): 691—699.
Kunstadter, P.
    1976 Do cultural differences make any differences? Choice points in medical systems
         available in Northwestern Thailand. *In* A. Kleinman et al (eds.) *Culture and Healing
         in Asian Societies.* Cambridge, MA: Schenkman.
Logan, K.
    1983 The role of pharmacists and over-the-counter medications in the health care system
         of a Mexican city. *Medical Anthropology 7*, 68—89.
Madan, T.
    1972 Doctors in a North Indian city: Recruitment, role perception and role performance.
         In S. Saberwal (ed.) *Beyond the Village: Sociological Explorations.* Simla: Indian
         Institute of Advanced Study.

Marriott, M.
  1976 Hindu transactions: Diversity without dualism. *In* B. Kapferer (ed.) *Transaction and Meaning: Directions in the Anthropology of Exchange and Symbolic Behavior.* Philadelphia: Institute for the Study of Human Issues.
Mauss, M.
  1954 *The Gift: Forms and Functions of Exchange in Archaic Societies.* London: Cohn & West.
Nichter, M.
  1981 Negotiation of the illness experience: Ayurvedic therapy and the psychosocial dimensions of illness. *Culture, Medicine and Psychiatry 5*: 1–27.
  1984 Project community diagnosis: Participatory research as a first step toward community investment in primary health care. *Social Science and Medicine 19*(3): 237–252.
  1986 The Primary Health Center as a Social System: PHC, social status and the issue of team-work in South Asia. *Social Science and Medicine 23*(4): 347–355.
Nichter, M. and Nordstrom, C.
  1989 *The Question of Medicine Answering: The Social Relations of Efficacy in Healing.* Forthcoming, *Culture, Medicine and Psychiatry.*
Parry, J.
  1980 Ghosts, greed and sin: The occupational identity of the Benares funeral priests. *Man* (N.S.) *15*: 88–11.
Parsons, T.
  1976 Epilogue to the doctor-patient relationship in the changing health scene. *In* E. B. Gallagher (ed.) *Proceedings of an International Conference* (pp. 78–183). Washington, DC: John E. Fogarty International Center for Advanced Study in the Health Sciences.
Synder, P.
  1981 Ethnicity and Folk Healing in Honolulu, Hawaii. *Social Science and Medicine.*
Van der Veen, K.
  1979 Western medical care in an Indian setting: The Valsad District in Gujarat. *In* S. Van der Geest and K. Van der Veen (eds) *In Search of Health.* Vakgroep Culturele Anthropologie, Universiteit van Amsterdam.
Weiss, M.
  1980 Caraka Samhita on the Doctrine of Karma. *In* W. D. O'Flaherty (ed.) *Karma and Rebirth in Classical Indian Traditions.* Berkeley: University of California Press.
Young, A.
  1983 The Relevance of Traditional Medical Cultures to Modern Primary Health Care. *Social Science and Medicine 17*(16): 1205–1211.

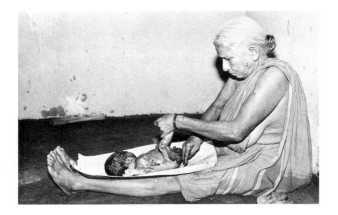

Grandmother's medicine: Folk medicine is most extensively used for infants and pregnant and lactating women.

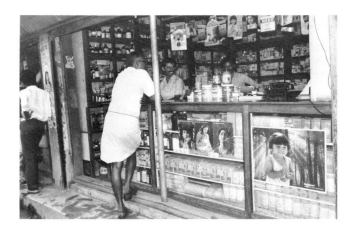

Eclectic medical resources: An allopathic pharmacy displays advertisements of a popular ayurvedic product for "women's complaints," tonics and patent medicines.

9. PHARMACEUTICALS, HEALTH COMMODIFICATION, AND SOCIAL RELATIONS: RAMIFICATIONS FOR PRIMARY HEALTH CARE

The most important myth is the myth of progress or in other words, the business of "onward ever onward." And the first problem that arises from this myth for advertising is that "newer", "bigger", "better", "stronger", "richer" products are put forward in the market and a "still better tomorrow" is envisaged. Nobody has bothered to ask "better than what?" I am still doubtful whether Mexaform or Entero-vioform is more effective than the indigenous herbal medicines dished out by our grandmothers 40 or 50 years ago. But we take so easily to Mexaform because we live in a "pill" age and wish to have recourse to convenience rather than consult a physician or the village healer which involves loss of time. (D' Penha 1971)

The country's drug policy is in utter chaos. It has been promoting a "drug culture", the culture of reaching out for a drug on the slightest pretext. This pharmaceuticalisation of health opens up the country for loot by drug companies (Ghosh 1986).

One cannot ignore the long term effects of encouraging a poorly educated population to develop blind faith in the infallibility of modern medicine and the magical properties of prescribed pills. In India, people who are too poor to buy rice are being led to believe that they need a cough mixture for every cough, an antibiotic for every sore throat, and a tranquilizer to solve the problems of everyday life. (Greenhalgh 1987).

In this chapter, I will discuss the growing trend toward the commodification of health through pharmaceuticals in India today. Considered is the manner in which pharmaceutical policy, production and marketing; polypharmacy prescription patterns and self help practices; cultural values and collective anxieties affect consumer demand for particular medicine products. A point emphasized is that what is being sold to the Indian public today is the notion that health in the short term can be derived through the consumption of medicines. At a time of increasing environmental deterioration (deforestation, erosion, pollution); rapid unplanned urbanization and industrialization; and related public health problems (Malhotra 1985), an emerging capitalist ideology is subtly reproduced in popular health culture. Underlying this ideology is the premise that one can buy back health and well being with a rising wage for labor. In other words, health has increasingly taken on an "exchange value". The working class tacitly accepts capitalist ideology through their efforts of private appropriation of commodified health. This ideology is being swallowed along with the pills that embody it. Health practices involving medicine taking and giving constitute an agency of socialization where relations of power, dominance, and dependency take concrete form.

Three sets of interactive factors need to be considered if we are to understand the relationship between changing patterns of medicine consumption sale and production in India. First we must explore the metamedical meanings associated with health products and the manner in which cultural

233

values shape the successsion of medical commodities developed to meet life exigencies as well as the market economy. Second, we must contend with coexisting and competing medical traditions as they have contributed to the commodification of health. Finally, we must examine health policy as it affects the profitability of marketing particular kinds of medicine.

A growing number of studies inspired by a world system approach to political economy have provided evidence of the strategies employed by multinational pharmaceutical companies seeking to secure new markets in developing countries for health products of questionable cost, relevance and safety.[1] A conspiracy of interests is portrayed with the health and growth needs of the global capitalist industrial body pitted against the health of inhabitants cum consumers. These firms, through affiliates and subsidiaries, promote medications with exaggerated claims while downplaying or omitting information about side effects and hazards (Osifo 1983; Poh Ai 1985; Silverman et al 1986; Zawad 1985).[2] The indigenous "lumpen bourgoise" are characterized in some accounts as agents of medical colonialization and underdevelopment who exploit and subject the interests of other classes in peripheral countries for the ultimate profit of capitalists in developed "center" countries. While there is much truth to these claims, the world systems perspective is limited. As Worsley (1985) has noted we need to look beyond studies of political economy to the agendas of real individuals and how they are influenced by economics and the social relations they entail. To understand pharmaceutical behavior in India we will explore the motivations and meanings underlying the use and sale of medicines. These issues are little appreciated but are crucially important for international health (Hercheimer and Stimson 1982).

Toward this end, I will focus both on health products designed to meet culturally constituted health problems, and on the local marketing initiative of indigenous pharmaceutical companies which operate in a context of intensive competition and increasing government regulation. In the last ten years allopathic medicines have been the subject of regulation attempts responsive to both national and international health lobby efforts.[3] Within this environment, I will examine the proliferation of an increasing number of commercial patent ayurvedic medicines, a range of medicines which John Laping (1984) has aptly referred to as "Ayurpathic medicines". I will consider reasons why these drugs are growing in popularity among both practitioners and consumers, and how their proliferation fosters health commodification.

In addition to drawing attention to the forces influencing medicine production, the social relations entailed by health commodification need to be explored. It is necessary to look beyond the economics of medical practice to consider health commodification in relation to the compartmentalization and decontextualization of health "problems" as well as people. Here, I wish to address ramifications of a growing illusion of false security rendered by medicine fixes among the middle and upper classes. My concern is that without raising consciousness about the relationship of health to the environment at large, false consciousness in the form of a false sense of health security is fostered by the inflated claims of medicines, and un-explained preventive health fixes. The false consciousness generated by health commodification serves to undermine the impetus to participate in ecological-environmental based popular health movements in a context where they are of crucial and immediate importance.

AN OVERVIEW OF THE PHARMACEUTICAL INDUSTRY

Medicalization is not as dependent on the monopolization of the health sector by any one type of medical practitioner or medical tradition so much as on the microeconomic and political structure that facilitates the penetration of modern prepackaged pharmaceutical products, their use by a variety of medical practitioners and by townspeople in curative and preventive regimes. (Ferguson 1981: 127)

Let us first gain an overview of the magnitude of the pharmaceutical industry in India. In India, pharmaceutical policy at once attempts to limit domination by multinational pharmaceutical firms, yet fosters the proliferation of medi-cines in the medical market place in the name of free enterprise. Estimates of the number of pharmaceutical companies in India jumped from 3,600—4,000 in 1980 to 8,000 in 1986 (VHA 1986).[4] Fifteen companies, however, continue to dominate 80% of the formal pharmaceutical market.[5] The Government of India supports scores of small scale production units through fiscal incentives (Gothoskar 1983), a policy partially implemented to break the monopolies of transnational corporations. This has resulted in a market where the production of medicine products has escalated. In comparison to most western countries where between 10,000—30,000 medicine formula-tions are available for sale,[6] approximately 60,000 commercial medicine products were estimated to be available in India in 1986 (VHA 1986).[7] These include standard allopathic medicines, "illogical combinations of medications,"[8] and over-the-counter patent medicines marketed, if not devel-oped, to appeal to popular health concerns.

Competition between pharmaceutical companies is keen. Promotional expenses are comparable to those found in the West and exceed 5% of total drug turnover revenues.[9] This figure is well in excess of government allocations for medications to primary health centers designed to serve the population at large. Rather than quote national figures to highlight this point, let me cite local data from South Kanara district on expenditures by pharmaceutical companies on the activities of their pharmaceutical repre-sentatives in the fields. Bear in mind that my estimates are conservative and do not include advertising costs and promotional gifts.

In South Kanara in 1974, approximately 70 pharmaceutical representa-tives (reps) routinely visited doctors as well as several urban and 30 town chemist shops. In 1986 the number of reps canvassing the district had increased to 300, with an additional 200 reps occasionally visiting the district. Reps visited an estimated 1000 doctors and 109 (54 in towns) chemist shops now found in the district.[10] Data was collected on the activities of reps from in-depth interviews and observations of their chemist visitation patterns in one town (pop. 15,000—20,000) in 1976, 1980, and 1986. In 1980 most reps of small companies spent half a day meeting popular doctors and chemist shop owners in the town, while reps of major companies expended one full day. On average, each chemist shop was visited by 10 reps per day. Given 25 work days per month, at least 100 working days per month were invested in this town by reps of various pharmaceutical companies. The starting salary for reps was approximately Rs. 40 per day (an experienced rep being paid twice this), plus Rs. 35 for travel and maintenance expenses. This means that Rs. 7,500 a month (Rs. 90,000 a year) was expended on the interpersonal selling activities of reps in a town where the local hospital is allocated approximately one third (Rs. 30,000) this amount in drugs for the year to treat an outpatient load exceeding 150 patients per day.

THE COMMODIFICATION OF HEALTH

The term "commodification" has been used in a variety of different ways in the social science literature.[11] Let me therefore be specific about what I mean by the commodification of health. What I am referring to is the tendency to treat health as a state which one can obtain through the consumption of commodities, medicine. This entails an objectification of the body, the decontextualization of sickness as disease (Young 1982), and an economy primarily based on "exchange (labor) value" in contrast to "use value". In its extreme form, health becomes dependant on medicine. It is broadly recognized in India that an individual's health is contingent upon their constitutional endowment and circumstance. The latter is determined by one's physical environment and sociomoral relations as well as the qualitiative state of a changing cosmos; all of which are interactive and multidimensional. While one's constitution can not be altered beyond the changes which occur in one's life cycle, it may be managed through regimes which counterbalance excess, calm, correct for deficiency, and facilitate the processes of flow within. Circumstance can likewise be mediated both externally and internally. Where one's external environment is unhealthy, those able to cash in labor value for health giving medicine products are able to obtain short term health as a form of wealth.[12] This exchange relationship has social significance beyond that of health of the individual body per se.

To some degree, this characterization oversimplifies the associations perceived by South Indians of health with prosperity and sickness with trouble. Health and illness are often deemed to be signs of more general sociomoral states not states in and of themselves. For the present, however, I may focus on more immediate "functional" perceptions of health (Kelman 1975). This will enable me to highlight health commodification as a process responsive to particular health concerns elaborated upon by marketing strategies which play upon collective anxiety and index cultural values.

In present day India, health commodification has been fostered by a rising concern about adulteration and environmental deterioration especially prominent among members of the low-middle to upper classes drawn toward a more cosmopolitan style of life. The upper classes in India, as everywhere, have the capacity to insulate themselves from an increasingly noxious environment. They have the means to create a separate personal environment; acquire imported foods from far off places where the rivers run pure, and purchase tonics to fill deficiencies and cleanse the blood. Among the less well to do, a concern about adulteration is well founded in physical reality. It also serves as an expression of latent anxiety about alienation from cultural perceptions of a "normal body" defined in terms of routine body signs (physical body) and social relations (social body).[13] These signs and relations constitute prototypical knowledge of the parameters of well being from a time past, an unobtainable state of well being in a context of rapid change and modernization. This loss of a multidimensional sense of well being is articulated in many ways.

For example, a loss of well being is often communicated through discourse about food, the substance from which health is derived and social relations constituted. The act of eating and the institution of taking meals are events over which one exerts some sense of control in a universe where humans are subject to multiple influences ranging from gods and planets to sorcery and the economic fluctuations of the international market place. While control is realized through the routine of meal taking as a symbolic as well as a physical act, alienation is articulated through complaints about digestion (Nichter 1987).

Digestion problems serve as a natural symbol for the metaphorical expression of social problems entailing family integration, feelings of passive aggression, and powerlessness, etc. Improper digestion displayed through breaks in one's habitual diet further index a concern about blood impurity in a culture maintaining what Mariott (1978) and more recently Daniels (1984) have described as a fluid sense of self. In India, a hydraulic model of ethnophysiology coexists with a dominant ideology where purity is equated with status, well being and power. Consequently, concern about digestion, weakness and impurity articulated by medicine use, indexes sociomoral relations as well as physical states. "Gastritis" constitutes a somatic idiom of distress.

I point this out to argue that the commodification of health has not simply come about as a result of pharmaceutical agents peddling products of dependency or doctors trained to use expensive, rarified foreign products in the treatment of disease at the expense of the poor. The situation is far more complex. A broader cultural context must be taken into account. As Emiko Ohnuki-Tierney (1986: 77) has noted of Japan, commercialization does not occur in a vacuum: it plays upon deep seated cultural concepts and practices. The pharmaceutical industry has responded to, built upon, and perpetuated cultural health concerns and somatic idioms of distress.

PHARMACEUTICALISATION

In a context where functional health, (the ability to perform work roles in the short term) is increasingly taking precedence over experiential health (proto-typical preconceptions of the healthy life), the popularity of technical fixes grows in an environment of alienation. The proliferation of commercially prepared pharmaceuticals and a concurrent rise in medicine consumption is a concrete expression of health commodification. It entails the commodification of health to a point where medicine fixes to life's immediate problems increasingly "appeal" to the public. Health commodities do not have to be pushed, they are demanded. The appeal of medicine is not simply the product of pharmaceutical marketing campaigns.[14] It is part of a much larger phenomenon represented by other fixes and fantasy escapes such as alcohol, movies, romance magazines and television. Just as the non-astrological variety of movie stars in India are prone to fetishization by the masses and are even worshipped as gods, so medicines have likewise been attributed "powers" beyond their active ingredients. I refer here to their ability to render health and protect against sickness in general. In the words of one patron of a Bangalore city chemist shop:

Whenever I feel an illness has come, I take antibiotic and Liv 52 for one or two days and I am protected. Whenever I feel weakness I take tonic and when I can not sleep I take Calmpose and Gastrogin. I have done this for five years and have no need for any doctor. It is cheap and the best way to stay healthy. I am satisfied.

The need for magic in an uncertain world is fodder for pharmaceutical companies who sell medicines to both consumers off the street (through chemist shops) and to practitioners who require some amount of mystification to survive in a competitive medical marketplace. In a context where medicine is freely available over the counter, there is continual need for doctors to offer something new to patients. One marketing specialist of a large multinational drug company explained the situation to me as follows:

You see it is all a case of brand vitality and *brand fatigue*. We introduce a medicine and it is popular for some time among practitioners who are our good customers. In many cases. sales peak, level off and then decline. Brand fatigue has set in. The public purchases the drug, but doctors purchase less because it is a known thing. We monitor sales continually. When brand fatigue occurs a new product will be marketed. Sometimes this drug will be constituted out of a combination of popular products. Brand fatigue drives a market where a limited number of pharmaceutical compounds are differentiated largely by claims, names and images of potency.[15]

The pharmaceutical industry happily supplies practitioners a steady stream of new medicines complete with inflated promises, research testimonials and statistics. The development of new products provides the illusion of progress and breakthroughs. The industry is in turn supported by a state apparatus attempting to nurture a "healthy economy" and create an image of improved health through the increased availability of medical resources. Medicines constitute visible and tangible proof of increasing well being. Commodified health plays an important role as a fetish of modernization. On this note it is worth mentioning that the regulation of pharmaceuticals in India does not fall under the direct authority of the Ministry of Health (dealing with physical bodies), but the Ministry of Petroleum, Chemicals and Fertilizer which has a vested interest in the health of the country's industrial body and the exchange of goods in a world system.

THE APPEAL OF MEDICINE ADVERTISEMENTS

Medicine advertising in India exploits popular imagery associated with modernization, grass roots nationalization, group fantasy and anxiety. Its success lays largely in presenting products in such a manner as to interpellate existing health concerns, perceived needs, and tacit desires. Medicines are associated with metamedical values through key symbols and images evoking networks of semantic meaning. As Good (1977) has clearly demonstrated in Iran, illnesses are imbued with cultural meanings. Advertising overdetermines the capacities of drugs with exaggerated claims which address symptoms, popular health concerns, and associated cultural meanings. This fosters the process of pharmaceuticalisation, a term designating the appropriation of human problems to medicines. The latter may be distinguished from medicalization where appropriation by the medical profession gains monopoly power and increased social control in territories of human experience.

In India, the medical profession's monopoly power is weak. Doctors are administrators of medicine and subject to a client dominant competitive health care arena (Friedson 1970) where catering to patients' wishes and expectations keeps one in business. Peer review is weak. As such, doctors are more closely tied to the pharmaceutical industry which offers them the resources to remain competitive. The range of products made available is significantly influenced, if not largely determined, by the profit needs of the industry, not the health needs of the country as defined by epidemiological or nutritional data.[16]

The advertising industry has the task of creating for the medical profession, even more than for the lay consumer, an illusion of progress. The illusion is that there are products available capable of broadly treating common symptom sets which doctors face with limited means of diagnosis in a competitive marketplace with rising patient expectations. One doctor noted:

We are not fools, but we want to be fooled. We need to believe that we can do wonders in an impossible situation. I know better than to believe in these broad spectrum antibiotics and tonics, the wide use of steroids, and other such things. But the nature of my practice, the demands on my time, the limited understanding of patients leads me to give what I am told is best by the companies with the biggest names. Then I can say I am recommending the most prestigious medicines to a patient. And the patient is happy. As a doctor I must diagnose not only the disease but the prestige and the pocketbook of my patients. Definitely, I am influenced by the advertising. That last patient, the Muslim woman who attended with the baby and a two year old child, has been either nursing a child or pregnant for the last five years. Her husband is a timber contractor. She is anaemic and weak but tonight her husband will come to her. I could give her ferrous sulfate tablets and offer her advice about diet, and if I did she would never be back and I will have lost a client. So, I recommend a new forte tonic called "Mother's Milk" and I give her a B12 injection and I think yes, she needs these things and the tonic may have some trace minerals she needs. We all feel better. The tonic costs Rs. 20 but her husband can afford it. In fact, that beautiful bottle with the picture of a blossoming mother will be shown to all in his house and they will think her husband is a wonderful chap for purchasing it and praise me.

The symbolic importance of medicine, especially tonic will be addressed shortly. For the moment, let me raise concern about the fetishization of medicine by way of a case vignette. A few years ago while visiting a friend in rural South Kanara, I observed a young man aged 20 diligently reading a medicine advertisement in a newly arrived weekly magazine. He marveled at this advertisement for an analgesic which promised to relieve pain in minutes. This advertisement showed the transformation of a somewhat cranky mother-in-law into a kind, doting woman inquiring into the welfare of her daughter-in-law after using the product. My inquiries into his interpretation of the advertisement led him to discuss other medicines he had read about and intended buying. These included a tonic to give him increased strength through better digestion, a blood purification medicine, a glucose solution named Electrose which he described as "electronic solution" for tiredness (advertised as a glucose solution supplemented by electrolytes "not recommended for diarrhoea"), flatulence tablets to take when travelling, liver tablets for giddiness, and other assorted products.[17] From my conversation with this boy and several other high school educated rural youths, I came to realize that claims of medicine efficacy were often accepted quite literally. Medicines promised magic. As with magic, some medicines were deemed to be authentic sources of power while others were considered to be the bogus product of some imposter trying to dupe the public. In principal, the claims of popular commercial companies were believed especially if they were foreign. Foreign medicine was held in high esteem, for after all, had not western peoples even travelled to the moon, a fact known to every schoolboy!

A curious request during my stay led me to consider the fetishism of medicine more personally. One day I was asked by my friend if I would administer a medicine and prepare a talisman for this young man against his fear of the dark. His fear was so severe that it prevented him from leaving the house to urinate at night. My friend's request had to do with the young man's deep seated belief in medicine advertisements and foreign products. Visits to local exorcists had already failed and the family did not wish the stigma attached to bringing the boy to a psychiatrist. My friend had told the boy that I had studied exorcism as part of my research from a renowned exorcist prior to his death. This was partially true in that I had observed his practice for several months as part of my initial fieldwork. To make a long story short, a talisman was prepared according to the procedure documented by my field notes and was offered with one 5 mg. tablet of valium removed from my "overnight bus ride survival kit". The treatment proved to be temporarily effective for a radius of 20 feet from the house — just far enough to reach a suitable tree behind which to urinate. Fearing being labeled an American exorcist, the young man was sworn to secrecy about the entire incident.

My reason for introducing this story has little to do with mental health and is somewhat embarrassing to me professionally. I share it to emphasize three points. First, although I had been studying medicine consumption behavior for several years, I had not comprehended how concretely advertisements were interpreted by a population which had less exposure to them and therefore were less critical of their exaggerated claims. Following up on this incident I found a notable absence of social science research on cultural interpretations and constructions of medicine advertisements.[18] A second point is that the request for me to give the boy medicine as well as a talisman was in itself indicative of local recognition that the two work well together. An increasing number of exorcists employ medicines with sacred verse (mantra) and talismans in South Kanara. In the 1970's most exorcists I observed were covert about their use of medicines. Some exorcists used commercially available rauwolphia serpentine tablets (sold in Ayurvedic chemist shops) ground up with a mixture of tumeric and lime paste presented as a substance embodying the power/presence of a deity associated with the exorcist. I was only once told about this practice directly and discovered its wider prevalence through research at two popular ayurvedic medicine supply shops in Mangalore city. By the 1980's the situation had changed. Three of the six exorcists I had the opportunity to visit during short field trips in the mid 1980's openly displayed boxes from which medicines were taken and promotional gifts from pharmaceutical companies acquired from chemist friends.

A third point underscored by the story reconfirms Alland's (1970) observation that it is often western medicines rather than "Western medicine" which appeals to nonwestern populations. The boy's own perceptions of the cause of his fear of the dark were strictly humoral and spirit linked. They were associated with the shock from a scare he had experienced in the night during a high fever when he saw spirits hovering outside waiting to devour his flesh. Medicines promising to control fever and pain, reduce anxiety and supply confidence appealed to him, not a medical system per se. Indeed, among his wish list of medicines to purchase included a mixture of ayur-pathic, homeopathic and allopathic drugs. As he gazed into my first aid kit one evening, he sighed and told me that with such medicines one could go anywhere without fear.

CONFLICTING INTERPRETATIONS OF MEDICINE AND "DOUBLE THINK"

Not everybody reads advertisements as concretely as this young informant nor ascribes special positive powers to that which is distant and modern. As Ewen and Ewen (1982) have noted in their study of advertising in the West, consumers do not necessarily or uniformly take in the meaning and sales pitch of advertisements. Indeed, in order for the flow of commodity capital to be maintained a constant stream of new products must appear which challenge the action of previous products. These products make claims of being unique or praise the virtues of past products of which they are a new and improved scientific reincarnation. In India, the virtues of both tradition and bioscience are being promoted, and coopted.

An underdevelopment perception of modern medicine coexists in India which is just as popular as a modernization perception represented by the young man described above. As noted in Chapter 7, many people envisage allopathic medicines to be powerful but unpredictable, affording illness management at the cost of long term health. For some, modern medicine constitutes a symbol of underdevelopment, of short term gains followed by negative side effects. For these people, ayurvedic medicine comprises a means of embodying traditional values in a commodified form. Taking ayurvedic medicine constitutes what I have described elsewhere (Nichter 1981b) as a medicinal rite de passage, a return to a life of proper digestion, purity, proper flow and a transformed sense of self. In this instance, meta-medical dimensions of culture emphasized by researchers such as Obeysekere (1976) are approached through the symbolic act of health care seeking.

Life is pervaded by paradoxes; by both continuities and discontinuities. Many people long for both the modern and the traditional, a condition the late J. P. Naik characterized as "double think". The pharmaceutical industry has responded to this paradox in two ways. Modern forms of traditional medicine have been marketed as the wisdom of past ages reaffirmed as scientific through the use of biochemical terms and Latin nomenclature. Modern medicines, on the other hand, have been marketed to accord with traditional values.

Commodified answers to "double think" have taken on regional charac-teristics. Each region and cultural group has had its own share of entre-preneurs who have been ready to maximize popular imagery. They have also appended to caste affiliation in their efforts to sell commodified answers to health problems in a changing world. Affiliation has itself been commodified.

Just as Evans Pritchard once wrote that the Nuer consume the soil of their place to maintain a metonymic relationship with land, so South Kanarese migrants to Bombay, Bangalore, and the Middle East consume locally manufactured traditional medicines as a means of embodying affiliation. This is illustrated in the following interview with a South Kanarese informant who relocated to Bombay.

Anthropologist: You have just told me you use *draksha arishta* (an ayurvedic tonic) made by the Shastri family in Mangalore. Is this the only company from whom you purchase this medicine?

Informant: Yes, I use this tonic only. The tonic is sent to me by my elder sister, or sometimes I purchase it here from a chemist who is also from South Kanara. I buy other medicines from Germany, England, Bombay and Calcutta. But the *draksha aristha* we use and the *dasamoola aristha* used by my wife after her delivery are always Shastri brand.

Anthropologist: Are there other brands of these medicines which are of good quality?

Informant: There are many good companies and *vaidya* who prepare such medicines.

Friend of informant: He waters his roots with his Kanarese medicine! (Laughter follows . . .)

Informant: Yes, it is true. It is of my place. My sister also sends me *kodi madhu* (a traditional herbal home remedy) to give to my children at the time of year when new buds appear on the trees at home. We are protected by these things. They are from our place. Our people have taken them for many long years.

In this interview a relationship between home (*mulla sthana*) and present place of residence is established through the consumption of medicines having "use value" and associated with well being, nurturance, recovery and vitality. In a sense, this comprises a secular act complementary to the sending of *prasada* (blessed substances) from rituals at local South Kanarese temples to the homes of those living outside by kin within the district. At times of vulnerability, *prasada* from home deities is consumed for health and protection. The gift of medicine and *prasada*, articulates social relations involving affiliation, care, reciprocity and social support.

FACTORS PROMOTING THE COMMODIFICATION OF HEALTH

The competitive marketing and manufacture of commercial medicines in India began in the 19th century, but it was not until post independence that the medicine market experienced rapid growth (Leslie 1988). Market expansion was no doubt fostered by the setting up of a national health service placing the public in closer contact with doctors and the remarkable demonstration effect of antibiotics. In the last two decades, several factors have increased public acceptance of, if not dependence on, commercial medicines. As noted in Chapter 8, the very fact that practitioners are paid on the basis of a distribution of medicines encourages polypharmacy for each and every ailment.[19] This has led people to become accustomed to receiving medicines for all health problems. The somatic expression and physiomorphic experience of distress (Nichter 1981a) as well as cultural conventions fostering the metacommunication of affect also render states of psychosocial disease treatable by medicine. While this often entails the consultation of practitioners for medicines, a multitude of medicine products are now available in the market place for the home treatment of illness and distress. These medicines have come to constitute new symbolic resources available for articulating metamedical messages from the body of one experiencing distress to significant others.[20]

Consistent with the growing popularity of the term "psychosomatic", practitioners have increasingly begun utilizing mild tranquilizers in the treatment of vague body states associated with somatization. Over the past decade, four chemist shops which I have been observing during brief yearly/ biyearly visits to South Kanara, all report significant rises in the amount of Diazepam used for patient care in the 1980's.[21] For example, in one chemist shop observed in a small crossroads town in 1986, diazepam sales averaged 500 tablets a day compared to sales of 150 tablets a day in 1983. The shop did not report a significant rise in mean clients per day and was not identified as a special source for this common medication. Several doctors whom I have observed over the years now routinely administer Diazepam and vitamins to patients complaining of general somatic complaints. Five to ten years ago, they treated such complaints with vitamin tonics alone. The brand name Calmpose is becoming familiar among the rural population.

A case study may highlight the use of tranquilizers and antidepressants as a fix for patients presenting what appears to the allopathic practitioner as vague somatic complaints. In 1987 I visited the household of a former neighbor, a robust woman in her late 40s whose wit and playful scolding I remembered well. Upon entering her house I was struck by her lassitude and awaited a tale of tragedy. Instead, I found that the family's fortune had improved. The daughters with whom the woman was close had been married nearby, a daughter-in-law had given birth to a happy grandson who busily played in the courtyard, and the family's debts had been paid off. Inquiring about the woman's health she spoke of a set of symptoms she had presented to me seven years before, symptoms characteristic of anemia and riboflavin deficiency. She stated:

Your medicines helped me the most. They cured the cracking (angular stomatitis) at the corners of my mouth and gave me blood. The doctor's medicines I take daily give me good sleep and a good appetite but I am weak and can not work as I did before. I eat rice gruel and sit quietly but my mouth is always dry and I am constipated.

Upon examining the woman's medication I found that she was taking an antidepressant and had been doing so for over a year. Yet, a long discussion with her family, whom I knew well, revealed little evidence of anxiety, sadness, nor physical symptoms associated with depression. I became curious as to why this woman had been prescribed this medication and interviewed the practitioner who had prescribed it as well as family members who had accompanied the woman to the doctor. The practitioner had last seen the woman two weeks prior to my visit and recalled the woman as continually complaining of weakness, heat sensations, and slowly moving blood. His diagnosis was that she was suffering from psychosomatic problems related to menopause. During an interview with family members and the woman, it was revealed that she had attributed her weakness to the ending of menstruation associating this state with blood impurity and sluggishness. Initially presented with complaints which the women related to a hydraulic notion of ethno-physiology, the doctor interpreted them as indicative of a psychosomatic problem as distinct from a cultural conceptualization. The woman's notion of a somatic imbalance in her body was taken as a mental imbalance which the doctor wrongly assumed was linked to unhappy social relations at home. She was treated accordingly and the effect of the medication she was taking reinforced her cultural notions about her failing health. Paradoxically, she came to depend on the medication for health. Her state of health became redefined in relation to good sleep and appetite. Minimal health was now purchased.

The commodification of health is not influenced by the medicine giving practices of practitioners and somatization alone. Some ailments are increas-ingly being anticipated as the price one pays for working in a cosmopolitan environment. For example, digestive complaints are reported to be on the increase by almost all of my long-term lay and practitioner informants. Contributing to this increase may well be the frank adulteration of food; insecticide residue poisoning; increased consumption of hotel food exposing a greater number of people to disease transmission by food handling; and incomplete absorption of antibacterial drugs (eg. penicillin, ampicillin, tetra-cycline) commonly mis-prescribed and often misused. Irrespective of the biomedical causes of digestive complaints, they are commonly interpreted by the lay population in humoral terms. This has led many people to routinely consume medications to clean their blood, remove gas (*vayu*) and improve digestive power as a means of obtaining health in an unhealthy environment or work situation. Another example of this commodified preventive health reasoning is the purchase of tonic by beedie cigarette rollers as a means of promoting health while engaging in a vocation recognized to be unconducive to health. The allocation of resources for tonic to beedie rollers to some extent mitigates the concern of household members when a beedie roller member displays lassitude associated with the monotony of their work. Here we find a commodified expression of concern vis-à-vis medicine, a relation-ship of care articulated through medicine as a symbol as well as a resource.

I will focus attention on tonic use below. At present I may point out that the practice of consuming medicines as a means of promoting health is not new. What is new is the range of products available for this purpose and increases in disposable income making the purchase of these products possible among a growing percentage of the population. The range of problems targeted for the marketing of medicine has also expanded. Curi-ously, medicine products have emerged on the market that not only profess to purify the blood following the consumption of adulterated food, or in times of environmental stress, but following the consumption of allopathic medicines and the use of birth control methods. For those who perceive cosmopolitan medicines as rendering the blood impure, products like "Liv Up" specifically advertise to appeal to constipation and weakness "resulting from antibiotic use." Charles Leslie's observation two decades ago is even more apropos today:

There is a joke in India that says it doesn't matter whether you consult a hakim or a doctor, you will get penicillin anyway. But the joke could be turned around to say it doesn't matter whether you consult a doctor or a hakim, your penicillin will be supplemented with a regimen and tonics of unani or ayurvedic origin (Leslie 1967).

TONICS: A SPECIAL CASE OF HEALTH COMMODIFICATION

A majority of the population surveyed have the erroneous view that daily consumption of tonics is essential to health. It is necessary to remember that nutrition can not be built across the pharmacy counter . . . (Krishnaswamy 1983)

Tonic consumption constitutes a clear case of health commodification. A pharmaceutical company executive once described India to me as "a nation addicted to tonics". There is a long tradition of liquid tonic use in India associated with ayurvedic restorative and rejuvenation, *rasayana*, medicines. Pharmaceutical companies have responded to the popularity of tonics by competing for a market share of this profitable sector. Their marketing strategies have included extensive mass media advertising campaigns as well as intensive interpersonal sales efforts aimed at practitioners and chemists. Interpersonal marketing has been deemed especially important given that tonics are fairly similar and that brand loyalty for tonics among doctors often carries over into self purchase behavior by satisfied patients.

Arduous attempts to win over practioners to specific brands of tonic are understandable considering that before regulation changes in 1983 vitamin preparations were allowed a 100% markup over production costs in comparison to a 40% markup for essential drugs. New regulations reduced potential profits to 60% over production costs. In 1983, vitamin sales accounted for nearly two thirds of Pfizer's in-country profits and one third of Abbot's total production of medicines. These companies joined with Glaxo, the country's largest producer of non standard vitamin combinations, in protest of the new regulations which reduced their profits significantly. A spokesperson for the pharmaceutical companies was quoted as stating that: "If profitable areas of operation became unprofitable then present subsidized production of essential drugs would inevitably stop, leading to scarcity and increased imports".[22]

In this context it is worth noting that roughly 10% of drug formulations in India are vitamins, accounting for 15% of total drug production costs. More than 800 micro and macro nutrient supplements are listed in the Indian Pharmaceutical Guide. While in the early 1980's there was a decline in the total percentage of drugs produced in India classified as life saving and essential drugs, there was an increase in the production of tonics and non-essential drugs. Ironically, the content of popular vitamin tonics often does not match the country's nutritional deficiencies and tonics have been criticized as being an enormous economic waste. JayaRao (1977) and more recently Krishnaswamy (1983) and Greenhalgh (1987) have pointed out that B-complex drugs which are widely prescribed and self purchased in India are often not warranted:

Combinations of B complex containing B1, B2, B6, B12 and other vitamins rank first among sales, whereas vitamin B2 and iron deficiency anaemia are most often encountered in the population. Vitamin B-complex in various combinations and forte preparations are being used without any scientific rationale. These preparations are one of the five largest selling drugs in the country. (Krishnaswamy 1983).

My interviews with consumers engaged in the self purchase of B-complex preparations leads me to suspect that the action of this medication is widely interpreted in terms of popular images of the liver and bile (*pitta*) strongly influenced by humoral medical tradition. Doctors and chemists are not simply prescribing or suggesting tonics to "humor" patients. There are economic incentives at stake. These incentives range from promotional gifts to high profit margins when tonics are directly sold.

Let me briefly present data from South Kanara on the rise in tonic use. In 1979—80, approximately three quarters of 82 poor to low-middle class households participating in a community diagnosis project (Nichter 1984a) reported that tonic had been prescribed to one or more members by a doctor during the previous year. In a majority of cases, informants stated tonics were recommended each time they received a prescription chit from a practitioner. During the same time period, two town chemist shops under observation reported that approximately 10% of their sales were for liquid tonics involving 20% of their customers. This amounted to the sale of 20—30 bottles of tonic a day. The large majority of tonics purchased were prescribed. During a short field visit to the district in 1983, I interviewed members of some of the same households. The following table summarizes the data collected on bottles of tonic (ayurvedic and allopathic) actually purchased by these households (as distinct from bottles prescribed) during 1979 and 1983.

TABLE I. Percentage of Households Purchasing Tonic.

Locale	Sample Size	1979	1983
City	20	90%	100%
Town	20	65%	85%
Village	20	25%	55%

In each of the three samples of poor-low middle class households, tonic users had increased over the four year period of time. Increases were especially significant among town and village households. Additionally, it was found that between 1979—1983 the mean number of bottles of tonic consumed by user households rose from slightly less than 2 bottles to over 3 bottles at an average cost of Rs. 45 in 1983 as compared to Rs. 26 in 1979. One week observational studies of the two chemist shops in 1983 revealed that approximately 20% of their total sales and 45% of prescriptions involved nutritional supplements — a doubling over a 4—5 year period of time.[23] In 1986, an estimate of tonic sales was secured from a representative of a large pharmaceutical company who has worked in the district for over a decade. According to his sales figures, there has been a 25% rise in the sale of tonics between 1978—86. Between 30—40% of his total sales are for tonics with another 25% of sales accounted for by antibiotics. Questioned as to what were the three fastest rising sales items, he noted tonics, antacids, and antiamoebics.

During interviews with chemists and physicians in 1983 and 1986 I was continually told that tonic had "become a fashion" at a time when money was more readily available. One young doctor interviewed just after completion of his rural based social and community medicine rotation stated:

These people do not place importance on changing their diet once a sufficient amount of rice is eaten. When they are ill they consume less for some days which we have learned will interfere with immunity and catch up growth among children. We tell them to eat eggs and to take milk and fruits and they say, "we are poor people, we can not afford these things." But sir, I do not believe this is the truth. These people will buy tonic for Rs. 15 or 20 and feel happy if we prescribe it. They will not change their diet for more than a few days, if that, and then only because they think diet is necessary for the medicine they are taking. I used to scold them and then I returned to my family home and observed the tonic bottle "worshipped" there too! I have been blind to this. My mother has some *aristha* cure all and my brother's wife her "forte" vitamins and glucose packets, and my younger brother takes ayurvedic capsules for strength. Tonics have become a fashion. In the old days perhaps there were not many different types to choose from, but today there are so many. Just as people have become more interested in different fashion clothes, they are now interested in different fashion tonics.

Discussions in a town and village area with laypersons in the process of purchasing tonics suggested other reasons for their increasing popularity. A town informant noted the following:

I buy a bottle of tonic every couple of months and it lasts for two weeks. For health I should drink it daily, but usually I buy a bottle when I need strength or my wife feels weakness or there is some sickness. Five years ago I took tonic only when I was sick and the doctor gave me a chit to bring it. Now it is a common thing among the people. Why? Life has changed. It's like fuel for cooking. Five years ago, we used firewood. Then the price rose and we used kerosene and then there was rationing so we changed to gas and now my wife even has an electric hotplate. At first I did not like the change, the food had less taste, but cooking was easy. Food tastes better when it is cooked in mud pots over firewood, everyone will tell you this in India even if they are a rich person. But now aluminum and stainless steel pots and gas or kerosene are used for cooking because it is easy and quick. It is like that with tonic. Ten years ago, even five years ago, good quality local rice was available here. Now, nobody grows and hand pounds local rice for sale. Today I go to the shop and buy a mixed thing — chinese rice, IR-8 — a hybrid rice, and rice from upghats (other districts in the Deccan plateau). I am not sure of this rice. It does not have the taste of the rice I ate as a boy nor the strength, but it is available and I buy it because it is easy. So I take tonic for strength, it is also easy. After some time of taking it you develop a habit for it and then you feel you need this tonic to be healthy. Now we are a country of tonic drinkers.

On the same topic, a low-middle class villager noted:

My daughter has complained of weakness and heat since winter season when she was in hospital and was given medicine for fever. That medicine was very powerful. The fever was cured but a red rash fell to her skin when she went in the sun and she became weak. Now she needs tonic every month. English medicine is like the new hybrid rice strains we receive from your country. They mature faster and give bigger yields but when we use them it is necessary to add other things to the field or troubles come. These things were not necessary for local rice. Like that, we used English medicine for my daughter for two weeks and now she must have tonic for her health. To remove the fire from her body left by the medicine, a *vaidya* told me it would take one month of ayurvedic medicine. My mother says I should give her this medicine. But with tonic she has strength. When there was fever, ayurvedic medicine did not cure. Ayurvedic medicine does not have the strength it did when I was a child because of chemical fertilizers. My daughter will need to take English medicine again and so it is better that she become habituated to this medicine.

Revealed by the statements of the latter two informants is a sense that tonics are needed more today because of a decline in the quality of life. Tonics are an easy way to compensate for deficiencies resulting from an impoverished diet perceived in terms of the quality of staple foods. Concordant with this impression, a high level pharmaceutical marketing executive noted to me that nutrient supplements like Horlicks and Bournvita sold much better in South India where people perceived the quality of their foodstuffs as questionable and felt some "deficiency." For this reason his firm recommended the advertising of products to fill this "food gap." I was told that in North India more blood purifying tonics were sold. In the opinion of this informant, this was because the North Indian population was concerned about the quality of their blood as affected by non-vegetarian foods. Whether this impression is true or not, his firm advised companies accordingly and these concerns were played upon in regional advertising campaigns.

Another reason for tonic popularity revealed by the two interviews was the feeling that modern life entailed reliance on allopathic medicines for short term functional health. This required tonic use to compensate for extra demands on the body. Tonic use becomes the price one pays for the use of modern medicine. Several informants spoke of tonics as a "habit" not simply a fashion, a habit in the sense of a dependency. For the capitalist system, the ultimate measure of success is to have a population not only desire a product which sustains a mode of production, but a population which feels that they "need" and "depend" on this product for their well being. Health is redefined in relation to the commodity elixir. This is a clear illustration of the embodiment of capitalist hegemony. In the U.S. one could point to other illustrations. A poignant example would be our increasing use of the terms "dependency" and "addiction" to describe and mitigate responsibility for our market behavior. Compulsive shopping is described by some people as an "addiction" as well as something one does to feel better. This constitutes a powerful ideological statement.

The use of tonics has altered over the last two decades. During my initial fieldwork in the mid 1970's, I collected data on tonic use during a study of pregnancy and postpartum related behavior. Among the poor-low middle class, tonic was considered an important felt health need during the post-partum period and following any surgical operation. Aside from these specific times, tonic was purchased as a kind of medicine at the recom-mendation of a doctor.[24] Today, vitamin tonic sales are as commonly pur-chased without a prescription as with one, and tonic is as likely to be purchased for health as for illness.[25] Tonic use has come to reflect a sense of prosperity as well as an act of health promotion. Tonic sales peak just after harvest season among agricultural laborers, a time when food is more plentiful. A rise in over the counter tonic sales also signals a broad change in attitudes toward the use of commercial medicines. In India, there has been a marked increase in the substitution of patent medicines for home prepared herbal medicines. I will return to this point shortly.

For years practitioners have prescribed tonics for general bodily com-plaints presented by patients in accord with physical sensations, felt health concerns and perceptions of body processes. Practitioners often reason that these symptoms are linked to some kind of malnutrition and feel that tonics "might help and can't hurt" in a situation where something has to be given as a tangible form of care and a means of collecting payment. Over time, tonics have come to be expected by the public. Today, the Indian population both requests prescriptions for tonics and uses them for self care for an increasing variety of bodily complaints. Interviews on the action of tonics identified them with: strength, vigor, blood quantity, blood quality, blood circulation and distribution, the liver, digestion, a balancing of humors and hot/cold, and among some educated informants, acid and alkaline blood. Given a wide range of tonics from pluralistic medical traditions, a variety of options exist for managing health problems through tonic use. If one tonic does not produce desired results, there is always another one to try. Let me cite an example illustrating how the range of tonics can influence patterns of health care seeking.

On one memorable occasion I observed a patient request tonic for bloodessness from a doctor for a case involving hookworm infestation resulting in acute anemia. "Doctor," the woman implored, "tonic please." The doctor struggled to convince the patient not to rely on tonic as a cure for her weakness. He prescribed medicine to remove the worms and ferrous sulfate tablets. An experienced health center peon informed the doctor that local people avoided worm medicine during monsoon season. During this time of climatic extremes it is considered dangerous for deworming especially when one was ill and weak. The doctor thought for a moment and then told the woman that if she drank tonic the worms would only drink the tonic and grow fat increasing their hunger causing them to become even more troublesome. She was told that the worms must be removed and was given the prescription. I sent my field assistant to find out what in fact she would do. She left and immediately visited an ayurvedic compounder asking for a tonic to give her strength, but one which was bitter, one which would not be consumed by worms which preferred sweet things. A medicine tonic answer to her immediate problem was invented concordant with her ideas about health, risk and the nature of worms.

Two last points need to be made concerning the rise in tonic use as it pertains to the commodification of health. It is necessary to point out that tonic exchange is a means of articulating concern and care. As noted earlier with reference to beedie cigarette rollers, offering tonic to a family member articulates social relations and personal expressions of affect. On a number of occasions I witnessed a husband express affection and concern for his wife or mother through the gift of a bottle of tonic. In critiquing tonic as an economic waste, we must not be so hasty as to neglect the psychosocial dimensions of tonic exchange and the importance of tonic as a symbol. Our focus must not be strictly reduced to a biomedical gaze of disease and must extend to a consideration of the experience of illness (Eisenberg 1977), distress (Nichter 1981a), and caretaking behavior.

A related point may be raised with regard to the meaning of tonic. In one of the interview vignettes presented, a man purchasing tonic remarked that he did so when he required strength or when his wife suffered from weakness. Based on interviews and a preliminary assessment of tonic promotionals, it appears that a cultural theme, that of female vulnerability and male strength, is being reproduced through advertising campaigns.[26] In a study in an ayurvedic medicine shop in Mangalore, 15% of medicines sold were to women for tonic associated with weakness with an additional 5% being sold for leukorrhea associated with weakness. On the other hand, 13% of sales were for male rejuvenation tonics for increasing strength and general vitality. While it may be argued that the tonics were actually being promoted for the same complaint (i.e. weakness), differences in marketing strategy are noteworthy for they perpetuate gender stereotypes.

A final point to be made with respect to tonic use involves children. An important sector of India's expanding tonic market is comprised by children's tonics. Glucose powder has long been marketed in India as tonic for children as well as those convalescing. Today, glucose is being superceded by products advertised as more modern sources of health and vitality which active children require. Middle class parents who once purchased an occasional packet of glucose or a monthly can of Horlicks or Bournvita food supplement to augment "poor diet and a child's special needs" are now the advertising target of an increasing variety of tonics. A growing number of products are marketed to improve child health and brain power in a competitive world. Among these products is electrolyte solution marketed not for dehydration but energy. Presented with a box of Electrose brand oral rehydration solution most informants interviewed associated it with sports and power. As noted earlier, a popular name for this and similar rehydration products was "electronic solution". In a world where increasing emphasis in the media is being directed toward computers and where satellite dishes are appearing in villages, electronic solution represents the embodiment of modernity in contrast to the balancing of humors, or for that matter, electrolytes.

SELF TREATMENT, CHEMIST SHOPS AND THE COMMODIFICATION OF HEALTH

Let us return to the observation that home preparation of raw herbal remedies are rapidly being replaced by commercial medications in South Kanarese households. Home treatment has traditionally played an important role in health care in South Kanara for a wide range of ailments. Home care is more extensive in some castes and among some groups of people than others. Survey research carried out in 1975 and again in 1979 revealed that among poor to lower middle class non-Brahmans, home care is most prevalent among women, preschool children and the elderly.[27]

The form of home care is rapidly changing. In the mid 1970's, the use of commercial medicines in the home was fairly limited and primarily observed in nuclear two generational households where elders were rarely present. During a household survey in 1975, I found that members of such households often remembered the function of local raw herbal preparations, but were vague about preparation details and dosage. They were twice as likely to have purchased ready made ayurvedic and cosmopolitan medicines than those living in three generational households. Today, this distinctive pattern has diminished. Greater contact with medicine distributors (chemists, provision shops stocking medicines, ayurvedic medicine distributors) has led to increased familarity and active experimentation with commercial products guided by the suggestions of friends and shopkeepers alike.

In the 1980's, commercial medicines have rapidly become popular home care resources for many common illnesses including diarrheal and respiratory conditions. Informants speak of the ease of taking prepared products as opposed to the time consuming boiling of decoctions which require dietary regulations. Use of commercial products is often rationalized by statements to the effect that raw herbal products no longer have the power they once did due to pesticides, insecticides, and chemical fertilizers. Increased familarity with a larger number of chemist shops has been facilitated by better transportation, more patent medicines available at provision shops, a growing recognition of medicines prescribed time and again, and rising literacy opening new eyes to advertisements. All of these factors have had an influence on self help patterns.

Increased cash flow and disposable income in the 1980s have enabled more vigorous health consumerism. Pharmaceutical companies have recognized this change in the rural medicine market. I was told by a high level pharmaceutical marketing specialist that the rural sector was given minimal attention before the mid 1970s. With agricultural change and new wealth in rural areas, pharmaceutical marketing efforts were stepped up. He estimated that in India as a whole, rural per capita medicine expenditure in 1981 was Rs. 20 and that current expenditure was two to two and a half times this. This estimate, across classes, is remarkably close to my own approximations based on household survey data.

We may briefly consider changes that have occurred in medicine purchasing behavior by viewing data collected at three South Kanarese chemist shops. At one rural chemist shop observed in 1984 for three days in winter season, nearly 41% of clients purchased medicines without a prescription. Twenty five percent directly presented a symptom, 5% requested a drug by name and another 10% presented a medicine label or name scribbled on a piece of paper. The shopkeeper noted that over-the-counter purchases of medicine had steadily been increasing over the last ten years. In a second shop observed for the same duration, 28% percent of clients purchased medicine over-the-counter. At this shop only 10% presented symptoms to the chemist, 18% directly asking for a drug by name. Clients of this shop considered the owner more a vendor of medicines than a practitioner in contrast to the first shopkeeper. At both shops, a wide range of medicines were requested without a prescription (other than tonics and vitamins). In order of commonality these included: analgesics, antipyretics and anti-inflammatory drugs (45% sold without a prescription), drugs for flatulence, upset stomach, and diarrhea; cough mixtures; topical preparations; and antibiotics.[28]

In urban areas, over-the-counter purchase of medications appeared even higher than that reported in rural towns. The third chemist shop observed was a city chemist shop in Mangalore. Over 55% of customers over a three day period of time in 1984 conferred with the chemist about their symptoms. The chemist offered them advice about medicines; substituted generic for more expensive brand name drugs when poor clients were unable to purchase prescribed products; and convinced those with means to buy products maximizing his profit margin. Many clients referred to the chemist as "doctor". Several openly told me that the chemist was the best practitioner to consult for routine problems because he knew more "company pharmaceuticals" than doctors. Moreover, he was willing to listen to their past experience with drugs (not just symptoms) enabling him to suggest new medicines when results from medicines already used were unsatisfactory or side effects manifested.

Important to highlight is that a number of customers noted to me that urban living required their taking medicines to maintain health, not just cure disease. A cost of urban living was a need for more medicines. They discussed these medicine needs with the chemist. Medicines purchased for this preventive/promotive health purpose included tonics, digestive aids, liver medicines, vitamins, sleeping tablets, menstrual regulators, medicines for constipation and diarrhea, and eye inflammation. Once again, these medicines were for problems which customers anticipated as a consequence of rapid urbanization and life style change occurring in Mangalore.

The data from this urban South Kanarese chemist shop takes on greater significance when viewed in relation to a large study on medicine purchase behavior carried out by scientists attached to the National Institute of Nutrition in Hyderabad (Krishnaswamy and Kumar 1983; Krishnaswamy et al. 1983). This important yet little known study (in the West), may be highlighted to illustrate the rising prevalence of self treatment utilizing commercial products. In the study, data was collected on drug purchasing behavior in 10% of all retail chemist shops in the twin cities of Hyderabad and Secunderbad (pop. 2.5 million). Six trained investigators observed the activity of druggists at 330 shops for two hour periods for four days over a four month period. Data was collected on over 26,000 sales involving the purchase of nearly 45,000 drugs. Both prescription and over-the-counter drug purchases were monitored. The following medicine purchasing patterns were noted:

1. Nearly half (47%) of all medicines purchased were for self care. Of these, 58% were for scheduled drugs which were supposed to be dispensed only with a doctor's prescription.
2. Ninety two percent of the prescriptions filled were from private doctors. A majority did not contain the patient's name, provisional diagnosis, dosage schedule, or duration of therapy.
3. The profile of drugs purchased by clients on their own and patients with prescriptions were remarkably similar.
4. Nutritional products (tonics) headed the list of medicines prescribed by doctors. They accounted for 27% of all prescriptions with B-complex accounting for 42% of nutritional products prescribed. Among self purchases, nutritional products accounted for 19% of purchases.
5. With respect to other categories of drugs, Table II (see below) provides a brief summary of the percentages of prescription and self help purchases comprised by various types of drugs.
6. Types of sedatives and tranquilizers as well as antidiarrheal drugs and antihistamines were self-purchased to the same extent that they were prescribed.
7. Broad spectrum antibiotics were used indiscriminately within the urban area. More than 30% of doctor's prescriptions contained antibiotics as

TABLE II.

Therapeutic class	Doctor's prescription	Self purchase
sulfa/antibiotics	16%	9%
analgesics antipyretics anti-inflammatory	13%	24%
gastrointestinal	9%	12%
respiratory	8%	11%

did some 13% of self purchases. The researchers suggested that the "public was adopting an antibiotic mentality similar to that of doctors".

8. Only 18% of self purchasers and 40% of prescription holders purchased a full course of antibiotics. Thirty percent of self purchasers purchased only a one day supply of an antibiotic requested.

The data collected in this large study complements my own intensive observational studies in South Kanarese chemist shops with two exceptions. First, self purchase for antibiotics in Hyderabad was more common than observed in South Kanara. The second difference is that in the Hyderabad study, less than 2% of drugs were purchased at the recommendation of the chemist after symptoms were presented — a finding the researchers admit may well be an artifact of the investigator's presence. In South Kanara, chemist consultation and medicine recommendation were very common among some, but not all, chemists.

Another reason for highlighting the Hyderabad study is that it provides ample evidence that the medicine taking behavior initiated by doctors, for a complex of reasons, has influenced popular health behavior. The influence of prescription patterns has not only made an impact on illness related self help behavior, but medicine taking associated with health promotion and illness prevention.[29]

COMMERCIAL AYURVEDIC PATENT MEDICINES

Little research exists on the commercialization of traditional medications despite the growth of an impressive herbal medicine industry in countries such as Japan, Indonesia, and India. In India, Leslie (1988) has pointed out that the history of commercial ayurvedic drugs extends from a period of time when revivalistic ideology fostered the manufacture of traditional medicine as an expression of Indian civilization, to the present where pharmaceutical companies foster "double think" modern traditional medicines for profit.

The revivalist rhetoric that appealed to several generations of Indian nationalists grew stale with repetition, and finally began to appear ridiculous. But this does not mean that the ways people experienced their bodies or their humoral understanding of these experiences changed. The commercially sophisticated and well managed companies that produce Ayurvedic and Unani medicines appeal to these experiences and understandings, and their stylishly packaged products appeal to the middle class conviction that modern appearing things are valuable on their own account (Leslie 1988: 22).

In India there has been a steady rise in the number of companies marketing both commercial quality "standard ayurvedic" preparations and "patent ayurpathic" products. By commercial quality medicines, I refer to mass produced medications in contrast to those produced by traditional (*shastric*) production techniques which are labor, time, and fuel intensive as well as imbued with a symbolic dimension to medicine preparation. Ayurpathic products are new, commercially produced, modern herbal patent drugs described as ayurvedic and thought of by the public as acting on body humors. Estimates as to the size of the ayurvedic drug market are difficult to come by. Leslie (1988) cites Dr Kurup, a WHO adviser on Indian Systems of Medicine, as estimating that in 1980, 3000 private companies manufactured ayurvedic pharmaceuticals worth in excess of Rs. 50 million in addition to ayurvedic products (soap, hair tonic, etc.), a major source of profit.

The growth of a commercial ayurvedic pharmaceutical industry has had a tremendous impact on the local production of ayurvedic medicines, the practice of medicine and home treatment. Let us first consider how large commercial ayurvedic medicine companies have effected the local production and availability of ayurvedic medicine. Over the last decade I have seen a number of small traditional ayurvedic medicine production units go out of business due to significant price hikes in raw herbs and fuel as well as an inability to compete with the commercial rates and sales incentives offered to shops and practitioners by large ayurvedic pharmaceutical companies. Just as companies selling allopathic medicines have engaged in intensive marketing campaigns, pharmaceutical representatives of large ayurvedic companies have been assigned aggressive marketing programs. In many instances, they offer more attractive incentive schemes than companies of allopathic medicines.

Let me briefly consider the case of one established ayurvedic medicine company in South Kanara using traditional production methods. In 1985 the company sold a 400 ml. bottle of *dasamoola arishta*, a standard ayurvedic tonic, for Rs. 25. Several out of district companies sold commercial *dasamoola aristha* for Rs. 14. The company, which had an excellent reputation, folded in 1986 after three generations of medicine production. The owner, who also manages a medicine shop, decided it was more profitable to sell commercial products than to produce a quality product at a price deemed unreasonable by a growing number of his customers. During an interview he noted the following:

My profit on a bottle of ayurvedic *aristha* last year was Rs 2-3 when all expenses were accounted for. If I sell commercial brands I make Rs. 4-6 and get one free bottle of medicine as an incentive for each 10 that I sell. Not only that but most companies will give me 30 days of free credit and a bonus if I become a steady customer. I get more profit; I also get a guilty conscience. I know medicine and the products I now sell have little medicinal value compared to the medicine I produced. But then they are used incorrectly anyway. People come in and want a peg of *aristha* to make everything better. They are not following the advice that used to go with the medicine. Look, that rickshaw driver came in here to get a peg of *arishta* for his upset stomach. He comes in everyday. There is no cure for his problem because he is being bounced around in the heat all day, he breathes in smoke and fumes, eats hotel food, drinks tea to stay awake and arrack to go to sleep. He doesn't expect a cure, he just wants some relief to get him through the day, or at least something to make him feel he is doing something good for health. It doesn't matter whether he takes a commercial or a shastric prepared *aristha* for his purposes. Chalk powder would be just as good for him. I feel badly that I am selling this inferior quality medicine, but that is what people are interested in. Actually, it is a *pāpa* (sin), but at least I am only selling it and not making it. To do that would be to dishonor my father and the medicine business he built. My son wants me to mass produce medicines, using electric current instead of firewood, and sugar instead of honey. But I will never do it. Now I am like other chemists. I sell the company which makes me the most profit. So I stock 200 ml. bottles of commercial *ashoka arishta* which I sell for Rs. 7 and I make Rs. 3 profit. But, if my customer is not an old client, I say, "Look here, I have a new product called Vanitaplex and I sell it to him for Rs 9.50 and make even more profit. It's the same ingredients with an English name. That is the future of ayurvedic medicine. This is what will spoil ayurveda, not allopathic medicine. Business has never been better!

Let me elaborate on this informant's last point, that the proliferation of patent ayurpathic drugs with English names is the direction of contemporary ayurveda. To do this I need to consider the plight of new ayurvedic medicine production units. Popular demand for ayurvedic medicines has been increasing due to a number of factors including a growing concern that powerful allopathic medicines (such as antibiotics and injections) are hard on the body and produce a variety of side effects reduced by ayurvedic medicines. Local companies have emerged to meet local market demand for familiar products at the same time that national companies have intensified regional sales campaigns. While some established local companies have gone out of business due to their inability to offer competitive prices for standard medicines, new companies have arisen to meet the challenge of large companies on home turf by mimicking their sales strategies and price schedules.

Two strategies are available for making a profit. First, a local company can maintain its operations in a rural area where labor and firewood charges are low and raw herbs, oil, honey, ghee, etc. are locally available reducing transportation costs. A medicine of equal or superior quality to that of large commercial companies can be produced cashing in on the renown of a patron practitioner and local affiliation. Some profit may be made in this manner, but a proliferation of alternative competitively priced medicines keeps market prices low.[30] The second strategy is to produce a few quality traditional products to maximize the reputation of a patron practitioner and then market a new patent product which fetches a handsome profit and is advertised as being unique.[31]

The latter strategy adds to the proliferation of patent ayurvedic products in India, but why English names? In the first place it need be noted that the marketing of unique patent medicines is not a local phenomenon, but a national pattern well established since the 1950's and capitalized on by such companies as Himalaya and Charak.[32] English names for ayurvedic medicines have increased in popularity because of a general ascription of "quality" attached to a new, modern and foreign sounding name. Two other factors have popularized English names. First, a price ceiling has been placed on an increasing number of allopathic medicines which serves to limit and control profit margins. Medicines labelled ayurvedic are not as subject to price control and taxation as allopathic medicines.[33] This is one reason that a number of allopathic medicine companies (e.g. Franco India, Walter Bushnell, Sandhu Bros., Dattatraya Krishna) have begun producing modern ayurpathic products and perhaps the reason that one finds the words "ayurvedic medicine" written in small letters on the bottom of Vicks Vaporub containers. Whereas chemists and doctors purchase most allopathic medicines for 8—15% below retail price, they may purchase ayurvedic medicines for 30% or more below retail price. The economic incentive for selling such products is obvious.

The second factor is that many MBBS doctors are reluctant to prescribe ayurvedic medicines with Sanskrit names despite the fact that patients look favorably at the inclusion of ayurvedic drugs in their treatment regime. One doctor described his view as follows:

If a patient comes to me and I say here is a chit for a medicine which you can get from the village vaidya, the patient will question why he should see me, since I charge more and he gets the same thing he could have obtained in his village. What he doesn't realize is that I have diagnosed his problem correctly and find this ayurvedic medicine a good medicine to be used with other medicines. There have been great practitioners in Indian history and some of the ayurvedic products developed are useful, but then many are nonsense also. To prescribe traditional products is to support ayurveda as a whole and this I will not do. Also many traditional preparations have not been prepared in a hygienic manner. But what I can do is prescribe an ayurvedic product sold with an English name prepared by a standard company in a scientific way. I can prescribe R compound for arthritis which is actually *Maharogaraja googalu*, Hepril instead of *Kumari Asawa* or Feedal instead of *Ashwaganda Aristha* as tonics. These medicines are known to me and used by my family also. For the new name I will be respected, patients are happy because the medicine is modern and ayurvedic, and I am not supporting other quack medicines included in ayurveda. Everybody is satisfied.

The sentiments expressed by this practitioner were echoed by several other doctors whom I interviewed. A growing number of allopathic doctors as well as recent graduates of ayurvedic schools who wish to be seen as modern are eager to use ayurvedic patent medicines which have attractive profit margins and popular appeal established through advertisements.

Responsive to their enthusiasm is an ayurvedic drug industry which has produced popular medicines with such English names as:

R compound (arthritis)
Kitt's pulmo tone (respiratory diseases)
hormoprin (inflammatory catarrhal conditions)
gastogen (gastric disorders)
Liv 52 (prevents hepatic damage, promotes hepatocellular regeneration, stimulates appetite and growth)[34]
Liv up (constipation and disorders due to antibiotic usage)
Bonnisan (baby tonic)
Mustang (male rejuvenator)
Vim fix (male rejuvenator)
Tri sex (male rejuvenator)
Hincolin cream (stimulates blood supply to the penis)
Tentex forte (depressed libido)
Geriforte (anti stress)
Gasex (flatulence)
Septilin (infections and congestions)
Pause (abortive, menstrual regulator)
Famopolin B (menstrual regulator)
Masturin (women's health needs)
Osteon D (tonic for the total development of children)
Haemocleen (blood purifier for all skin diseases)

Two observations may be made with respect to the products listed. First, many are tonics which are marketed to address popular health concerns which index collective anxieties underscored by humoral associations. Second, and paradoxically, the insert information and packaging of these medicines is presented in metascientific language complete with biochemical and biomedical terms followed up by testimonials from doctors and vague references to research. My intent here is not to discredit these medicines, for I happen to think ayurveda contains many valuable medicinal resources. I rather wish to highlight the manner in which these medicines are marketed, and the messages they convey. In my interviews with practitioners, I rarely met anyone who paid much attention to promotional literature beyond a description of what the medicine was for. What was important was not the content of this literature, but the manner in which it served as a symbolic resource making the practitioner and user appear scientific and modern.

In most insert literature, the user is instructed to check with their doctor before using the over the counter ayurvedic product. In bold black letters the information provided is specified for registered medical practitioners only. This is mere rhetoric to make the medicines sound important. While some trepidation exists about using allopathic medicine, this is certainly not true for ayurvedic medicine. The overwhelming impression among the population is that "ayurvedic medicines have no side effects." This is an impression fostered by practitioners and the advertising industry alike, yet a statement identified as dangerous by four ayurvedic pundits whom I interviewed. I was reminded that even too much water could kill a thirst stricken man or that honey and ghee mixed in the wrong proportions could imbalance the humors and lead to death. What the statement meant, I was told, is that ayurvedic medicines are not poisons like allopathic medicines. This is not however, the layperson's interpretation which I encountered.

Ayurvedic medicines were widely deemed safe to try as are homeopathic medicines. Homeopathic medicines were described to me as being "only milk sugar and harmless medicine". Two issues may be raised. While many herbal medicines may be, or appear to be, harmless in their traditional form, little is known about the long term effects of newly introduced medicines having different concentrations of essential ingredients, altered rates of absorption etc. The label ayurvedic leads the public to trust a new product and exercise less caution in using it. The second issue involves the implicit "fix" ideology propagated in humoral terms. Is the ideology of health commodification underlying widespread medicine use harmless?

Over the last few years I have observed an increasing number of people consuming commercial ayurvedic drugs with impunity both as curative medicines and as promotive health resources. Recall the ayurvedic medicine distributor who noted that people take these medicines nowadays without the dietary and behavioral regimes that once accompanied them. My observations suggest that he is correct. An increasing number of people whom I have interviewed in the last few years are clearly looking for ayurpathic fixes for health; fixes which are easy, in tablet or capsule form and which do not require life style change. While it is true that many people still inquire about what kind of diet to take with medicine purchased, an increasing number swallow the pill or tonic and return to life as usual. Commercial ayurvedic medicine is for these people "cosmopolitan medicine". It is also, "cosmopolitical" medicine. Pfleiderer and Bichman (1985) have used this term to denote the role of western medicine in establishing and maintaining the interests of former colonial powers and those of third world elites. My usage is somewhat different indexing more subtle dimensions of capitalist ideology associated with the maintenance of health through medical products and the exchange of labor capital for well being in a cosmopolitan world. Medicines are cosmopolitical in that they are a conduit for the embodiment of capitalism.

The commodification of health has been advanced by a wealth of ayurpathic products which promise health to the consumer with regular use. Product appeals have aroused collective anxieties and deep fears about vital essences, impotency, impure breastmilk, poor mental concentration, and one's inner worth as well as outer complexion. Medicines have appeared in new forms, with new names and with both old and new locus of operation. The action of many, if not most have been shaped by cultural concerns. One of the reasons these drugs are so popular is because they are developed and/or marketed to act on a combination of symptoms recognized in popular health culture to coexist in complexes (eg. headache, weakness and improper bowel function).[35] New concerns about cancer and heart attack are linked to these familiar complexes. The product lists of pharmaceutical companies continue to expand as catalogues of concern, hope, and commodified answers to life's problems.

One more point needs to be made with respect to the popularity of commercial ayurvedic medicines. To understand the market and consumer demand for ayurvedic medicines one must consider coexisting medicine resources and medicine regulation policy. Let me cite an example. During the 1970's I was struck by the misuse of E. P. Forte, a combination of estrogen and progesterone (Chapter 7). Designed as a treatment for amenorrhea and as a hormonal test for pregnancy, I found the drug commonly being used in Mangalore as an abortive and morning after pill by women who believed that if a low dose could bring on one's period, a high dose could either prevent pregnancy or cause an abortion. Numerous studies in the U.S. and Germany found the use of these drugs dangerous and they were taken off the market in the West. Despite impressive research in India,[36] it was not until 1983 that the drug was banned. Soon after the drug was banned by the Drug Controller of India, two manufacturers of these products obtained a stay against the ban arguing that it "denied women their rights to a valuable medicine" (Shiva 1987). Notably, there was a temporary shortage of these products in South Kanarese chemist shops during this time. What is important to highlight is that the E. P. Forte drugs had created, or rather developed, a consumer need. When these drugs became scarce in the market, the demand gap was soon filled by ayurpathic patent medicines such as "Pause" and Famoplin".

COMMODIFICATION AND COSMOPOLITAN MEDICINES

Health commodification is fostered by a cosmopolitan life style characterized by consumerism. The term cosmopolitan used in this context refers less to space (urban areas) than to an orientation toward time and a dependency on commercial goods produced by a growing industrial complex. In the example noted above, there is no conceptual difference between the allopathic and ayurpathic medicines sold for menstrual regulation. They both constitute "cosmopolitan drugs" to stretch Leslie's original formulation of the concept beyond allopathic medicine. In chapter seven, I made the point that the layperson does not simply view medicines in terms of the ayurvedic and allopathic medical tradition, but in terms of illness and age specific prefer-ences for specific medicine forms. It is also necessary to recognize that ayurvedic patent drugs with English names and allopathic drugs are both viewed as "cosmopolitan" medicines offering convenient short term fixes for health problems or sources of immediate vitality. Notable, with a mix of allopathic and ayurpathic medicines commonly being prescribed, patients are not sure which kind of shops stock the medicines they need. Sitting in a commercial ayurvedic medicine shop in Mangalore in 1986, I noticed that over one quarter of the clients who walked through the door with a prescription were looking for allopathic drugs and did not know they were in the wrong type of shop. One third of the prescriptions presented which did require ayurvedic medicines were written by an allopathic doctor. While sitting in allopathic medicine shops over the last decade, I have observed an increasing number of ayurvedic medicines being prescribed. Because these medicines yield large profit margins, shop owners are stocking a greater variety of commercial ayurvedic drugs.

Ten years ago a town chemist whom I observed, sold a few bottles of a popular ayurvedic *aristha* each week from a stock kept in the back room. Five chemists interviewed in 1986 reported between 10%-20% of their total sales being commercial ayurvedic medicines. Promoting such sales are the reps of national ayurvedic companies who canvas the same practitioners and chemist shops as reps from multinational pharmaceutical companies.[37] Chemists commonly obtain a 30% profit margin from ayurvedic medicines. Given this high rate of return they are keen to recommend them to clients who ask for advice. Because the products are "ayurvedic", chemists can state they are safe and have no side effects. In this way, I have observed several customers frequenting chemists for minor complaints introduced to patent ayurvedic tonics or medicines like Liv 52.

RAMIFICATIONS OF HEALTH COMMODIFICATION FOR COMMUNITY HEALTH

The abuse of antibiotics is not an answer for infections and is not a replacement for sanitation and hygiene (Krishnaswamy 1983a).
    Western allopathic medicine has found itself to some extent in a cul-de-sac, striving over-exclusively for the entirely technological "breakthroughs" so beloved of journalists and so usually untrue, misreported or ephemeral. The need is rather to appreciate the high value of Western linear medicine as one part of wider possibilities ... The idea is slowly percolating that most disease is not due to one agent but to many circumstances in combination (Jeliffe and Jeliffe 1977).

A false sense of security has emerged from the exaggerated claims of curative and preventive health fixes. At a time of environmental deterioration, rapid urbanization and industrialization, a mystification of health has occurred resulting in a depreciation of social responsibility for the conditions of health. Health has been decontextualized and medicalized. It has been turned into an individual pursuit in which commodified health is purchased in the form of medicine and doctor-patient encounters are reduced to an exchange of drugs as the measure of a meaningful transaction. Embodied in such a transaction is an ideology consistent with a set of values associated with consumerism and the growth of the capitalist state. In community health terms, the cost of such growth is high.

To appreciate the possible ramifications of health commodification in India and elsewhere in the third world, it is instructive to briefly review the history of public health in Europe in the early to mid 1800's. If one looks at the history of public health in Europe at the time of the industrial revolution it is quite evident that environmental and sanitation reform did not come about for purely humanitarian reasons despite the religious and moralistic rhetoric of the day.[38] In frank terms, it was associated with the growth of an urban middle class and their fear of contamination from the poor raised to a fever pitch at a time of multiple epidemics when a miasma (malevolent airs) paradigm of disease etiology was prominent. Public health was not politically neutral, it was championed by the middle class at a time when the political power of this group was increasing. Environmental sanitation reform was initially extreme with the poor treated like powerless children. A medical police model of public health control was enforced against an impoverished labor force deemed purveyors of filth, and in Calvinist terms, the "damned". Notably, it was at least three decades, from the 1830's to the late 1860's, before the working class took an active part in the public health movement.

In the third world today, the false security rendered by a proliferation of medicines for health as well as illness reduces the impetus of both the middle class and the poor to actively mobilize for environmental health, sanitation and hygiene. The medical value of such proven public health resources as tetanus toxoid vaccinations merge with the inflated claims of tonics, and the misuse of antibiotics. As a composite they offer compartmentalized protection, quick fixes and a means toward health which does not rock the boat or deal with the muddied water. At a time of cholera there is always the magic, if not the science, of cholera vaccinations to rely on (Nichter 1989) and when a new disease associated with deforestation emerges, like Kyasanur forest disease (Nichter 1987), there is always the vaccination just around the corner to place one's faith in, a fix for all seasons. And yet a look at the disease patterns in India leads one to quickly recognize that an increasing number of diseases are emerging as diseases of development and underdevelopment, rapid urbanization, pollution and environmental deterioration at the micro as well as the macro level. Consider for a moment the potential danger rendered by a pattern of over prescription and excessive consumption of antibiotics:

Indiscriminate prescribing of antibiotics adds needlessly to mounting pressures for resistant organisms. It may seem an overstatement to describe it as environmental pollution, but when the full and ultimate consequences of the manner of use are grasped, it is less of an exaggeration than might at first appear. (Whitehead 1973)

In the last two and a half decades an increasing number of studies have reported the emergence of antibiotic-resistant strains of bacteria.[39] Given present medicine taking behavior in India, popular antibiotics may soon be of limited medical value for a number of resistant pathogens. A class division may be rearticulated through access to new and most likely more expensive alternatives to antibiotics rendered ineffective by misuse or overuse. The pharmaceutical industry has everything to gain from such a scenario. For the pharmaceutical industry, resistant strains mean new business and new markets.

I have gone to some length in considering the ways health consumer behavior is effected by political economic, cultural and social relational factors. One of my reasons for doing so is to call for a reconsideration of primary health care in relation to existing medicine consumption behavior and those factors influencing this behavior. There is a need to look below the surface of medicine consumerism, and the marketing of medical goods, knowledge and services. Changing medicine consumption practices must be viewed in relation to socialization, the embodiment of tacit knowledge, and changing perceptions of health. Implicit meanings are conveyed by medicines explicitly marketed as short term fixes. These meanings support an individualistic short sighted approach toward well being which undermines community health mobilization.

Given this reconsideration of primary health care, health education must be interlinked with consumer education. Without appropriate conceptualization (Fuglesang 1977) of what medicines are and are not, chances of inappropriate use are increased, and mystification sets the stage for inflated claims and false expectations.[40] What emerges is medicine taking as a habitual response to ill health, weakness and distress. One learns to reach for the medicine bottle, injection, or vaccination and little more. A critical consumerist posture toward medical fixes needs to be developed which weighs the merits and costs of alternative means of health enhancement and illness management.

Let me specify what I mean here. The commodification of health is already a strong trend in India, the pharmaceutical market is markedly overdeveloped and widespread self treatment has been documented. Provision of knowledge about alternative forms of basic medicines, (how much they cost, for whom and when they are appropriate etc.) constitutes a concrete subject through which change facilitators may confront health commodification setting the stage for comparative shopping and community activism directed toward: 1) proper administration and equitable distribution of public medical resources for identifiable health problems; 2) cooperative purchasing of commonly used generic medicine resources; and 3) the consideration of alternative health maintenance and disease control strategies.

It may be argued that providing information to the community about medicines goes against medical ethics and will increase self treatment practices. In countries where drugs are freely available over the counter, self purchase is already high, and prescription practices are grossly inappropriate, this argument is academic and more commonly advanced by constituencies having economic than humanitarian motives. The issue is that inappropriate patterns of self care and prescription behavior presently exist. They need to be identified and addressed. There is no excuse for the poor wasting scarce resources on multiple doses of antibiotics for scabies, viral respiratory ailments or watery diarrhea when cheap appropriate medicines exists. Compiling a list of misguided treatment patterns for common ailments is a first step (VHA 1986). As a second step, documentation of the prevalence of such patterns might provide those monitoring the activities of pharmaceutical companies evidence for lobby efforts aimed at curtailing misleading advertising.

Sending health educators out with tired slogans and boring film shows to compete with marketing firms is much like sending David to fight Goliath and await a miracle. Deployment of marketing techniques for social marketing purposes constitutes a useful strategy so long as it is recognized that the end is not just the sale of more appropriate products, but the provision of knowledge making for a more informed and critical consumer. For their part, those involved in international health need to pay closer attention to the ramifications of alternative means of introducing medical fixes. Biotechnical resources need to be introduced in a way which is responsive to a broader concept of development than that offered by an ideology of health commodification.[41]

CONCLUSION

In South Indian Hindu culture, health and prosperity are bestowed upon the household, family, and kingdom, for conformity to the sociomoral order by ancestors, gods and patron spirits. The living maintain reciprocal relationships with these agents. Properly worshipped they protect and reward. Not appropriately respected, their power may turn to wrath manifest as illness, a form of misfortune as well as a sign of breach in the sociomoral order. In modernizing India, the social order is in transition, and unfulfilled obligations to the living as well as the supernatural are rife. These breaches are consonant with changes in social relations fostered by an increase in cash-based contractual labor relations.[42] Needed at this juncture has been a form of magic to ease anxiety, and provide a source of immediate security at a time when cultural norms are being violated in increasing measure. Cosmopolitan medicine is being marketed as powerful impersonal magic.[43]

As a form of power rendering immediate demonstration effects, allopathic medicine has become a fetish for an emergent capitalist ideology in need of a symbol of progress. However, while immensely popular, allopathic medicine has been perceived as a source of danger and impurity as well as power. In chapter seven, I noted a complementarity in rural South Kanara between fast acting allopathic medicines and powerful but somewhat rash *bhuta* spirits. In contrast, ayurvedic medicines are more closely associated with the qualities of Pan-Indian Brahmanic deities.[44] Recall for a moment the informant who spoke of his daughter suffering from bloodlessness after being treated by allopathic medicines and having to consume tonic both during and sub-sequent to treatment. Two images may be juxtaposed. The first is that of the girl drinking tonic and the second, devotees feeding patron *bhuta* spirits with blood offerings. Both constitute acts maintaining a positive relationship with a form of power to which one has entered a dependency relationship. Blood offerings are made to *bhuta* as external sources of power and tonic is taken to replenish the blood once allopathic medicine has extracted its "blood toll" for curative actions. I would claim that in part, allopathic medicine are under-stood culturally in terms of preexisting ideas about power and dependency. While modernization has been accepted, its cost has been comprehended in physical terms through cultural perceptions of blood and digestion. This has in turn increased the market for tonics and ayurapathic medicines promising to restore a lost sense of health. Paradise lost has been made available for the cost of a modern elixir based on an ancient formula.

The commodification of health needs to be considered in relation to relationships of dependency as well as a process which Bateson (1972) has described as schizmogenises. Schizmogenises entails an uncorrected positive feedback loop wherein (to use the case of medicines) increased conscious-ness about a medicine (like tonic), increases demand for the product. This in turn fosters an increased supply which in turn increases consciousness and felt need. An accelerated cycle of medicine need and supply has been set in motion in India. How iatrogenic this cycle is remains to be documented.

In this chapter I have argued that factors contributing to the commodifi-cation of health in India today include market forces and pharmaceutical policy as well as cultural factors including tacit, largely unconscious, sources of motivation which influence consumer demand. To account for this range of factors it has been necessary to consider medicine prescribing and consumption behavior as practices which have at once explicit and implicit meaning. Implicit meanings need to be discerned in relation to core cultural values; changing perceptions of well being consonant with changing modes of production and the social relations they entail; group anxieties as well as displacements of these anxieties; and attempts to mediate paradox in a world of competing ideologies given expression in coexisting modes of medical treatment. The implications of health commodification for primary health care are considerable. They impact on the health of individuals, the com-munity and the micro as well as macro environment.

NOTES

1. A few examples of such studies are Evans (1981), Gustafsson and Wide (1981), Lilija

(1983), Medawar (1979), Pradhan (1983), Phadke (1982), Shiva (1987), Silverman (1976), Silverman, Lee and Lydecker (1982), Victoria (1982), VHA (1986) and Yudkin (1980).

2. Studies on the promotional and insert information of medical products in developing countries note that they often do not include or play down side effects and make recommendations for use among age groups where risk is high. In India, Silverman et al. (1986) note that although significant corrections in drug promotional literature have been realized between 1973—1984, warnings still do not appear on dipyrone products (analgin) and Imodium products — two commonly used and abused medications.

3. The regulation of pharmaceuticals in India has been called for repeatably. For example, the Hathi Committee Report of 1975 recommended a change from brand to generic names for drugs to be implemented in a phased manner. In June of 1979, the Central Government published a notice that five drugs including analgin, aspirin, chlorpromazine, ferrous sulfate, and piperazine salts were to be marketed only with generic names. This order was aborted when the Delhi High Court ruled it was against the free enterprise system. Drug labeling rules introduced in 1981 made it mandatory to include the generic name of drugs in a "conspicuous" manner next to their tradename and to use generic names for newly introduced single ingredient drugs. This practice has not been widely implemented.

4. Rohde (1988) has more recently noted that 16,000 registered pharmaceutical firms presently exist in India in contrast to 12,000 primary health centers.

5. It may be noted that in the world pharmaceutical market, six countries control over 70% of pharmaceutical production. While no single firm controls more than 20% of any national market, the top 10 pharmaceutical companies control 25% of the world's pharmaceutical trade (Faizal 1983). Many of the large multinational companies have extended their power base in India through subsidiaries and joint ventures. The VHA (1986) report presents a list of these companies, their subsidiaries, the percentage of their trade constituted by essential and nonessential drug formulations and market share.

6. The number of medicine products in Sweden is approximately 2,000 and in Germany 30,000. In 1980, 8,000 medicine products were listed in the American PDR guide to pharmaceuticals. Two hundred of these drugs accounted for 70% of market sales. Of the 8,000 drugs, 1,000 were defined as "basic chemical entities," the remaining drugs constituting a range of dosages and combination (Morgan and Kagan 1983). In 1977, there were 757 manufacturers of "ethical drugs" in the U.S. Of these, 292 employed more than 20 workers. Estimates of all types of commercial medicine products available in the U.S. is approximately 30,000.

7. On January 16th, 1988 India's health minister was quoted in the Indian Express Cochin, as admitting that India had no list of essential drugs nor did he have an idea as to the number of drug formulations manufactured in the country. The Drug Controller of India speaking at the all-India Institute of Medical Science was quoted as stating that in his opinion the number of formulations available was not excessive. By Japanese standards it is not. Ohnuki-Tierney (1986) notes that over 100,000 medicine products are available in the Japanese market. In 1983 there were approximately 2,500 pharmaceutical companies in Japan, 90% of which employ less than 50 people (Pradhan 1983).

8. In 1980 the Central Drugs Consultative Committee composed of members of central and state drug control organizations examined a group of fixed dose drug combinations and in over two thirds of cases no therapeutic rationale was found for their existence. Half were deemed frankly harmful. These included combinations such as antihistamines and tranquilizers, antihistamines with antidiarrheals, vitamins with analgesics, antiinflammatory agents with tranquilizers, and antibiotic combinations such as chloramphenicol and streptomycin as well as penicillin and streptomycin. A report by the Drugs Technical Advisory Board appointed by the Consultative Committee flagged 22 combinations of drugs covering 350 products to be removed from the market. Of these as many as 300 were produced by Indian companies. The pharmaceutical industry argued that these

combinations enhanced therapeutic efficacy through increased bioavailability and therapeutic synergism; reduced side effects; increased compliance; and the list goes on to the point of increasing absurdity. While 16 drugs were banned by the committee in 1981 the ban never went into effect and the governments legal power to ban ineffective drugs has been directly challenged in court. See the debate between Jayarman (1986) and Phadke (1986) as well as Greenhalgh (1987) for further details.

9. Of promotional expenses, Pradhan (1983) has estimated that some 40—50% goes to maintaining a sales and intelligence force comprised by "detail" personnel or what I have termed "representatives". Pradhan cites evidence that detailing is the most effective of all promotion strategies.

10. This figure includes only MBBS doctors and the most popular registered medical practitioners (RMP) with licentiate diplomas. I have pointed out elsewhere (Nichter 1981c: 232) that the pharmaceutical industry has maintained a significant financial interest in the RMP. In 1976, of 206 practitioners in five rural taluks of South Kanara visited by the rep. of a major pharmaceutical company, 48% were RMP. Of their best clients, rated in terms of medical sales, 36% were RMP. In 1987, interviews with rep. suggested that the importance of RMP in terms of their sales was decreasing, but still substantial.

11. My use of the term 'health commodification' draws upon several sources. Central is Marx's concept of exchange value as it relates to self constitution. 'That which exists for me through the medium of money, that which I can pay for, i.e., which money can buy, that am I, the possessor of money', (Quoted in Williamson 1978). This concept is further developed by Althusser (1970, 1971), who equates consciousness with an ideological state, and Lacan (1968) whose theory of mirror-phase describes the drama of identification and alienation. Marx's concept of alienation is relevant for just as workers lose control of the products they create, so too they come to lose control of their production and perception of health. Functional health comes to replace experiential health (Kelman 1976). People come to embody a state of "normality" discussed by Gramsci (1971), Althusser (1970, 1971), Foucault (1973, 1975, 1977) and others in relation to a dominant ideology and the process of hegemony. This subtle process is more concretely discussed by Bourdieu (1978) in relation to habitus, the embodiment of ideology through habitual practice. "Commodification," as I use the term is an example of the process by which "health" purchasing habits in the market place subtly reproduce capitalist ideology. In contrast to the above theorists, however, I do not view this process as complete. Following Raymond Williams (1977), I acknowledge the presence of coexisting ideologies given expression through coexisting voices (Bakhtin 1981). Elsewhere (Nichter and Nordstrom 1989) I argue that a precapitalist perception of healing efficacy counterbalances notions of curative efficacy underlying health commodification.

12. On discussing this theme with an ayurvedic chemist shop owner he pointed out to me that the idea of transferring wealth to health was very old. This was done on one plane by the performing of rituals. On another plane people could ingest valuable minerals for their health giving attributes. He pointed out that gold and silver coated pills were extremely popular in ayurveda. Gold is believed to have special health giving properties as well as being the purist (in a ritual sense) of metals. A gold ring worn on the right hand while eating is said to convey health giving properties to the food consumed.

13. Douglas and Wildavsky (1982) in their study of the social conditions underlying societal concern about environmental pollution, claim that alienation and failed confidence in the state foster concern about adulteration.

14. This has been the theme of several sociological studies of the advertising industry and consumer behavior in the West (Ewen 1976, Ewen and Ewen 1982, Fox 1985, Schudson 1984 and Williamson 1978, to note just a few). In each of these studies it is pointed out that advertising is as much a "mirror as a mind bender." Advertising reinforces as much as it imposes. This is not to underestimate the power of advertising to shape demand and

desire, but to call for an assessment of culturally constituted forms of desire, their underpinnings and the manner in which goods are sold as available, substitutable, commodified forms of desire.

15. On this issue in the U.S., see Goldman and Montagne (1986).

16. Consider for example India's deficit of medicine for T.B. and leprosy while having a proliferation of vitamin tonics (Shiva 1987). Only half of India's minimum requirement of anti-T.B.drugs and one third of anti-leprosy drugs are produced a year. Among vitamin supplements, vitamin A production has gone down in spite of a shortage of supply. For supporting medicine production figures see Rane (1982) and VHA (1986).

17. At a time when a concerted effort is being made to popularize oral rehydration for diarrhea management in South Asia, no attention has been directed at the marketing of "rehydrant" products that detract from the dehydration-diarrhea message. A number of such products are marketed with the image of sports and vigour as a central theme. For example, packets of "Staminade" are marketed as a body salt rehydrant for sports and the label on Electrarose specifically states it is not to be used for diarrhea management. This is precisely the situation which Green (1986: 365) cautioned against in his consideration of alternative social marketing possibilities for ORS in Bangladesh.

18. While I agree with Smith (1978) that villagers are not brainwashed fools bedazzled by full color advertisements, advertising must not be underestimated as a generator of knowledge as well as secondary desire. James (1983) has likewise questioned the extent to which the "discounts" of a skeptical western public are applied by the public in developing countries when presented with advertisements. James presents data on infant formula as a case in point.

19. This pattern of over medication associated with microeconomics of fee collection is not a strictly Indian phenomena. Variations on the pattern described in chapter eight include doctors giving samples of medicines acquired from reps. as promotional gifts to patients to enhance relations through commodity exchange in a competitive marketplace. Another pattern emerges in countries where doctors are reimbursed for their services in accord with a system where they are given incentives for the ordering of medicines. For example, Emiko Ohnuki-Tierney (1986: 83) notes that in Japan doctors are given points for reimbursement for prescribing medications, a system leading to *yakugai*, medicine pollution.

20. I have described the metamedical messages conveyed by states of ill health elsewhere when considering idioms of distress (Nichter 1981a, b). At present my emphasis is on polyvalent symbolic meanings conveyed by medicines. For example, acquisition of ayurvedic medicines such as Tripaladi oil (a well known medicine for sleeplessness, anxiety, and mental coolness) conveys a silent but well articulated message to others about one's state of being. Use sets in motion changes in interactional relations. Addition of new medications to popular pharmacopeia is also the addition of new expressive symbolic resources.

21. Kapur (1979), has noted the indiscriminant use of minor and major tranquilizers by practitioners in South India suggesting that practitioners are guided by the representatives of pharmaceutical firms. In addition to pharmaceutical representatives and promotional literature is the mimicking of teachers and colleagues. For example, one doctor known quite well to me noted that he began using diazepam more commonly after seeing doctors use the drug liberally during family planning camps. He was advised to prescribe the drug with analgesics if women complained of general side effects after the camps. Complaints were set up to be deemed psychosomatic.

22. A study quoted by Singh (1983) as "initiated by the National Council of Economic Research" found that 23 drug companies lose money on the production and marketing of essential drugs. The implication is that they must sell vitamins at a good profit to stay solvent. A similar argument has been raised with respect to the subsidizing of research costs spent in developing new medicines. Companies claim that they must sell OTC drugs to be

able to afford research. In fact research on medicines for tropical diseases has been meager while developing countries spend between $15—$20 billion dollars a year on pharmaceuticals. Research on new pharmaceuticals is primarily directed toward the diseases of developed nations where 75% of world drug consumption takes place (Patel 1983, Taylor 1986).

23. Greenhalgh (1987) found that nutritional supplements accounted for 23% of drugs prescribed by general practitioners in a sample of large Indian towns. Sixty-seven percent of patients were prescribed supplements. She further reported that half of all money spent on over the counter preparations went on vitamin, protein or carbohydrate supplements.

24. Ironically, those who most often need therepeutic doses of vitamins and minerals are the least likely to comply with doctors orders to consume mega (forte) tonics. A perception exists among the very poor in village South Kanara that tonics while yielding strength require milk to control their effects. If funds are not available to obtain milk, tonic use is questioned.

25. I have used the term "vitamin" tonic because little recognition is given to minerals in popular health culture. Indeed, a distinction between vitamins and minerals is not commonly made.

26. This remains a field impression. Future fieldwork need be conducted on both the kinds of tonic purchased by gender, reasons for purchase, and a content analysis of tonic advertising using male and female stereotypes.

27. Parker et al. (1978) reviewed surveys on home health care in South Asia conducted during and following the Johns Hopkins Functional Analysis project (1966—1977). They have noted that of the field sites surveyed self care was higher in South India than North India or Nepal. A Karnataka based survey found that over a two week period, 9% of the sample population and 42% of those reported to be ill engaged in self care. In general, more higher than lower caste men and children engaged in self help initiative, while more lower than higher caste women engaged in self help. Self help was noted to be particularly common for fever, upper respiratory track infections, diarrhea, skin ailments and muscular problems. Approximately 40% of the self help efforts reported involved the use of allopathic medicines.

28. Mark Fallon, a M.D. graduate researcher from the University of Arizona medical school, conducted a small study of medicine procurement in a Tamil Nad town and village in 1986. Of 410 interactions at chemist shops he found that 47% of drugs were by prescription. The largest single category of drug in self medication was analgesic, anti inflammatory and antipyretics constituting 44% of the total. The second group was antibiotics and other anti-infectives constituting 16% of the total.

29. As I have argued elsewhere (Nichter 1983), illness prevention has local meaning. It often incorporates the notion of preventing an already existent illness from becoming worse. This state of illness may be manifest or latent. In South Kanara illnesses such as *tamare* (chapter six) and T.B. are believed by some people to exist in latent form becoming manifest in times of weakness or overheat. This concept overlaps with biomedical literature on subclinical disease and the relationship between nutrition and infection.

30. I am not addressing the production of *shastric* (pure) ayurvedic preparations by vaidya themselves for use in their own practice. A renowned vaidya may charge handsomely for a home prepared medication which is imbued with his person as well as the herbs he uses. Patients will spend more on such products and view them in a different manner. Due to their national reputation companies such as Kottakal are also able to fetch higher prices for their products.

31. It may be noted that while there are several hundred patent herbal (ayurvedic) drugs sold in India, only a few have large regional market shares. However, in India, even a small local market share translates into a significant number of sales. The unique product may be a rediscovered traditional ayurevedic medicine like *tambula asava* or a newly discovered patent medicine.

32. In some instances new herbal preparations with English names were not introduced as ayurvedic although assumed to be so by the public. Himalaya Pharmaceuticals for example markets its products as composed of ancient medicines manufactured by modern processes to yield high quality.

33. The profit differential in marketing a patent drug as ayurvedic is substantial. Consider the example of Iodex, a patent medicine recently taken to court by the grassroots consumer group Consumer Forum. Iodex was orignally marketed as an allopathic medicine. When the essential ingredients of the medicine were price controlled, the manufacturer marketed it as ayurvedic. This allowed the company to maintain a Rs. 8.5 unit price instead of having to drop the price to Rs. 3.5 in accordance with price control regulations. Moreover, by labeling the medication as ayurvedic the medicine was exempt from a 15% central government tax and an 8% state tax in Karnataka.

34. Himalaya drugs sells in excess of 60 million units of Liv 52 a year. This company employs more than 400 pharmaceutical representatives, 24 of whom operate in Karnataka State.

35. It would be interesting to analyze some of the seemingly irrational combinations of medicines sold in India to see whether a cultural logic did not underlay their locus of action.

36. On the hazards of using this drug see an editorial in The Antiseptic entitled "Hazards of Hormonal Pregnancy Tests" Volume 80: 4, 1983. Research is reviewed including that of Prof. K. Palaniappan who found an incidence of hormonal drug use of 31% among the mothers of 52 deformed babies.

37. I interviewed representatives from both a large ayurvedic and allopathic company canvassing the same region of South Kanara. The latter visited 320 doctors and 90 chemist shops while the former visited 250 of the same doctors and 80 of the chemist shops.

38. I am not arguing that moralism did not contribute to the public health movement. There is little doubt that public health reform acts in England in the 1840's were motivated by images of immorality and promiscuity occurring in the mines where men and women worked naked to the waist and where illegitimacy was deemed to be rampant. On the history of public health see Rosen (1958).

39. On the issue of antibiotic misuse and resistant strains of bacteria see Simmons and Stolley (1974), Phillips (1979), Nature (1981), Altman (1982), Levy (1982), Hossain, Glass and Khan (1982), WHO (1983) and Kunin (1983, 1985). On resistant strains in India see Jajao (1982) and summaries of reports reviewed in Greenhalgh (1987).

40. For example in chapter six I discuss the disappointment of Sri Lankan villagers in ORS which they came to perceive as a medicine for diarrhea, not dehydration.

41. Two criteria of an ideology are (1) the objective concealment of contradictions and (2) a body of ideas which serve the interests of the dominant class.

42. I am not suggesting that obligations to deities were always fulfilled in the past during precapitalist times for I doubt this was true. Based on a number of interviews with informants at the time when land reform was being implemented, it became abundantly clear that outstanding vows and obligatory rituals were more the norm than the exception. However, post land reform the frequency of breaches increased and took on new dimensions.

43. I recognize that my use of the term impersonal is not entirely satisfactory. Modern medicine while a secular source of power is not strictly impersonal. It may embody the attributes of the person giving the medicine which in turn effects its capacity to "take" to the afflicted. This is the subject of a separate paper (Nichter and Nordstrom 1989).

44. This dichotomy is somewhat artificial in that pan-Indian deities are incorporated into the local cosmos and given locale specific attributes. In other words there is not simply Shiva but Shiva of such and such place, Shiva of that big tree!

REFERENCES

Alland, A.
  1970 *Adaptation in Cultural Evolution: An Approach to Medical Anthropology.* New York: Columbia University Press.
Althusser, L.
  1970 *Reading Capital.* New York: New Left Books.
  1971 Ideology and Ideological State Apparatuses'. In *Lenin and Philosophy and Other Essays.* New York: New Left Books.
Altman, L.
  1982 New Antibiotic Weapons in the Old Bacteria War. *New York Times,* Sunday, January 10.
Bakhtin, M.
  1981 *The Dialogic Imagination.* Austin: University of Texas Press.
Bateson, G.
  1972 *Steps to an Ecology of Mind.* New York: Ballantine Books.
Bordieu, P.
  1978 *Outline of a Theory of Practice.* Cambridge: Cambridge University Press.
Daniels, E. V.
  1984 *Fluid Signs.* Berkeley: University of California Press.
Dannhaeuser, N.
  1987 Marketing Systems and Rural Development: A Review of Consumer Goods Distribution. *Human Organization 46*(42): 177—185.
Douglas, M, and Wildavsky, A.
  1982 *Risk and Culture: An Essay on the Selection of Technological and Environmental Dangers.* Berkeley: University of California Press.
D'Penha, H. J.
  1971 Promise and Influence of Government Advertising. *Promotion 5*: 1, 3.
Eisenberg, L.
  1977 Disease and Illness: Distinctions Between Professional and Popular Ideas of Sickness. *Culture, Medicine and Psychiatry 1*(1): 9—24.
Evans, P. B.
  1981 Recent Research on Multinational Corporations. *Annual Review of Sociology* Vol. 7: 199—223.
Ewen, S.
  1976 *Captains of Consciousness: Advertising and the Social Roots of the Consumer Culture.* New York: McGraw Hill.
Ewen, S. and Ewen E.
  1982 *Channels of Desire.* New York: McGraw Hill.
Faizal, A.
  1983 The Right Pharmaceuticals at the Right Prices: Consumer Perspectives. *World Development 11*(3): 265—269.
Ferguson, A.
  1981 Commercial Pharmaceutical Medicine and Medicalization: A Case Study from El Salvador. *Culture, Medicine and Psychiatry 5*: 105—134.
Foucault, M.
  1973 *Madness and Civilization: A History of Insanity in an Age of Reason.* R. Howard (Trans.). New York: Vintage.
  1975 *Birth of the Clinic: An Archaeology of Medical Perception.* A. M. Sheridan Smith (Trans.). New York: Random House.
  1977 *The History of Sexuality, Volume I: An Introduction.* R. Huxley (Trans.). New York: Vintage.

Fox, S.
1985 *The Mirror Makers*. New York: Vintage Books.
Friedson, E.
1970 *Profession of Medicine*. Harper and Row: New York.
Fuglesang, A.
1977 *Doing Things Together: Report on an Experience of Communicating Appropriate Technology*. Uppsala, Sweden: Dag Hammersjold Foundation.
Goldman, R. and Montagne, M.
1986 Marketing "Mind Mechanics": Decoding Antidepressant Drug Advertisements. *Social Science and Medicine 22*(10): 1047—1058.
Good, B.
1977 The Heart of What's the Matter: The Semantics of Illness in Iran. *Culture Medicine and Psychiatry 1*: 25—58.
Ghosh, S.
1986 Drug Policy Needs: A Sea-change. *Hindustan Times*, Saturday, March 8.
Gothoskar, S.
1983 Drug Control: India. *World Development 11*(3): 223—228.
Gramsci, A.
1971 *Selections from the Prison Notebooks*. London: Lawrence and Wishart.
Green, E.
1986 Diarrhea and the Social Marketing of Oral Rehydration Salts in Bangladesh. *Social Science and Medicine 23*(4): 357—366.
Greenhalgh, T.
1987 Drug Prescription and Self Medication in India: An Exploratory Study. *Social Science and Medicine 25*: 3, 307—318.
Gustafsson, L. L. and Wide K.
1981 Marketing of Obsolete Antibiotics in Central America. *The Lancet*, January 3: 31—33.
Hercheimer, A. and Stimson G.
1982 The Use of Medicines for Illness. *In* Richard Blum (ed.) *Pharmaceuticals and Health Policy*. London: Crown Helm.
James, J.
1983 *Consumer Choice in the Third World*. New York: St. Martin Press.
Jaya Rao, K.
1977 Tonics: How Much an Economic Waste. *In* A. J. Patel (ed.) *In Search of Diagnosis*. Wardha: Medico Friends Circle Press.
Jajoo, V.
1982 *Misuse of Antibiotics*. New Delhi: Voluntary Health Association of India, Document No. D10.
Jayaraman, K.
1986 Drug Policy: Playing Down Main Issues. *Economic & Political Weekly*. June 21.
Jeliffe, D. and Jeliffe, P.
1977 The Cultural Cul-De-Sac of Western Medicine. *Transactions of the Royal Society of Tropical Medicine and Hygiene 71*(4): 331—334.
Kapur, R. L.
1979 The Role of Traditional Healers in Mental Health Care in Rural India. *Social Science and Medicine 13b*: 27—31.
Kelman, S.
1976 The Social Nature of the Definition in Health. *International Journal of Health Services 5*: 4, 625—642.
Krishnaswamy, K. and Kumar, D.
1983 *Drug Utilization: Percepts and Practices*. Nutrition News. Hyderabad: National Institute of Nutrition 4: 5.

Krishnaswamy, K., et al.
   1983   Drug Usage Survey in a Selected Population. *Indian Journal of Pharmacology*
          15(3): 175—183.
Lacan, J.
   1968   The Mirror-Phase as Formative of the Function of the I. *New Left Review 51*: 71—
          77.
Laping, J.
   1984   *Ayurveda: Its Progressive Potential and Its Possible Contribution to Health Care*
          Today. Second International Congress on Traditional Asian Medicine, Sept. 2.
          Surabaya, Indonesia.
Leslie, C.
   1967   Professional and Popular Health Cultures in South Asia. *In* W. Morehouse (ed.)
          Understanding Science and Technology in India and Pakistan. New Delhi: Foreign
          Area Materials Center, University of the State of New York.
   1988   Indigenous Pharmaceuticals, the Capitalist World System and Civilization. *Kroeber*
          Anthropological Society Journal, forthcoming.
Levy, S.
   1982   Microbial Resistance to Antibiotics. *The Lancet,* July 10. 83—88.
Lilja, J.
   1983   Indigenous and Multinational Pharmaceutical Companies. *Social Science and*
          Medicine 17(6): 1171—1180.
Malholtra, K.
   1985   *Changing Patterns of Disease in India with Special Reference to Childhood Mor-*
          tality. Paper, Wenner-Gren Symposium on The Health and Disease of Populations
          in Transition, October 19, Santa Fe, New Mexico.
Mariott, M.
   1978   Toward an Ethnosociology of South Asian Caste Systems. *In* K. David, (ed.) *The*
          New Wind. The Hague: Mouton.
Medawar, C.
   1979   *Insult or Inquiry: An Inquiry into the Marketing and Advertising of British Food and*
          Drug Products in the Third World. London: Social Audit.
Medawar, C. and B. Freese
   1982   *Drug Diplomacy.* London: Social Audit.
Menon, A. K.
   1983   Drugs: An Unhealthy Trend. *India Today,* Nov. 15, p. 90.
Morgan, J. and Kagan, D.
   1983   *Society and Medication: Conflicting Signals for Prescribers and Patients.* Mass.:
          Lexington Books.
Nature
   1981   Saving Antibiotics from Themselves. August 20, 661.
Nichter, M.
   1981a Idioms of Distress: Alternatives in the Expression of Psychosocial Distress: A Case
          Study from South India. *Culture, Medicine and Psychiatry 5*: 379—408.
   1981b Negotiation of the Illness Experience: The Influence of Ayurvedic Therapy on the
          Psychosocial Dimensions of Illness. *Culture, Medicine and Psychiatry 5*: 5—24.
   1981c Toward a Cultural Responsive Rural Health Care Delivery System in India. *In* Giri
          Raj Gupta (ed.) *The Social and Cultural Context of Medicine in India.* New Delhi:
          Vikas Publishers.
   1984   Project Community Diagnosis: Participatory Research as a First Step Toward
          Community Involvement in Primary Health Care. *Social Science and Medicine*
          19(3): 237—252.

1987   Kyasanur Forest Disease: Ethnography of a Disease of Development. *Medical Anthropology Quarterly*, December.

1989   Vaccinations in South Asia: False Expectations and Commanding Metaphors. *In* J. Coreil and D. Mull (eds.) *Anthropology and Primary Health Care*. The Netherlands: Kluwer Academic Publishers.

Nichter, M., and Nordstrom, C.

1989   The Question of Medicine Answering. *Culture, Medicine and Psychiatry*, forthcoming.

Obeysekere, G.

1976   The Impact of Ayurvedic Ideas on the Culture and the Individual in Sri Lanka. *In* C. Leslie (ed.) *Asian Medical Systems: A Comparative Study*. Berkeley: University of California Press.

Ohnuki-Tierney, E.

1986   *Illness and Culture in Contemporary Japan*. New York: Cambridge University Press.

Osifo, N. G.

1983   Our Promotion of Drugs in International Product Package Inserts. *Tropical Doctor 13*: 5—8.

Parker, R., Shah, S., Alexander, C. and Neuman, A.

1979   Self Care and Use of Home Treatment in Rural Areas of India and Nepal. *Culture, Medicine and Psychiatry 3*: 1, 3—28.

Patel, M. S.

1983   Drug Costs in Developing Countries and Policies to Reduce Them. *World Development 11*(3): 195—204.

Pfleiderer, B. and Bichman, W.

1985   *Krankheit und Kultur: Eine Einfuhrung in die Ethnomedizin*. Verlag: Berlin.

Phadke, A.

1982   Multinationals in India's Drug Industry. *Medico-Friend Circle Bulletin*. January-February. Pune.

1986   Drug Policy: Industry's Misleading Arguments. *Economic and Political Weekly*. May 10.

Phillips, I.

1979   Antibiotic Policies. *In* D. Reeves and A. Graves (eds), *Recent Advances in Infection, Vol. I*. Edinburgh: Churchill Livingston.

Poh-ai, T.

1985   Ciba-Geigh's Cover-Up. *Multinational Monitor 6*(11): 1—3.

Pradhan, S. B.

1983   *International Pharmaceutical Marketing*. Westport, Connecticut: Quorum Books.

Rane, W.

1982   Why don't our drugs match our diseases. *Science Today*, October.

Rohde, J.

1988   Good health makes good politics. *Economic and Political Weekly*. March 26, pp. 637—38.

Rosen, G.

1958   *A History of Public Health*. New York: M.D. Publications.

Schudson, M.

1984   *Advertising: The Uneasy Persuasion*. New York: Basic Books.

Shiva, M.

1987   *Towards a Healthy Use of Pharmaceuticals*. New Delhi: Voluntary Health Association.

Silverman, M.

1976   *The Drugging of Americas*. Berkeley: University of California Press.

Silverman, M., Lee, P. and Lydecker, M.
    1982 *Prescriptions for Death: The Drugging of the Third World*. Berkeley: University of
          California Press.
    1986 Drug Promotion: The Third World Revisited. *International Journal of Health
          Services. 16*(4): 659—667.
Simmons, H. and Stolley, P.
    1974 This is Medical Progress? Trends and Consequences of Antibiotic Use in the
          United States. *Journal of the American Medical Association 227*(9): 1023—1028.
Singh, C. V.
    1983 Drug Manufacturers: Rising Temperature. *India Today*, October 31, p. 106.
Smith, R.
    1978 *Kurusu: The Price of Progress in a Japanese Village, 1951—1975*. Stanford: Stanford
          University Press.
Taylor, D.
    1986 The Pharmaceutical Industry and Health in the Third World. *Social Science and
          Medicine 22*(11): 1141—1149.
Victoria, C. G.
    1982 Statistical Malpractice in Drug Promotion: Case-Study from Brazil. *Social Science
          and Medicine 16*:707—709.
Voluntary Health Association (VHA)
    1986 A Rational Drug Policy. New Delhi: VHA Press.
Wagner, R.
    1981 *The Invention of Culture*. (Revised ed.) Chicago: University of Chicago Press.
Whitehead, J.
    1973 Bacterial Resistance: Changing Patterns of Some Common Pathogens. *British
          Medical Journal 2*: 224—228.
Williams, R.
    1977 *Marxism and Literature*. Oxford: Oxford University Press.
Williamson, J.
    1978 *Decoding Advertisements: Ideology and Meaning in Advertising*. London: Marian
          Boyars.
Worsley, P.
    1984 *The Three Worlds*. Chicago: University of Chicago Press.
Young, A.
    1982 The Anthropologies of Illness and Sickness. *Annual Review of Anthropology 11*:
          257—285.
Yudkin, J. S.
    1979 Provision of Medicines in a Developing Country. *The Lancet*, April 15: 810—812.
    1980 The Economics of Pharmaceutical Supply in Tanzania. *International Journal of
          Health Services 10*(3): 455—477.
Zimmerman, F.
    1987 *The Jungle and the Aroma of Meats*. Berkeley: University of California Press.
Zawad, K.
    1985 The Fight to Bar Bogus Drugs. *Multinational Monitor 6*(9): 1—3.

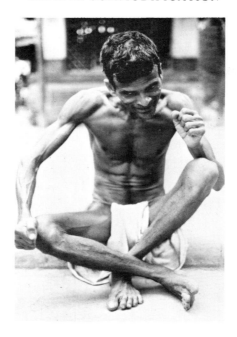

The characteristics of children's illnesses are communicated bodily through the acting out of symptoms and sounds as well as through the use of illness terminology.

SECTION FOUR

HEALTH EDUCATION

INTRODUCTION

Anthropology has an important role to play in contextualizing health education and transforming it from the passive handmaiden of a reductionistic biomedical tradition to a decentralized approach to community health problem solving. I have suggested in previous essays that an anthropologically informed health education will better be able to convey meaning and engender trust by: 1) addressing popular images of ethnophysiology; 2) acknowledging popular health concerns; 3) working within local illness classification systems and established patterns of folk dietetics; 4) maximizing cultural resources (both material and conceptual) and 5) identifying perceived and biomedically recognized risk factors for disease. I have also highlighted the role of the health educator in consumer education. Patterns of self treatment and over-the-counter drug use need to be identified and assessed culturally as well as biomedically.

In this section two additional contributions of anthropology to health education are noted. The first is the evaluation of existing health messages and how they are interpreted. The second contribution is helping health educators communicate health concepts more effectively. I suggest that health educators need to build upon the familiar to describe the new. As distinct from linear didactic teaching, an analogical method of health communication is proposed.

10. DRINK BOILED WATER: A CULTURAL ANALYSIS OF A HEALTH EDUCATION MESSAGE

How are public health messages interpreted by people in developing countries? Messages that fail to take the lay health culture into consideration are open to misinterpretation, compartmentalization and desensitization to priority issues. My purpose is not to preach the importance of a cultural perspective in health education since the literature is riddled with this sermon. But I would like to present a case to illustrate the point. The example concerns the most basic of health messages, 'boil drinking water'.

Three decades ago Wellin (1955) published a frequently cited account of water boiling education in Peru. Demonstrating how this behavior was influenced by the culture, he wrote:

> A trained health worker can perceive "contamination" in water because his perceptions are linked to certain scientific understandings which permit him to view water in a specially conditioned way. A Los Molinos resident also views water in a specially conditioned way. Between him and the water he observes, his culture "filters in" cold, hot or other qualities that are as meaningful to him as they are meaningless to the outsider.

The present case from Sri Lanka complements Wellin's ethnography of Peru. In contrast to Peru, 90% of the men and 82% of the women in Sri Lanka are literate. They are also within easy reach of health facilities, with the average person living within three miles of one or another clinic. Over the last two decades, the country has experienced a notable decrease in infant mortality, which is presently 37 per 1000 births. Even so, diarrhoeal diseases remain a leading cause of morbidity and mortality, accounting for 53% of all infectious disease deaths in 1979. In the same year, they were the third leading cause of death for the population at large, with 44.9 deaths per 100,000.[1] One study (Pollock, 1983) has indicated that deaths from water-borne diseases increased by 49% in the 5 years between 1971—1976.[2] Reviewing existing morbidity/mortality data, Pollack observed:

> The trend of decreasing disease specific mortality in hospitals without parallel decreases in morbidity, suggests that, for specific diagnosis (e.g. gastroenteritis, typhoid fever, and malnutrition), there is an awareness of the availability of curative intervention, but the preventive intervention components have not been emphasized or have been unsuccessful.

To learn why preventive intervention has been unsuccessful for water related diarrhoeal diseases, I studied the main forms of behavior associated with the spread of these diseases: defecation habits, hand washing, food handling and drinking water. This paper is confined to the latter variable.

Public health inspectors and family health workers have encouraged people to drink boiled water for well over three decades. Despite their efforts, field workers know that the message is largely unheeded. One health inspector with whom I spent considerable time in the field, estimated that less than 10% of the rural families he visited regularly used boiled drinking water. Why do literate Sri Lankan people pay so little attention to this health precaution? Health workers who urge boiling water have a respectable status in the community,[3] so it cannot be that they are dismissed as outsiders. Let us consider two other possibilities:

1) Is the underlying issue one of fuel scarcity? In some areas of Sri Lanka this may be an important variable, but it was not important in the Horana-Ratnapura region of southwest Sri Lanka. Firewood was available, and even wastefully used.

2) Is the underlying issue that the local culture does not attend to the qualities of water? This certainly is not the case anywhere in Sri Lanka. Indeed, one of the few material possessions a Sinhalese Buddhist monk is prescribed to carry is a water filter, and everywhere the taste, smell and inherent qualities of water are important concerns. Villagers are keen to see the source of their drinking water. This is one reason that closed wells are not popular. Another reason is that a limited amount of sunlight is considered necessary for keeping water fresh. Drinking water of unknown origin is considered a hardship. In fact, one way a villager expresses to a friend the hardship of having to remain in Colombo city for a period of time is to exclaim "ayyo! pipe water — you have to drink and bathe in it!"

While daily commuting to Colombo from a village, I observed passengers in crowded buses jostle their water bottles and lunch packets. Bringing lunch packets was easy to understand in relation to micro-economics, but water? My commuter friends explained that they did not trust Colombo 'pipe water'. They spoke of pipe water as *marana vatura* — dead water or *kivul vatura* — water tasting of iron and associated with urinary problems. They disliked the 'medicinal' smell of chlorinated water. On the other hand, they felt that boiled water was tasteless,[4] so they preferred to transport small bottles of unboiled well water an hour and a half by crowded bus. Why did they ignore the public health advice, which they all knew very well, to boil their drinking water?

Before considering why people do not do something, it is more prudent to consider why they do what they do. In the present case, I talked to people about my observation that boiled water was routinely prepared for ill people, but not consumed by other members of the household. The reason offered to me by public health colleagues seemed insufficient, for they reasoned that because the advice to drink boiled water was originally introduced and most adamantly repeated during epidemics of cholera, typhoid and gastroenteritis, people associated the practice with illness.[5]

I identified three reasons for boiling water in discussions with lay people. The first requires an appreciation of indigenous water management. The qualities of water from different sources affect the purposes for which it is used. When water is plentiful villagers use different sources for drinking and bathing in accord with the clarity of the water, the depth from which it comes and its exposure to the sun. When water is scarce, an available source is used for many purposes, but efforts are differentially expended to transform the qualities of water used for drinking. Strong and healthy people are little concerned about the water they routinely use, unless its color, smell or taste changes. When people are ill or in a transitional body state, e.g. infants and pregnant women, the qualities of water are tended to. For example, water from a deep well is thought to have a cooling quality that is harmful to someone who is suffering from or vulnerable to illnesses associated with coolness, such as stiffness and pain, or with an excess of phlegm (Nichter, 1987). On the other hand, water directly exposed to the sun is said to be 'sun baked' (Karunadasa, 1984) and inappropriate for someone who is suffering from or prone to heating illnesses. When these are the only sources of water, healthy people use them without giving the issue much thought. When water from these sources are the only ones available for ill or vulnerable people to drink, then it will be boiled in an attempt to mitigate its properties. For bathing, traditional prescriptions that specify appropriate times will be more rigorously followed.

Water is also heated to reduce its shock affect on ill or vulnerable people. Shock is an important health concept in South Asia. Emotional distress like fear, and hot or cold physical distress may cause or compound illness. Shock occurs when a person in a vulnerable state is subjected to an excess of hot or cold. People at risk to phlegm problems will not consume cold liquids on hot days. Similarly, ill people only consume and wash with tepid water. Villagers interpret advice to drink boiled water in relation to the concept of shock.

Because villagers do not associate boiling water with killing bacteria, they place more emphasis on administering tepid water to the ill than on fully boiling it. They may boil water for the ill or vulnerable person, and then recontaminate it by adding cool unboiled water to make it tepid. Nevertheless the point not to be lost sight of is that the preparation of water is an act of caring accorded positive social value. This introduces some irony into the context of hospital care, where tepid water is not available even though patients and their families feel that they need it. This fact is cited by laypeople as an example of the poor care in public health institutions.

Another idea associated with boiled water involves the Sinhala concept of *sehellu*, lightness. Digestion is a central health concern in Sinhalese popular culture, and in the learned system of ayurvedic medicine. Dietary regulations vary in accord with the ascribed characteristics of different illnesses. Regardless of the specific characteristics of an illness, however, a general restriction will prevail against the consumption of heavy, *bhara*, foods. A light diet helps to restore normal digestion to an ill person. Indeed, it is fundamental to balancing the humors, and the restriction against heavy foods includes a conception of heavy water. Well water is considered to be heavy unless it is boiled. Boiling causes water to lose some quality or residue that renders it light. The heaviness of unboiled water is considered good for health when one is in a normal state. Clear unboiled well water, *hondai vatura*, is said to satisfy thirst better than light boiled water. Furthermore, unboiled well water is considered 'fresh', 'full of life' and 'having strength' in contrast to pipe water, which is 'dead', and boiled water, which lacks strength. In one informant's words:

> The *guna*, character, of water is like the *guna* of green leafy vegetables. When you eat them fresh, they have life. If you pluck them, transport them and keep them for sale, they lose their life and wilt. When you cook vegetables, they lose their freshness rapidly. It is like that with water. When water is running or in a well exposed to the sunlight, it is fresh. If you collect it and transport it through pipes it is *marana vatura*, dead water, if you boil it water loses its *guna*, its strength.

Except in the evening, when it may be health promoting, drinking boiled water is associated with illness. Some cooling foods are also avoided in the evening. Since heavy food and heavy water are relatively difficult to digest, some people regularly drink 'light' tepid water in the evening. Their reasoning reflects a general concern that digestion is weakest during inactivity and sleep. The advice to drink boiled water is thus interpreted by some villagers in accord with the concept of *sehellu*, and deemed most relevant for people who have a weak digestive capacity. This interpretation, like that involving shock is supported by the advice about food that ayurvedic practitioners give to pregnant women, the mothers of infants and ill people.

CONCLUSION

In Sri Lanka the advice to drink boiled water is understood in the context of illness and vulnerability. Public health workers emphasize this advice during epidemics, and it is associated with ayurvedic advice to take a light diet when ill. Underscoring lay interpretations of these messages are folk health concepts; ideas about the qualities of water, shock, and digestive capacity. Thus, for a health message as simple as drink boiled water to be communicated effectively, careful observation of customary behavior and the analysis of cultural systems is essential. The analysis may also generate innovative ideas by health educators. For example, the concept of *sehellu* might be used in a program to persuade parents that children under three years old are vulnerable to illness and should consume boiled water.[6] Such a program might support the notion that *sehellu* foods, including boiled water, are best for a child's developing digestive and immune systems.

NOTES

1. Among infants, a rate of 242 deaths per 100,000 is reported and among children 1—4 year olds, 16% of deaths are directly related to diarrhoeal diseases with many more likely

to be indirectly related. During the period 1971—1979 of the ten leading causes of infant mortality, only diarrhoeal diseases showed no downward trend after 1975. Statistics on diarrhoeal diseases were gleaned from the reports of Gaminiratne (1984) and Pollack (1983). It should be noted that district standardized death rates due to diarrhoeal diseases differ significantly. These range from 10.1 in Trincomallee and 16.5 in Matara to 127.3 in Batticaloa and 90.8 in Amparai. Percentage deaths due to these diseases range from, 1.5% in Kalutara District and 2.9% in Matara to 15.1% in Amparai and 12.6% in Batticaloa. To correct any misconception that urban conditions contrast markedly with rural conditions, it may be noted that the Colombo infant mortality rate due to diarrhoeal diseases is 158% the national average — although for all age groups it is considerably lower than the national average.

2. A study, conducted by the Sri Lankan Department of Health Services, quoted in the Marga Institute report; *Intersectoral Actions for Health*; (Colombo 1982) notes that in the Mahaveli Development region, diarrhoeal disease accounts for some 40% of all persons seeking medical treatment and that the latter are largely related to contaminated water sources.

3. Public health inspectors and family health workers enjoy social status in Sri Lanka equivalent to that of a secondary school teacher. As Wellin reported of Peru, advice by the latter to alter health related behavior carries significantly less weight than the same advice offered by a doctor. This weight was more evident in respect to immunization and family planning, technical fixes, than in respect to water boiling as a long term enterprise related to preventive health. On this point I may note that in India boiled cooled water is not regularly used even by the educated. In a personal communication, Charles Leslie noted that drinking boiled cooled water is uncommon among New Delhi academics. He was told by a Professor of Social Medicine at Benares Hindu University that the highest rate of typhoid in Varanasi in the early 1970s was among faculty and students living in University housing.

4. I do not wish to underplay tastelessness as a factor negatively influencing water boiling behavior any more than time or the cheap availability of fuel. My purpose is rather to identify other cultural factors impacting on water boiling behavior.

5. Routine water supply testing is not performed by Public Health Inspectors and attempts at well purification are only done during epidemics.

6. Generalizing the *sehellu* rationale might even prove helpful in marketing a weaning food less likely to be shared in the family than the present weaning food, Triposha, which people ascribe both a strength giving and neutral quality suitable for general consumption. For a short discussion of the CARE weaning food, Triposha, see Nichter (1987). A new supplementary weaning food might be marketed as *sehellu*, just what a child needs for its developing or weak digestive system. I am suggesting this idea as an example of how cultural concepts might be used as health resources in social marketing. I do not claim that this particular idea would prove effective, but suggest that it would be worth looking into.

REFERENCES

Gaminiratne, K. H. W.
   1984 *Causes of Death in Sri Lanka: An Analysis of Levels and Trends in the 1970's.* Department of Census and Statistics, Colombo, Sri Lanka.
Karunadasa, H. I.
   1984 *Domestic use of water and sanitation: A behavioral study.* National Water Supply and Drainage Board, Colombo, Sri Lanka, 1984.
Nichter, M.
   1987 Cultural dimensions of hot, cold and sema in the Sri Lankan health culture. *In* L. Manderson (ed.) *Hot-Cold Conceptualization: A Reassessment.* Special Edition, Social Science and Medicine 25, 4: 377—387.

Pollack, M.
    1983   *Health problems in Sri Lanka: An analysis of morbidity and mortality data*. Report, USAID, Colombo, Sri Lanka.
Wellin, E.
    1955   Water boiling in a Peruvian town. *In* B. Paul (ed.), *Health, Culture, and Community*. New York: Russell Sage Foundation.

11. EDUCATION BY APPROPRIATE ANALOGY

Why should we expect the illiterate villager to adjust to the way of thinking of the educated man? Why should he alter his perception of the world to understand us? . . . Is development a one-sided process of duplication? . . . It is perfectly possible for an educated man to adapt to the concepts used by the illiterate villager, but he has to study them. (Fuglesang 1977, p. 96)

A Kannada proverb of South India states that "The plant in the courtyard is not a medicine," meaning that what is familiar and close is often overlooked as a valuable resource. This proverb is an appropriate beginning for this paper for what will be discussed is not a new method of education but rather a use of the familiar to explain the new — education by analogy.

In the field of health education far more time, energy and resources have been expended identifying what a population does not know or do than in assessing what a population does know and the way in which it is known. What is often neglected is a consideration of those concepts of health and images of body processes which underlay the layperson's health promotion and illness prevention practices. Due to this lack of appreciation of indigenous health behavior and the tacit knowledge (common sense) upon which it is based, cultural resources are underutilized by health educators. Also overlooked is the use of analogy as a mode of communication. The value of this mode of communication is that it facilitates contextual as opposed to decontexualized learning and conceptual integration as opposed to the compartmentalization of information. In contrast to introducing new "bits" of health information into a culture irrespective of preexisting knowledge and experience, new information is introduced within a context of existing associations, experiences and health concerns.

Described analogically, the premise of this essay is that a good analogy is like a plough which can prepare a population's field of associations for the planting of a new idea. If the field of associations is not adequately ploughed to accommodate new ideas, it is difficult for such ideas to take root. Indeed, simply introducing ideas irrespective of local culture is much like scattering seeds in the wind. As much effort need be put into preparing the field and improving the plough as perfecting the spread of seed.

Metaphorical communication and juxtaposition of imagery is a fundamental mode of human communication and a basic form of human understanding.[1] Susan Langer has described this mode of "reasoning" as a primary step in conscious abstraction:

Every new experience or new idea about things evokes first of all some metaphorical expression. . . . It is in this elementary presentational mode that our first adventure in conscious abstraction occurs (1942: 125).

287

The very process of scientific understanding may be characterized as "starting with metaphor and ending in algebra" (Black 1962).[2] All too often the health educator has attempted to introduce "algebra", nutrition messages based upon nutrient equations for example, into a villager's world before facilitating an appropriate metaphorical stage of understanding.[3] A need exists for health educators to take stock of the "commonsense rationality" (Schutz 1964) of the villager. Although ideas expressed through analogy, metaphor and proverb may not be logical in a strictly scientific sense, they shape the inchoate giving it a familiarity which enables actors to adopt a strategy for dealing with a new situation. Analogies may also serve to enhance rapport and problem solving from within the layperson's world.[4]

BANKING VERSUS THE NEGOTIATION MODE OF EDUCATION

During anthropology of health research, we observed a range of interactions between laypeople and health professionals including both trained government health staff and indigenous medical specialists. While observing these interactions, we were struck by the general ineffectiveness of health and nutrition education monologues "delivered" to villagers. These attempts to introduce new health ideas were largely ineffective because 1) they did not address people's health concerns, 2) they were introduced without any reference to local illness categories or ideas about etiology and folk dietetics, and 3) advice was not tailored to the economics of subsistence or the practicalities of village life. Reality was more often ignored than worked with and villagers were asked to blindly accept new health ideas.

To borrow an analogy from Paolo Friere (1973), information was introduced via a "banking mode of education". That is information was deposited into a villager's mind verbatim as if the account (i.e. the mind) were empty: the assumption being that interest would accrue over time. The bankruptcy of this type of education in rural South India and Sri Lanka was clearly evident in the dividends it yielded; namely, the compartmentalization of new information and frank inertia on the part of villagers to integrate new ideas into everyday life.

While living with primary health care fieldstaff, we observed that they themselves did not utilize much of the information they were teaching to others in their own lives on a day to day basis. This is not to say that they did not encourage their own family members to be immunized or to visit a doctor when ill. Their lack of adoption of promotive health ideas was evident in their unaltered dietary habits and their inability to express to friends and relatives why nutritional advice should be followed beyond the laconic statement "it is good for health". In discussions with health staff about their training, it was apparent that they had not received advice, let alone instruction, on how to bridge the conceptual gap between the two cognitive universes in which they lived and worked. There seemed to be a tacit assumption on the part of health trainers that once health workers were supplied information, they could then pass it on to villagers in a suitable manner. Training in interpersonal communication skills was largely overlooked as a subject in both primary health worker and community health worker training programs.

In a review of India's Community Health Worker manual, Srivastava (1980) highlights the ramifications of this oversight:

> The work of the CHW requires an extensive facility in self expression. The manual and the training programme do not consciously generate opportunities in the acquisition or development of such an ability. Simulation exercises recorded by the project team indicate that the CHWs tend to over awe the patient by an excessive use of borrowed terms and associative explanations. The speech interaction is largely one way ... The exposure of the CHWs to terms in the medical sciences creates problems in communicating with the village population. (p. 46)

In contrast to the didactic approach to education utilized by health field staff, we studied the methods employed by popular religious leaders, indigenous medical practitioners, astrologers and politicians in communicating new information to villagers. What emerged from our observations was a keen appreciation for how analogies were effectively used to include the known while locating and often encompassing the new. We noted the enthusiastic response which villagers would give religious leaders when they juxtaposed the themes of traditional mythology with a popular movie to emphasize a moral principle; how traditional ayurvedic practitioners would convey information about the relationship of body humors by reference to the sun, wind and rain; and how astrologers discussed social relations with reference to the stars describing in turn the qualities of celestial forces by reference to body humors and kinship relations.[5] Politicians were likewise well received when they referred to India's past history, not only in an attempt to recall past glory, but in an effort to present new events in terms of known occurrences or myths which served as timeless charters.[6]

EDUCATION BY APPROPRIATE ANALOGY: A PARTICIPATORY RESEARCH APPROACH

Education by analogy draws from the popular patterns of effective communication noted above. The fundamental difference between an analogic and banking approach to education is that in the banking approach an educator starts out with an analysis of what a population does not know and then fills in gaps of knowledge as the professional sees them; the educator using an analogical approach begins by studying what a population *does know* conceptually and experientially. The educator-facilitator identifies areas of conceptual overlap between what is known/experienced in daily life and the new information. As opposed to simply depositing bits of information for recall, recall is engendered through cultural associations and whenever possible, through culturally relevant problem solving. Participatory research is essential to the generation and testing of appropriate analogies. Through participatory research, lay health concerns as well as images of health and illness are identified in context through a process which is reflexive.

Initially, an analogical message is developed which is deemed to be culturally relevant on the basis of preliminary research. It is posed to evoke a response leading to dialogue and feedback. Successful communication is measured by laypersons responding to an initial analogy through elaboration or the posing of what they consider to be more appropriate or alternative analogies. The latter are often anchored to local sayings, proverbs or stories. The generation of analogies by villagers either in support or in clarification of the original analogy serves as a check on comprehension. In addition, analogy posing serves as entertainment to villages by providing an environment in which individuals can share their wit as well as their knowledge.

To provide a more structured sense of the process involved in generating analogical messages, seven ideal steps in framing appropriate analogies for health education may be outlined briefly. This is followed by examples of how teaching analogies were developed in the field in southern India and Sri Lanka.

Steps:
1. The deconstructing of health/nutrition messages into underlying assumptions and concepts.
2. The collection of data on indigenous health concerns and lay preventive/ promotive health behavior; ideas about folk dietetics; indigenous categories of illness associated with states of malnutrition; identifying underlying assumptions and concepts of health.
3. Cultural free association about health themes in complementary domains of experience. For example, free association about child growth and crop growth among agriculturists; cooking and dehydration among women; night fishing and the collection of night blood for filiarisis testing among fishermen etc.
4. The identification of points of conceptual and experiential convergence between indigenous and biomedical thinking about health. For example, a common concern for blood quantity, digestive capacity, health as a state of balance, positive health, etc.
5. Compiling a list of familiar referential frameworks within the culture through the collection of common analogies, metaphors and proverbs.
6. The selection of analogies for an initial message which either 1) points out convergences between indigenous and new health conceptualizations: shared assumptions, health concerns, etc. or 2) uses experience in one domain of life to shed light on different domains, such as agriculture and health; cooking and health. Both cognitive models of abstract knowledge and knowledge in practice are recognized.

7. An analogical lead-in message is presented to a group of community members for their response. The message is rejected, refined, elaborated upon and/or alternative more appropriate analogies are generated. Linkage to proverbs and development of teaching stories strengthen the point being made. Positive and negative aspects of analogy use are examined.

We may illustrate the way in which education by analogy dialogues were developed in South Kanara and Sri Lanka and then review two projects wherein analogical approaches to immunization and family planning education were developed. The examples from India and Sri Lanka involved nutrition education and are framed around a traditional metaphor for development — the growing rice plant. Presented first will be the thinking which went into the development of a root analogy. This will be presented in outline form and will be followed by compressed rendering of analogical messages developed through guided dialogue.

CONSTRUCTION OF AN ANALOGICAL MESSAGE

Formal Nutrition Education Message

Eat a mixed balanced diet. Foods recommended by health workers are typically categorized into three or four groups based on nutrient content. The grouping of foods in this manner by health educators is not comprehended by villagers. Foods which nutritionists group together into one category are often classified by villagers in different categories having distinct properties in accord with folk dietetics (Nichter and Nichter 1981; Nichter 1986).

Background Information: Cultural Resources

a. The process of rice cultivation is well known to the villager. This process requires a proper balancing and regulation of fertilizer and water.
b. Rice is not only the staple crop and cultural superfood (Jelliffe 1969), it is a central metaphor for life used in daily conversation. For example, a growing child is referred to in colloquial speech as a budding or developing rice stalk.
c. Digestive capacity and blood quality/quantity are central health concerns.
d. Health as balance is an important cultural concept. Balance is expressed through a concern for states of hot/cold and body humors (*tridosha*).

Areas of Cultural Sensitivity Identified

The folk dietetic system underlies cultural common sense. Foods are classified in accord with their qualitative state of hot/cold, lightness/heaviness, and effect on body humors (Nichter 1986).

Root Analogy Initially Introduced

The need for a balance of the right kinds of fertilizer in the field is like the need for the right kinds of food in the stomach.
Analogical Message Developed through Dialogue:

When cultivating rice, what is necessary? Good soil, a properly ploughed field, leaf manure, cow dung and ash. What happens if there is too little manure, green leaf or ash? (A discussion typically ensues about crop height, seed head size, weight, rice illnesses and overall yield). Your body is like a field. If the proper mix of nutrients are not given to the field inside, your yield — your health — is poor and your blood weak.

The field needs to be well prepared to cultivate a good rice crop. Preparing the field so the earth can "digest fertilizer" is like enhancing the stomach's digestive capacity so the body can take food and turn it into blood.

Just as enough good soil is needed for rice growth in the field, so enough rice is needed in our bodies for energy and strength. To improve your crop — your health — other things are needed as well. Just as the field needs green leaf manure, so the body requires green leafy vegetables, but as in the case of fertilizer not all leaves are suitable for manure and the best leaves need to be identified in each season. Like dung in the field, the body requires strength giving foods like fish and grams. Like ash for the field, the body requires foods which when cooked by the stomach fire provide the body with ash minerals. As in the field, if too much of one item is used and not enough of another, balance is not obtained and when there is no balance, illness may come by many means.

The above analogical message was developed as an alternative to monologues on food groups presented to villagers by health staff. Once the referential framework of agriculture was introduced it was found that it could be extended to address other nutrition education issues as well. Two examples may briefly be cited.

EXAMPLE ONE: TONIC USE

In the last decade, health has increasingly become commodified and medicalized by medical practitioners and a thriving pharmaceutical industry in both the commercial ayurvedic and allopathic sector. A visible outcome is an increased consumption of vitamin tonics, the ingredients of which often do not match deficiencies. Nutrition educators are faced with the task of countering the growing idea that consuming tonic when one is weak is a better investment of scarce resources than investing in a better diet (Chapter 9). In discussions with agricultural field officers, we found that a complementarity existed between villagers' ideas about tonic and the agricultural fertilizer, urea. Some villagers used urea as a tonic for the soil, failing to heed advice about the importance of balancing urea with other nutrients. As distinct from tonics, however, villagers were rapidly gaining experience with urea and were beginning to see that if their soil was not balanced, their crop yield would not improve despite the healthy appearance produced by urea when applied to a field. The farmers were learning that using urea without other nutrients left the soil acidic — "hot" — and in a state of imbalance.

Analogic Message Developed: Health Like a Good Crop Cannot Be Purchased Through a Bottle of Tonic or a Bag of Urea

When urea is placed on a field the field turns very green but does the crop yield increase? The crop is green and taller but is the grain head any larger? Is there profit or is there just more "show" if urea is used without being balanced by phosphates and calcium? What happens if phosphates are added to the field but not balanced with urea or calcium? The grain head increases in size, but the plant is too weak to support the grain head and it falls to the mud and rots. A balance of fertilizer is needed for a good yield. So it is with the body. Just as urea makes the crop look green quickly, when tonic is taken one feels better quickly. But does one become healthy and strong for long by tonic alone? Urea and tonic can only help the rice field and the body when balanced with other necessary ingredients.

If you wait until you are ill and then run for tonic expecting health, this is like supplying your field with urea at the time of harvest when your crop looks weak. Should one wait until thirsty to start digging the well? (A local proverb)

The indigenous concept of *soku* was used in support of the analogical message introduced above. *Soku* connotes a state of "being all puffed up", of looking big and strong, but actually being bulky and without substance — "like a big vine spinach plant which when cooked reduces to nothing in the pot." A plant which is given too much fertilizer and grows large, but has less yield is described as *soku*. In one informant's words "it is as if the plants become intoxicated and forget their function." In dialogues with villagers, the process of a plant becoming *soku* through an excess of urea was compared to the behavior of a person who consumes tonic instead of a balanced diet. Balance was discussed in terms of both the field: stomach analogy introduced above and in terms of folk dietetics (Nichter and Nichter 1981).

EXAMPLE TWO: DIET DURING PREGNANCY

Background

Primary health center staff have been encouraged to instruct rural women to consume more food during pregnancy in an effort to reduce low birth weight babies. Unfortunately, the message of "eat more food to have a bigger, healthier baby" is not well received in rural South Kanara (Chapter 2). Two reasons for this are fear of a difficult delivery if one has a large baby and a desire not to have a big baby which is *jabala*, a state in humans corresponding to *soku* in plants. The issue became how to educate pregnant women that they needed to eat more (or at least not less) without directly referring to baby size and setting off a chain of negative associations. A plausible alternative was to address the health of the mother and to engage her in a discussion of how her health affected that of her baby after delivery.

It was necessary to identify popular health concerns, particularly among women. The first concern identified was "less blood", a condition often corresponding to anemia and the second loss of *dhatu* (a body substance) associated with strength and vigor. *Dhatu* is the quintessence of strength giving foods derived from successive processes of transformation and purification. Analogically, blood is refined to become *dhatu* just as milk is churned and boiled to produce ghee, clarified butter (Nichter 1986). Healthy breastmilk is thought to contain *dhatu*. When a breastfed baby becomes weak, women suspect that their *dhatu* is less. Other features of *dhatu* are that it is stored and it takes time to produce. A wide range of opinions exist however, as to just how long it takes food to become blood and blood to become *dhatu*.[7] We found through dialogue that the two previous nutrition messages could be adapted and conjoined to address the problem of diet during pregnancy.

Pregnancy and Diet Message

When you are thirsty is that any time to start digging a well? At or near the day of harvest if the rice crop looks weak, is that the time to think of adding manure to the field? So it is with a baby growing within its mother. A mother is like a field and her baby like a rice stalk. Just as the field needs fertilizer prior to harvest, so a woman needs to consume foods during pregnancy which will produce blood and dhatu. When a woman has enough blood and dhatu, her baby will grow strong in the womb just as a rice shoot grows strong in the field which is well fertilized. Like the field where dung, ash, and green leaf take time to be digested by the soil, so food takes time to be digested and become blood and dhatu. A pregnant woman needs to produce a stock of dhatu and blood. Why? Because a mother loses blood during delivery and because she shares her dhatu with her baby through breastfeeding. It is important for a woman to produce a good store of blood and dhatu during pregnancy for her health and the health of her baby.

Following this lead in message, dialogue was generated around the issue of which foods are considered blood and *dhatu* producing within folk dietetics (Nichter 1986). Nutrient rich foods advised for greater consumption were those foods deemed culturally appropriate to consume during pregnancy in addition to being affordable and accessible. Dialogue focused on the quantity as well as the quality of foods consumed associating these topics with blood and *dhatu* production.

THE USE OF ANALOGY IN SRI LANKA

During 1984—85, Mark assisted the Sri Lankan Bureau of Health Education develop a Masters Degree program in Health Education. As part of field training in anthropology and health communications, students conducted health ethnography research and used this data to develop a health education approach. Some chose to utilize an analogical approach to health message negotiation. The following account illustrates how this approach was applied by one health educator familiar with the South Indian nutrition messages discussed above. A similar theme, a comparison of the rice-field and the body was used by the health educator in Kurenagala, a rice growing area of Sri Lanka. Agricultural practices in this region entail the extensive use of chemical fertilizers in contrast to rural South Kanara where agricultural practices are more traditional. The Sri Lankan case presented illustrates a dialogical approach to working with analogy.

HEALTH EDUCATOR'S INITIAL MESSAGE: MATERNAL AND CHILD HEALTH

This morning, I will make a comparison (connection) between the growing paddy field and the growing child. The paddy plant is like a child. The needs of the paddy plant in the field are like a baby's needs in a mother's belly. When planting a paddy field, one needs to do this with good feelings, happiness and proper preparations if a good crop is to grow. In the same way, during pregnancy a woman needs to have good feelings and a happy home environment. One must care for the field as well as for the developing plant. If the field is not given proper treatment and enough fertilizer, the rice plant does not develop or germinate properly. A mother also must receive care and enough food so she will have sufficient blood so that the bady does not develop *mandama dosa*, (an illness associated with protein energy malnutrition).

The comparison between the child and the field underscoring the analogy frame was more clearly established by the health educator by asking villagers to draw correlations between the life stages of the growing rice plant and a baby. Through anthropological research, the health educator knew that local agricultural terms were used by laypersons to describe and discuss stages in the development of the fetus. For example:

Sinhalese term	Stage of rice development	Stage of human development
bitteravee	seed	egg
vela vee	germinated seed with root	fertilized egg in uterus
gayam phalleh	rice plant	pregnant woman
bandi[8]	flowering plant	pregnant woman in last trimester

Drawing upon the analogical framework described above and villagers' familiarity with rice agriculture, a discussion of vitamin/mineral supplements and immunization was facilitated:

Facilitator: You have learned through experience that a rice field requires fertilizer, weedicide and insecticide. Like that, a mother and infant require special medicines to protect them and make them strong. What kinds of fertilizer do you give the field and when do you apply them?

Villagers: We give minerals, *mandaposa*, and urea to the rice plant, *gayam palleh*. When the plant flowers, *bandi*, we give TDM fertilizer, *bandiposa*, to ensure a good crop.

Facilitator: In the same way it is necessary to give the field fertilizer, it is necessary to give a pregnant woman these mineral tablets (ferrous sulfate) and vitamins (folic acid, B complex). It is important to take these during the whole time the baby is growing to ensure good health.

You also use weedicides in your fields. These are like preventive medicines. There are many types of weeds that grow. Each kind of weedicide is for a specific type of weed. In the same way there are many different kinds of *visabija* (local term for germs). What kinds of things do you use to prevent weeds from spoiling a field?

Villagers: For *gayam palleh* we use two kinds of weedicides for the rice plants. At first we use Suropers, and later during *Bandi* when the rice is ripening we use Agroxion.

Facilitator: Just the way you use weedicides to protect the crop, so two immunizations (tetanus toxoid) are given to a mother to protect her baby during pregnancy from harmful *visabija*.

Facilitator: When do you use insecticides for the field?

Villagers: We mix less powerful insecticides in with fertilizer, like Kaberfuran, to protect the field against *keedewa* insects. Powerful insecticides (Andrex 20, Basa) are used only after insects have been seen in the field; These insecticides are dangerous and require careful handling.

Facilitator: Some medicines are like insecticides; they are used to control *visabija* and prevent sickness. Other medicines are only used when *visabija* are seen by doctors the way Basa is used only when insects appear. They are more powerful and need expert handling by a doctor. Although they can be bought at the chemist, they should not be used unless a doctor is consulted. Like insecticides used for difficult insects, there are different medicines for different kinds of *visabija*. If you use the wrong kind of powerful medicine or insecticide, it is not only a waste of money, it is harmful for the body, as it is harmful for the field.

Mark was present when this set of analogies was being developed and later had an opportunity to engage in a focus group discussion with eight villagers who had been presented with the analogical method of teaching. The group was composed of six females and two males ranging in age from twenty to sixty years old. The villagers stated that they had all been lectured to in the past by family health workers about nutrition, immunizations, and family planning. When asked the difference between previous talks and their recent experience, all said they found the "education by analogy" approach far more appealing. When asked why, they explained that instead of being treated like children who knew nothing, they felt respected for what they knew — agriculture. It was established that they were not ignorant villagers but astute observers of life. In this type of learning environment, they said they felt less afraid to speak their minds and ask questions. Expressed by the group was a sense of dignity from being able to share knowledge and experience with others. Given the opportunity to articulate their experience in rice agriculture — when and why various agricultural operations were conducted — set them up with a strategy for problem solving about health.

THE USE OF ANALOGIES FOR HEALTH EDUCATION IN KENYA

Adopting new ideas is easier and more dignified if they relate to existing knowledge systems. There has been a tendency for development work to carry out what one observer sees as "development by destruction" — destroying the very object of the development targets . . . Communication needs to be communication aimed at sharing and enhancing self-confidence and a sense of dignity in those whose quality of life is to be improved — that is, if the main objective is the development of the person, the people (Were 1985: 438).

Were, in her description of the Kakamega rural health project in Kenya describes a mode of health communication complementary to that developed in South Asia. She notes that priority health problems identified by the community and by health professionals were found to be very similar. In fact, agreement was higher than 90%. Despite the high level of agreement, however, compliance in health action was quite low. Investigation into this issue revealed that:

The tendency was that once a problem was recognized by the people and health staff, the health and other development workers immediately proceeded to expound on their understanding of the cause of the problem and would present their solution without paying attention to how the people explained causation and how they would go about getting to the solution. In spite of the common bricks of perceiving the same problems as problems, the bricks were not used for building further understanding and establishing a rapport. Instead, the next step was that the groups slid back into "those who knew" and "those who didn't know" and needed to be taught. (p. 433)

In an effort to rectify the communication problem between laypersons and health professionals, analogies were developed around a topic identified to be of critical importance, timely immunizations. Immunizations were difficult to explain to villagers because the terms needed to describe them could not easily be translated into the local language. As Were explains, it was not simply a matter of translating the words but actually finding a way of communicating the concept and rationale behind immunization that presented the problem. The problem of tailoring descriptions of immunizations to local knowledge and experience bases is worldwide (Nichter 1989).

An analogical message frame termed the "banana leaf model" was developed as a useful means of explaining the concept of immunization to mothers:

One of the uses of the banana leaf is to protect against rain. If one is outdoors and notices any sign of rain, one plucks a banana leaf well in advance. If one waits until the raindrops come, one may be drenched in the process of getting the banana leaf, which will render it useless. To keep dry, the banana leaf must be obtained in good time. This is the way it is with immunization. Waiting until a child has signs of infection of the feared disease before having it immunized does not protect the child. It has to be done well ahead of time, just as a banana leaf is obtained before the first drops of rainfall. (Were 1985, p.440)

The analogy was elaborated to explain to mothers why some children who had been immunized still experienced the disease, if a batch of immunizations had gone bad or if an immune response was incomplete.

Even if one does get a banana leaf well ahead of the rain, there are occasions on which one may inadvertently pick a leaf with a hole or a tear and the raindrops may still wet one's clothes. This does not mean that "banana leaves are useless in the rain" but simply that they don't always work 100% fo the time. (p. 441)

In both the banana leaf analogy and the fertilizer, weedicide, insecticide analogy utilized in Sri Lanka, familiar practices involving prevention in one domain of life experience were identified and extended. This served to legitimate an unseen relationship of cause and effect based on complementarity.

THE AGRICULTURAL APPROACH TO FAMILY PLANNING: THE PHILIPPINES

An educational strategy developed by the International Institute of Rural Reconstruction (IIRR) in the Philippines provides an example of how an analogical approach was used with farmers to facilitate understanding of new family planning concepts by reference to existing agricultural practices.[9] This project will be discussed in some detail as it is the only case where an analogical approach has been evaluated. Formal evaluation of a range of family planning education methods was conducted by the University of the Philippines Institute of Mass Communications (Maglalang 1976). Evaluating different forms of family planning education, it was found that increases in knowledge, comprehension and retention were highest in an analogical approach group while ambivalence and uncertainty of remembering were greatest among those who were lectured at without visual aids. A unique feature of the IIRR project was that after analogical messages were pretested for comprehension in several field areas, flipcharts and comic books based on analogical themes were generated and widely circulated.

Flavier (1979) describes how this approach was developed after several years of ineffective family planning compaigns among rural villagers.

I encountered an elderly woman, very respected, more learned than the usual and I confessed my problems . . . "I can't seem to put across the messages . . . How would you do it if you were in my place"? She was unsure and hesitant. She put it this way. "I do not know, but when you were explaining the whole family planning process, what kept coming into my mind were agricultural situations. You mentioned ovary, ovum, uterus, and frankly, they do not sound real to me, but I can understand them in terms of string beans whose seeds are pushed out and grow on fertile fields. (cited in Maglalang, 1976: 3).

Flavier found the grassroots analogy suggested by the woman attractive from both an illustrative and bioscience vantage point. Scientifically, just as the ovary is a human organ that has about 300 potential ova capable of replicating the human species, so a string bean is a vegetable with a pod with 12 to 15 ova capable of replicating the species. Assured of the analogy's scientific validity,[10] Flavier decided to return to the village the next week to discuss family planning in terms of string beans. He found that the beans provided relevant demonstration material particularly since they were a common vegetable crop in the area.

When I talked about the process, I could push the bean and a seed would come out; it was graphic and visual. They could see it externalized and could participate by bringing me string beans from their homes. If I pressed too hard, two seeds would come out and people would joke and say twins.

From this experience, Flavier came to appreciate the importance of making the abstract — in this case, the workings of a body organ, visible and concrete to rural villagers. Phrased another way, he came to appreciate the importance of providing villagers an "appropriate image" not merely a concept.

After his initial success with the string beans, Flavier began to search for other referential frameworks from which to generate analogies. He and his staff conducted a systematic study of indigenous farming methods and customs. They simultaneously conducted a survey to determine what villagers wanted to know about family planning. Flavier learned that villagers wanted practical knowledge about family planning, not only what family planning was, but how it worked. We may briefly review the way in which the IIRR working with Flavier proceeded to develop an analogical education program highlighting the teaching analogies developed.

IIRR fieldworkers opened discussions at small group meetings by asking villagers to talk about their agricultural practices in relation to specific topics such as the spacing of plants, what measures they took to induce a barren tree to yield, what they did to improve the quality of their fruits, etc. In the process of discussions, villagers were encouraged to draw pictures of what they were describing. Some of these pictures became the prototypes of flipcharts which presented two pictures — one depicting an agricultural operation, the other a family planning concept to which is was to parallel. The following are some examples:

The IUD. An IUD is like a fence which the farmer places around his fields to prevent animals from entering and destroying the garden. Placed inside a woman, an IUD prevents her from getting pregnant by preventing the seed from sticking in the uterus.

The pill. Horses are a necessity in the villages during the months of May through August to transport agricultural produce to the urban areas. If a horse becomes pregnant at this time, the farmer will suffer many difficulties. To prevent pregnancies, rice bran mixed with glutinous rice is fed to the horses. This mix renders the horse infertile. A woman, it is pointed out, can likewise become infertile by taking birth control pills.

The condom. To collect the *tuba,* palm wine from coconut palms, a bamboo tube which resembles a condom is placed at the top of the tree. The juice collects in the tube and when it ferments it becomes a drink. This tube is compared to a condom which collects the male juice. When the juice ferments it becomes a baby.

On the importance of practicing birth control. If a pomelo tree is laden with many fruits, it will produce fruits which are small and not so sweet. This is also true of the family. If there are too many young children, often they will be small and sickly. In order to avoid the crowding of too many fruits of the pomelo tree, the flowers are reduced and only the better quality flowers are left to grow into fruits. In the case of people, successive pregnancy can be avoided if one uses the methods of birth control.

On the concept of spacing. Rice seedlings grown in a seed bed grow slowly because the seedlings are near to each other. They need to have ample spacing to grow fast and for the stalks to be healthy. In the same way, a woman who has successive pregnancies has children who are small and sickly. That is why it is very important to give proper spacing in order to take good care of them as they grow.

DISCUSSION OF THE AGRICULTURAL APPROACH

In developing agricultural analogies, both the IIRR and ourselves endeavored to find appropriate images complementary to scientific rationales. This is not always possible and pragmatism often dictates practice. For example, the comparison of a fence around a garden is hardly representative of how an IUD works. Of ultimate importance is not the educator's perception of an analogy, but villager's perceptions and understanding within their own experiential universe. Analogy posing is no easy task and meaning can be misconstrued by an audience. This is the reason we have stressed participatory research and pretesting as important elements in developing analogical teaching messages.

CONCLUSION

In the mid 1970's a good deal of discussion emerged about the use of the folk media for development. Some communication researchers such as Ranganath (1976) described the folk media in terms of existing institutions (e.g. puppet shows, drama, folk songs) which were popular, non-elitist and available at low cost. They were presented as a social resource affording great potential for persuasive communication. To these researchers and others (Eapen 1976), the folk media was a ready resource for the propagation of modern health and development messages.[11]

What is uncomfortable about much of this literature is that it solely reflects a modernization approach to development. The folk media is presented as a familiar medium through which those in the "know" can inject messages to those "who don't know". Rather than being characterized as an arena in which community problem solving may be engendered, the folk media is coopted. Curiously, cultural performances which challenge development as "under development" and provide critical commentary are not acknowledged. Examples abound ranging from Shivaratri skits in India to community plays in Cuba. Little discussed in the folk media and development literature is the potential of cultural performances, both old and new, to engage community members in the act of consciousness raising in a context which permits critical thinking and the emergence of paradox. A very narrow view of the vitality of folk genres is depicted.

More sensitive non formal education researchers, such as Colletta (1975) have placed emphasis on looking beyond cultural forms as instruments for development to engaging folk media in the process of problem solving in cultural terms. He joins Fuglesang (1977) in arguing for "appropriate conceptualization" to complement appropriate technology. The process of deconstructing new ideas (products), negotiating knowledge and fostering critical thinking by posing analogies which ground as distinct from mystify, constitutes one method of facilitating appropriate conceptualization. Analogy posing is a means to initiate problem solving, not an end point. Analogies provide strategies for action which reveal as well as mask. Their use must be monitored and critically examined. This point follows from Chapter 9 where the marketing of health was considered in relation to the process of commodification.

We may illustrate the potential of analogy as a development resource initiating problem solving. In Sri Lanka, Mark was invited by two change facilitators to observe their work with groups of women coir producers in Galle and Matara Districts. Discussing his observations, we were struck by two things. The first was a group process which encouraged an airing of alternate views. The fifteen or so women in each group had to learn to engage in constructive criticism of each other's ideas without being defensive. This is a difficult enough task in any culture. It is particularly so in Sinhalese culture where an indirect verbal and non verbal communication style are in play which serves to minimize overt conflict. In Sinhalese culture, an attempt is made in all public occasions to defuse conflict and mask extreme emotions. This is one reason foreigners stereotype the Sinhalese as always smiling and why joking plays an important role in ritual healing.

The second thing which we noted was the problem solving frame employed by one of the groups. This strategy was based on an analogy between the activities of middlemen and the vendors of development schemes. The group of women comprising this group had followed the chain of coir production and sale from the purchasing of coconut husks and the leasing of soaking pits to the twisting of fiber, weighing in, transportation and market sale. By following this chain of events they had come to more effectively organize and bypass the middleman, *mudalali*, who once derived significant profit from their ignorance and powerlessness. These women were now in the process of extending their knowledge of coir and applying a "*mudalali* model" to other outsiders who came to their village. Included in their purview were development workers, health care workers, doctors, teachers, etc. Teachers were seen as the *mudalali* of education while doctors were considered to be *mudalali* of medicine and so forth. The womens' outlook was at once limited by their use of the coir analogy and an economic gaze, yet broadened beyond a former narrow "frogs in a well" perspective leading to powerlessness. The analogy provided them a strategy, someplace to begin, a framework in which to organize their thoughts and center dialogue.

Our discussion of the coir producers' "*mudalali* model" of dependency may appear to be somewhat distant from our initial discussion of education by appropriate analogy. Yet, it illustrates application of the principles of complementarity and elaboration basic to the analogical thought processes of South Asian villagers which may be maximized in development education. A South Kanarese proverb states "Telling proverbs is equal to Veda" (holy scriptures), *Gaḍegalu mathu vedakke sama*. This proverb highlights the importance given to objectified expressions of tacit knowledge gained through experience; knowledge propagated through teaching stories in the major religions of South Asia.[12] Commenting on our use of analogical messages for health education, one Sinhalese villager remarked, "This way of learning is Buddhist. The Buddha taught this way. It is like the Jataka tales which teach difficult moral lessons about life in a simple way." Perhaps what is lacking in village education today are modern Jataka tales, which in the words of an ayurvedic practitioner, "milk, churn, and boil down experience to its simplest clarified form."

NOTES

1. Our deployment of metaphors follows an interactional appreciation of metaphor as a construct used in the understanding and creating of reality as distinct from the describing of reality (Black 1962). Lakoff and Johnson (1980) in their popular book, *Metaphors We Live By,* have identified such metaphors as "conceptual metaphors" and have considered metaphor in relation to the production of knowledge. Köveseses (1986) has extended this analysis noting that prototypes of what something is or is about may be constituted by metaphors and analogical frames which structure vague domains of experience in relation to more familiar concrete domains. Accounts of conceptual metaphor often list inventories of interrelated metaphors. Missing is a sense of discourse — how metaphors are used in context. This is of paramount importance to the development of analogical teaching materials meant to contextualize learning. Fernandez (1974) for example points out that metaphor has at least three functions in discourse: the informative, declarative and persuasive. The use of metaphor and the introduction of analogy in speech may be associated with different voices and vantages. Use of metaphor may in itself denote a shift in voice or constitute a contrast to a more linear communication form indexing a particular form of social relationship. Choice of alternative metaphorical frames may likewise index social relations through subtle connotations.
2. As Toulmin (1972) has noted, science and to a greater degree the everyday understanding of the world, progresses less as a series of paradigm leaps — scientific revolutions —

than as an evolutionary process of reinterpretation and modification of existing knowledge and experience.

3. We have considered metaphor and analogy as complementary in this paper. We recognize that the function of these tropes may be distinct. For example, metaphor may be used to reveal complexity or offer poetic surprise while analogy may be used to simplify. Our focus is limited to the general means by which analogical reasoning is infused into the pragmatics of natural language such that correspondences between domains result in a sense of coherence. The literature on metaphor abounds with conflicting definitions and theories of usage some semantic and others pragmatic. Our thinking accords with a correspondence theory of metaphor well summarized by Levinson (1983). Herein emphasis is placed on the incidental and connotational rather than the strictly denotative characteristics of words and the factual properties of referents.

4. Burke (1954) has pointed out the strategic use of metaphor in his writing on the meaning of proverbs. See Fernandez (1986) for a discussion of metaphor providing an orientation for action.

5. For an excellent illustration of this process of encompassment vis a vis the use of analogy, see Trawick (1987). Trawick uses Indian data to refute Horton's (1967) depiction of traditional thought as uncritical of existing paradigms. She points out that ayurvedic epistemology is open not closed, or to use Levi Strauss' terms, hot not cold, to expansion.

6. The meaning of a message is, of course, only one factor involved in its acceptance. One must also pay credence to the social context in which this message is delivered and aspects of performance which lend it credibility.

7. We recorded a wide range of opinions as to how long it took food to become blood and blood to become *dhatu*. Questions as to how many drops of blood it took to make *dhatu* were rarely answered. Some informants believed it took seven days for blood to become *dhatu* and others sixteen days. Both numbers are symbolically associated with completion. Other informants spoke of this process being influenced by age or constitution, and still others perceived some foods as containing *dhatu* properties which immediately entered the blood after digestion.

8. Colloquially, the Sinhalese word *bandiya* means big belly, and is also used in reference to a pregnant woman.

9. Sumantha Banerjee (1979) has similarly argued for the use of analogies, proverbs and teaching stories based on folk knowledge as a means of teaching about family planning in India.

10. In some instances, analogies can be posed which maximize correspondences between local knowledge and what is considered biomedically correct (today). In other instances, an analogy or image may be presented which conveys a theme of public health importance. Examples are the theme of resistance/protection noted by Were in her banana plant analogy and more recently a set of images suggested by Bastien (1987) for introducing ORT in Bolivia. Among Kallaywayas in Bolivia, a complementarity exists between well being in the world and health within the body. Both are dependent on the continual exchange of fluids. This image was used in a set of health education messages addressing a hydraulic image of physiology and an Andean *ayllu* view of the universe.

11. Others such as Bordenave (1974) have argued quite the opposite. "As soon as the people realize that their folk songs, poems and art are being used for subliminal propaganda they will let them die." There is some truth to this fear. Development messages have more often than not been overtly as opposed to subliminally inserted into folk media. Audiences in South Kanara were not pleased to find family planning messages pushed at Yakshagana performances. In the northern part of Karnataka State, Yellamma songs — religious songs to a female deity — were altered to include family planning messages. Villagers rejected performances which incorporated these messages as being both inappropriate and sacrilegious. According to Lent (1982) use of the folk media backfired and villagers were alienated from the family planning program.

12. Health educators need to have on hand a stock of appropriate analogies and teaching stories and learn when and how to introduce them in the course of conversation. Much is to be learned from the study of communication styles of popular religious leaders, medical practitioners, midwives, astrologers etc.

REFERENCES

Banerjee, S.
  1979 *Family Planning Communication: A Critique of the Indian Programme.* New Delhi, India: Family Planning Foundation, Radiant Press.
Bastien, J.
  1987 Cross-cultural communication between doctors and peasants in Bolivia. *Social Science and Medicine 24*:12, 1109—1118.
Black, M.
  1962 *Models and Metaphors.* Ithaca, N.Y.: Cornell University Press.
Bordenave, J. D.
  1974 *Communication and Adoption of Agricultural Innovations in Latin America.* Proceedings of the Cornell-CIAT International Symposium on Communication Strategies for Rural Development, March 17—22, 1974. Ithaca, N.Y.: Cornell University.
Burke, K.
  1954 *Permanence and Change* (2nd edition). Los Altos: Hermes Publication.
Colletta, N.
  1975 *The Use of Indigenous Culture as A Medium for Development: The Indonesian Case.* Instructional Technology Report No. 12, September 1975.
Eapen, K. E.
  1976 Specific Problems of Research and Research Training in Asian and African Countries. *In Communication Research in the Third World: The Need for Training.* Geneva: Lutheran World Federation.
Fernandez, J.
  1974 The Mission of Metaphor in Expressive Culture. *Current Anthropology 15*: 119—145.
  1986 *Persuasiveness and Performances: The Play of Tropes in Culture.* Bloomington: Indiana University Press.
Freire, P.
  1973 *Pedagogy of the Oppressed.* New York: Seabury Press.
Fuglesang, A.
  1977 *Doing Things Together: Report on an Experience in Communicating Appropriate Technology.* Uppsala, Sweden: Dag Hammersjold Foundation.
Horton, R.
  1967 African Traditional Thought and Western Science. *Africa 38*: 50—71, 155—187.
Jelliffe, D.
  1969 *Child Nutrition in Developing Countries.* Washington, D.C.: U.S. Department of State, AID, Office of the War on Hunger.
Köveceses, Z.
  1986 *Metaphors of Anger, Pride and Love.* Amsterdam: John Benjamin Publishers.
Lakoff, G. and Johnson, M.
  1980 *Metaphors We Live By.* Chicago: University of Chicago Press.
Langer, S.
  1942 *Philosophy in a New Key.* New York: Mentor Books.
Lent, J.
  1982 Grassroots Renaissance: Folk Media in the Third World. *Media Asia 9*: 1, 9—16.

Levinson, S. C.
   1983   *Pragmatics*. Cambridge: Cambridge University Press.
Maglalang, D.
   1976   *Agricultural Approach to Family Planning*. Manila: Communication Foundation for
          Asia.
Nichter, M. and Nichter, M.
   1981   *An Anthropological Approach to Nutrition Education*. Newton, Ma.: Education De-
          velopment Center, International Nutrition Communication Service.
Nichter, M.
   1986   Modes of food classification and the diet-health contingency: A South Indian Case
          Study. *In* R. Khare and K. Ishvaran (eds.) *Aspects of Food Systems in South Asia*
          (pp. 105—221). Durham, North Carolina: Carolina Academic Press.
   1989   Vaccinations in South Asia: False expectations and commanding metaphors. *In* J.
          Coreil and D. Mull (eds.) *Anthropology and Primary Health Care*. The Netherlands:
          Kluwer Academic Publishers.
Ranganath, H. K.
   1976   A Probe into the Traditional Media: Telling the People Themselves. *Media Asia 3*:
          1, p. 25.
Schutz, A.
   1964   *Collected Papers* (Vol. 2). The Hague: Martinus Nijhoff.
Srivastava, R. N.
   1980   *Evaluating Communicability in Village Settings*. New Delhi, India: UNICEF Public-
          ations.
Toulmin, S.
   1972   *Human Understanding* (Vol. 1). Oxford: Clarendon Press.
Trawick, M.
   1987   The Ayurvedic Physician as Scientist. *Social Science and Medicine 24*: 12, 1031—
          1050.
Were, M.
   1985   Communicating on Immunization to Mothers and Community Groups. *Assignment
          Children*, Vol. No. 69/72.

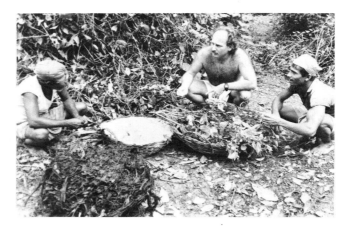

Teaching by analogy: Baskets of cow dung, green leaf and ash form the basis of a dialogue
about nutrition extending existing knowledge about rice agriculture.

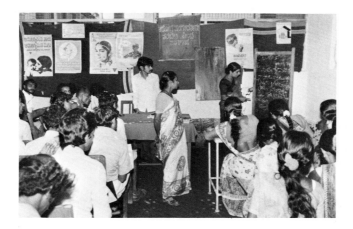

A didactic training session: Community Health Workers learn conventional health messages
but not the communication skills necessary to render them meaningful.

EPILOGUE

A Swahili proverb states that one can not see the soles of one's feet while walking. In addition to assisting those in international health develop health programs which make sense in context, anthropology facilitates reflexivity. I would like to end on this note by recounting a short field vignette.

"Health is not simply a physical or a mental state, it is a moral state, a state of balance and reciprocity." This was one of ayurvedic practitioner, *Vaidya* Ishwara Bhat's favorite messages. I would hear it time and again while sitting on his veranda reading the newspaper and waiting for the evening meal. One evening the front page of the local paper I was reading carried a lead story about U.S. aid to India. An American official was pictured shaking hands with an Indian official in front of what appeared to be a small mountain of wheat. Ishwara gazed over to me and said, "Your country is very lucky to have us to donate their wheat". I was mildly surprised by his comment, but because he was an avid reader of the paper, I assumed that the local press had at one time run a story on American farm subsidies and the international wheat market. In fact, I had completely misconstrued Ishwara's cultural interpretation of American aid. I offer his explanation, as I recorded it in my diary.

In India, it is believed that when a person has committed some pāpa (sin), looked to their own fame and fortune to the detriment of others or forsaken the gods in pursuit of personal gain or desire, the moral order of the universe is such that this action will eventually be counterbalanced. This is recognized by all people because a sense of justice is part of being human. America is young and reckless, like a teenager whose desires change with each new cinema. Yet, the American people sense this justice and you feel a need to give. America sends us aid and expects praise. In India, to lighten the weight of bad karma, offerings are made to those who may bear this karma and through good deeds burn this karma or dissolve this karma the way a salty solution may be made less salty by the addition of more and more fresh water. We give gifts of food or cloth to priests at a temple or beggars and feel that the weight of our karma has lessened. We are thankful to be able to give these things. It is for our own welfare even more than the welfare of the priest or beggar. We stoop to serve.

You send us wheat. It is your good fortune to have our people take this measure of the karma you have accumulated. By taking this food, by eating this food, our people lessen the load of karma that is yours. Without us, who would be there to lighten your load? And yet your people have not learned one important thing. You have not learned to stoop when giving. Have your people not learned that by giving they are helping yourselves?

Health is a state of balance in the body, the family, the village, the country, and the world. Disease is a hunger, food is a medicine for that hunger. For some, the hunger is in their belly, for others it is a hunger of desire, status, or power. For others it is a hunger to be seen as kind or to be forgiven. The patient who came to the *vaidya* in days past was given medicine to take and was prescribed a good deed, *seva*, to perform equal to the severity of the illness. The medicine, *seva*, special diet, and behavior changes prescribed were the foods necessary to

307

satisfy the hungers of the afflicted enabling this person to obtain the state of health possible for them.

That is the principle to be followed. Today, the principle is all but forgotten and the practice is to take medicine and give fees, to take aid from the government or from America and give praise in the newspaper. Are the conditions leading to disease removed in this way? When only one hunger is fed, one *dosha* (literally both humoral imbalance and trouble) quieted, another cries out and disease takes a new form. In your country has disease disappeared or have the faces of disease only changed? Each and ever day, one hears of new medicines and new development schemes. Whose hunger are they meant to satisfy, the poor or some politician or business person? Can any scheme, or medicine give health to the people? You must ask yourself these questions.

Doctors and donors can control the spread of some diseases and extend life; they cannot give health. Like the strength of cloth, health depends on the quality of the thread provided to the weaver, the care taken in the process of weaving, one's ability to preserve the cloth, and the conditions in which the cloth is worn over the years.

INDEX OF SUBJECTS